# BIOLOGICAL EFFECTS OF DRUGS IN RELATION TO THEIR PLASMA CONCENTRATIONS

# BIOLOGICAL EFFECTS OF DRUGS IN RELATION TO THEIR PLASMA CONCENTRATIONS

*Proceedings of a Symposium held by the British Pharmacological Society at the Royal Postgraduate Medical School, London, on January 4, 1972*

edited by

D. S. DAVIES

*Department of Clinical Pharmacology,*
*Royal Postgraduate Medical School, London*

*and*

B. N. C. PRICHARD

*Department of Clinical Pharmacology, Medical Unit,*
*University College Hospital*
*Medical School, London*

MACMILLAN

*First published 1973 by*
*THE MACMILLAN PRESS LTD*
*London and Basingstoke*
*Associated companies in New York*
*Dublin Melbourne Johannesburg and Madras*

SBN 333 13731 0

Printed in Great Britain by
Butler & Tanner Ltd
Frome and London

# List of Contributors


| | |
|---|---|
| ALEXANDERSON, B. | The Department of Clinical Pharmacology, Karolinska Institutet (Huddinge University Hospital), Stockholm, Sweden. |
| ÅSBERG, M. | Department of Psychiatry, Karolinska Hospital, 10401 Stockholm 60, Sweden. |
| BAKER, S. B. DE C. | Imperial Chemical Industries, Pharmaceuticals Division, Macclesfield, Cheshire. |
| BERTILSSON, L. | The Department of Clinical Pharmacology, Karolinska Institutet, Stockholm, Sweden. |
| BRECKENRIDGE, A. | Department of Clinical Pharmacology, and MRC Clinical Pharmacology Research Group, Royal Postgraduate, Medical School, DuCane Road, London, W12. |
| BRODIE, B. B. | Laboratory of Chemical Pharmacology, National Heart and Lung Institute, Bethesda, Maryland 20014, USA. |
| CHAMBERLAIN, D. A. | Royal Sussex County Hospital, Brighton, Sussex. |
| CURRY, S. H. | Department of Pharmacology and Therapeutics, The London Hospital Medical College, Turner Street, London E1. |
| DETTLI, L. | Department of Internal Medicine, Buergerspital, 4000 Basle, Switzerland. |
| DOLLERY, C. T. | MRC Clinical Pharmacology Research Group, Royal Postgraduate Medical School, DuCane Road, London W12. |
| FAIGLE, J. W. | Research Department, Pharmaceuticals Division, Ciba-Geigy Limited, Basle, Switzerland. |
| FENYVESI, T. | MRC Clinical Pharmacology Research Group, Royal Postgraduate Medical School, DuCane Road, London W12. |
| FORREST, J. A. H. | The Regional Poisoning Treatment Centre and University Department of Therapeutics, The Royal Infirmary, Edinburgh, Scotland. |
| FOULKES, D. M. | Imperial Chemical Industries, Pharmaceuticals Division, Macclesfield, Cheshire. |
| GARATTINI, S. | Istituto di Ricerche Farmacologiche 'Mario Negri' Via Eritrea, 62–20157 Milano, Italy. |

George, C. F. — MRC Clinical Pharmacology Research Group, Royal Postgraduate Medical School, DuCane Road, London W12.

Goldberg, L. I. — Department of Clinical Pharmacology, Emory University School of Medicine, Atlanta, Georgia 30303, USA.

Hedwell, P. — Research Department, Pharmaceuticals Division, Ciba-Geigy Limited, Basle, Switzerland.

Keberle, H. — Research Department, Pharmaceuticals Division, Ciba-Geigy Limited, Basle, Switzerland.

Levy, G. — Department of Pharmaceutics, School of Pharmacy, State University of New York at Buffalo, Buffalo, New York 14214, USA.

Lund, L. — Departments of Neurology and Phaımacology (Division of Clinical Pharmacology), Karolinska Institutet, S-104 01 Stockholm 60, Sweden.

Marcucci, F. — Istituto di Ricerche Farmacologiche 'Mario Negri' Via Eritrea, 62–20157 Milano, Italy.

Melmon, K. L. — Schools of Medicine and Pharmacy, Division of Clinical Pharmacology, University of California, San Francisco, California 94122, USA.

Morselli, P. L. — Istituto di Ricerche Farmacologiche 'Mario Negri' Via Eritrea, 62–20157 Milano, Italy.

Mussini, E. — Istituto di Ricerche Farmacologiche 'Mario Negri' Via Eritrea, 62–20157 Milano, Italy.

Mitchell, J. R. — Laboratory of Chemical Pharmacology, National Heart and Lung Institute, Bethesda, Maryland 20014, USA.

Mitchison, D. A. — Medical Research Council Unit for Laboratory Studies of Tuberculosis, Royal Postgraduate Medical School, DuCane Road, London W12.

Oates, J. A. — Departments of Medicine and Pharmacology, Vanderbilt University, Nashville, Tennessee, USA.

Orme, M. L'E. — Department of Clinical Pharmacology and MRC Clinical Pharmacology Research Group, Royal Postgraduate Medical School, DuCane Road, London W12.

Prescott, L. F. — The Regional Poisoning Treatment Centre and University Department of Therapeutics, The Royal Infirmary, Edinburgh, Scotland.

Price-Evans, D. A. — Department of Medicine, University of Liverpool, Liverpool 3.

| | |
|---|---|
| RIESS, W. | Chemical and Biological Research Laboratories of the Pharmaceutical Division of Ciba-Geigy Limited, Basle, Switzerland. |
| ROLINSON, G. N. | Beecham Research Laboratories, Brockham Park, Betchworth, Surrey. |
| ROSCOE, P. | The Regional Poisoning Treatment Centre and University Department of Therapeutics, The Royal Infirmary, Edinburgh, Scotland. |
| ROWLAND, M. | Schools of Medicine and Pharmacy, Division of Clinical Pharmacology, University of California, San Francisco, California 94122, USA. |
| SHAND, D. G. | Departments of Medicine and Pharmacology, Vanderbilt University, Nashville, Tennessee, USA. |
| SHEINER, L. | Schools of Medicine and Pharmacy, Division of Clinical Pharmacology, University of California, San Francisco, California 94122, USA. |
| SJÖQVIST, F. | Department of Clinical Pharmacology, Karolinska Institutet (Huddinge University Hospital), Stockholm, Sweden. |
| SPRING, P. | Department of Internal Medicine, Buergerspital, 4000 Basle, Switzerland. |
| TRAGER, W. | Schools of Medicine and Pharmacy, Division of Clinical Pharmacology, University of California, San Francisco, California 94122, USA. |
| TUCK, D. | Department of Psychiatry, Karolinska Hospital, 10401 Stockholm 60, Sweden. |
| WAGNER, J. | Research Department, Pharmaceuticals Division, Ciba-Geigy Limited, Basle, Switzerland. |

# Contents

**Session 3 Therapeutic Use of Antibacterial Drugs**

Chairman: Professor D. A. Price Evans



**Session 4 Therapeutic Use of Drugs Acting on the Central Nervous System**

Chairman: Professor F. Sjöqvist



**Session 5 When Ought We to Measure Plasma Concentrations in in Clinical Practice?**



Chairman: Professor C. T. Dollery

Panel: Professor L. Goldberg, Professor F. Sjöqvist, Professor D. A. Price Evans, Professor G. Levy

## ACKNOWLEDGEMENTS

The Organizing Committee wishes to express thanks to the Pharmaceutical Industry in Great Britain for their financial support of this symposium.

# Preface

The concept that the activity of a drug depends not on the dose, but the plasma concentration, was first put forward in the early 1940's. The subsequent discoveries of large inter-individual differences in steady-state plasma concentrations of drugs, largely due to differences in rates of metabolism, added force to the argument that therapy should be controlled by monitoring the concentration of drug in plasma. However, this assumes that the desired pharmacological response is achieved over a relatively narrow range of concentrations in different individuals. In recent years this assumption has been challenged. This appeared to be a particularly appropriate time for the Clinical Pharmacology Section of the British Pharmacological Society to organize its first symposium to examine the relationship between the biological effects of drugs and their plasma concentrations.

CTD
DSD
BNCP

**Session 1**

Chairman: Professor C. T. Dollery

ONE

# The Value of Correlating Biological Effects of Drugs with Plasma Concentration

BERNARD B. BRODIE AND JERRY R. MITCHELL[1]

*Laboratory of Chemical Pharmacology,*
*National Heart and Lung Institute,*
*Bethesda, Maryland 20014, USA*

## Introduction

The concept that the activity of a drug depends on its plasma concentration was first tested by E. K. Marshall with sulphonamides (Marshall, 1940), but the widespread application of this doctrine to rational drug therapy was firmly established during the clinical screening of antimalarials in World War II by Shannon and associates (Shannon, 1946).

The loss of quinine sources had created a crisis which made it crucial that potential antimalarial drugs be tested accurately using a small number of therapeutic trials. Initial studies revealed that the therapeutic effects of the four cinchona alkaloids could not be related to their dosage. Fortunately, their effects were found to correlate with their plasma concentration, making possible rapid screening for antimalarial activity. Subsequent studies showed a similar relationship between the antimalarial activity of synthetic substances and their plasma levels, and led to the effective use of mepacrine, a well-known compound that had been discarded as ineffective because it previously had been administered incorrectly (Shannon, Earle, Brodie, Taggart & Berliner, 1944).

Therefore the most important achievement of the antimalarial project

[1] Research Associate in the Pharmacology-Toxicology Programme, National Institute of General Medical Sciences, National Institutes of Health, Bethesda, Maryland 20014.

was not the development of new compounds but the development of new principles in drug screening.

## Kinetic Considerations Underlying the Use of Plasma Concentrations

A fundamental premise in pharmacology is that a drug response is determined by the quantity of drug fixed to sites of action. Since the concentration of drug in plasma can usually be measured, it is important to know whether changes in this concentration reflect changes in the amount of drug at its active site(s).

For drugs that act reversibly, the formation of drug-receptor complexes obeys the law of mass action. At equilibrium, the rates of formation and dissociation of drug-receptor complexes are equal. In general, the rates of association and dissociation are so high that changes in the number of drug-receptor complexes and in the intensity of response parallel changes in concentration of the drug in tissue water, which in turn is usually in rapid equilibrium with the drug in plasma.

Nevertheless, there are many instances when pharmacological effects are apparently not related to the plasma level of the drug. A therapeutic agent may be inactive itself but act through a bio-transformation product. In this case, the response will be related to the concentration of the metabolite in plasma. Whenever a response is clearly unrelated to the drug concentration in plasma, the possibility must be considered that the action of the drug is mediated through a metabolic product; a number of therapeutic agents have been discovered by the study of such relationships (Brodie, 1964).

In addition, other drugs act non-reversibly, i.e. the quantity of active agent attached to receptors is not related to steady-state plasma concentration. Such drugs often attach to their receptors and then bond covalently with them. A small amount of drug remains attached to these sites long after the rest of the drug has vanished from the body. Certain drugs, such as reserpine, act non-reversibly without bonding covalently, but they also are attached so tightly to receptors that they remain fixed to these sites after the concentration of unbound drug has declined to levels which are unmeasurable by our present analytical techniques.

Non-reversible drugs are inherently dangerous. Even when given in very small daily doses, the effects accumulate even though the drug apparently does not. Thus, they exert a persistent action and recovery depends on regeneration of the sites of action. Since plasma levels are not a guide to therapy, non-reversibly acting drugs must be handled with great care. Kinetic studies in animals will disclose whether a new drug acts non-reversibly; in fact, the clinical pharmacologist should insist on having this information before undertaking human studies.

**Extrapolation of Animal Data to Man: Plasma Concentrations as an Explanation of Biological Variability in Drug Response**

A major difficulty in drug development is the vast species variability in drug responses. This variability makes it difficult to extrapolate to man experimental results obtained in animals. Not long ago, species variability in drug responses was attributed to intrinsic differences in the responsivity of the target organ. This view was based on the assumption that the same dose of drug (in mg/kg) would attain the same concentration at drug receptor sites in various mammalian species. Recent years, however, have disclosed vast differences in rates of drug metabolism within and between species. This raises the possibility that variations in response may be due to differences in amounts of drug available at sites of action.

Consistent with this view is the fact that most drugs which elicit pharmacological effects of equal intensity after comparable doses in various mammalian species mainly are poorly lipid-soluble compounds which are not dependent on metabolism for elimination. For example, ganglionic blocking agents, many antibiotics, the thiazide diuretics and the adrenergic blocking agent, tolazoline, exert similar biological effects in animals and man. These drugs are disposed of by excretory processes that are essentially the same for all mammalian species. Hence, they attain similar plasma concentrations in most animals and show little species variability in drug response.

Even for drugs whose metabolism does show marked species differences, dependable predictions of activity are usually obtained if drug responses are related to plasma concentration rather than to dosage. This point is well illustrated by a few examples.

Despite great species differences in duration of action and rates of metabolism of several barbiturates, man and other animal species recover from hypnosis at similar plasma concentrations. In addition, variations in metabolism due to strain and sex differences are circumvented if activity is based on plasma levels (Quinn, Axelrod & Brodie, 1958). Similarly, the duration of sedative action of carisoprodol varies in four species from 0·1 h (in mice) to 10 h (in cats), but plasma concentrations are almost identical on recovery from hypnosis (righting reflex). Although hypnosis is three times as long in female as in male rats, and is markedly reduced by phenobarbitone pretreatment, plasma levels on recovery are similar (Gillette, 1971).

The compound ICI 33828 inhibits pituitary gonadotropic function at vastly different doses for a number of species. Despite a 200-fold variation in daily dosage, the inhibitory plasma level of each species is about 3$\mu$g/ml (Duncan, 1963).

To protect against glycerol-induced inflammation in the rabbit's eye requires 300 mg phenylbutazone daily. In man 5–10 mg/kg is required to exert an antirheumatic effect. In both instances, however, the plasma concentrations are 100–150 $\mu$g/ml. The marked difference in dosage reflects the biological half-life of 3 h in rabbits compared with 70 h in man (Burns, 1962). Again, the dose of N-isopropylmethoxamine that blocks the epinephrine-induced output of free fatty acids in man and dog is about 10 mg/kg and plasma concentrations are 3 to 6 $\mu$g/ml. In mouse and rat, the drug elicits no effects in doses up to 400 mg/kg, but the plasma levels do not rise above 0·5 $\mu$g/ml. Despite these apparent species differences, the antilipolytic effects of the drug are equally effective in isolated adipose tissue of rats and dogs (Burns, 1965).

## Drug Screening in Animals

As the above examples show, therapeutic agents are often metabolized much more slowly in man than in other animals. This raises the possibility that present methods of screening might well overlook many rapidly metabolized drugs that could be of therapeutic value to man.

The following are examples of drugs discovered in man that earlier animal tests would not have disclosed. Oxyphenbutazone has such a short half-life in animals (about 30 min in dogs compared with 72 h in man) that it would have been discarded if the investigators had not been aware of species differences in metabolism (Burns, 1962). The relatively short half-life of phenylbutazone in animals also caused it to be initially overlooked. The potent antirheumatic action of this drug in man was discovered by chance when it was used as a solubilizing agent for the parenteral injection of amidopyrine (Gsell & Muller, 1950). Likewise the antidepressant action (reversal of reserpine syndrome) of imipramine and its active metabolite desipramine would not have shown in rabbits or mice, since these animals rapidly inactivate both (Dingell, Sulser & Gillette, 1964).

## Drug Screening and Development of Optimal Dosage Schedules in Man

It is not generally recognized that a common cause of toxic reactions in man is 'overdosage' because of large person-to-person variability in rates of drug metabolism; in different subjects, the same daily dose of a drug may cure, cause severe toxicity or have no effect whatsoever. Clinical investigators whose experience has been confined mainly to polar drugs, such as the quaternary ammonium compounds and thiazide diuretics, may suspect that the importance of individual differences in metabolism has been grossly exaggerated. In contrast, researchers concerned with drugs having some degree of lipid solubility are aware of the wide divergencies in drug response but until recently have resisted the view that they are due to divergencies in drug metabolism. The individual variability in drug metabolism can indeed be large: bishydroxycoumarin and ethyl biscoumacetate, for example, show a fifteen-fold difference among various individuals. Many other drugs, including diphenylhydantoin, isoniazid, amidopyrine, antipyrine, desipramine, chlorpromazine and quinidine, are metabolized at widely different rates.

With such variability, how can a clinical pharmacologist be expected to evaluate a drug if, unknown to him, the plasma concentration progressively accumulates or oscillates between that which is ineffective and that which is toxic? Early information about the fate of a drug in man is needed to develop dosage schedules that will improve the efficiency of screening and reduce the danger of overdosage. With the imminent availability of $^{13}$C-labelled (non-radioactive) drugs and gas chromatography-mass spectrometry techniques, it should soon be possible, based on limited animal-toxicity studies, to evaluate in man the physiological fate of most drugs given in doses of only a few milligrams. From such studies, the degree of absorption of a drug can be determined from its concentration in plasma. If the plasma level is almost identical a few hours after both oral and parenteral administration, it may be assumed that absorption is rapid and complete. After intravenous administration, the biological half-life of the drug can be calculated from the slope of the exponential decline of the plasma concentration after diffusion equilibrium is reached. Such preliminary studies can decide whether a drug should be abandoned either because its absorption is inadequate or its excretion is too rapid.

Several examples show the value of these early studies.

1. A screening programme to find a barbiturate that would be rapidly metabolized in the body led to the discovery of a compound that was extremely unstable in dogs. After detailed and expensive toxicity studies, the compound proved to be the longest lasting barbiturate of all time when finally tested in man (Brodie, 1964).

2. Pethidine at one time was believed not to produce tolerance and addiction in man. This erroneous view arose from studies in dogs in which the drug has a half-life of a few minutes compared with 4 h in man (Burns *et al.*, 1955). The experiments in dogs only proved that it is difficult to produce tolerance and addiction to a drug that is not there.

3. Measurement of plasma levels would have shown that the 'special disease' by which chloramphenicol supposedly killed newborn children was simply overdosage due to chloramphenicol's slow metabolism in the neonate (Weiss, Glazko & Weston, 1960).

When optimal dosage schedules are developed, an attempt is made to maintain a drug at an effective concentration; that is, one that is above the therapeutic and below the toxic plasma concentration. Theoretically, a constant level can be maintained only by continuous intravenous infusion.

With oral administration, a compromise may be achieved by giving a priming dose of drugs large enough to produce the desired therapeutic plasma level followed by maintenance doses given at appropriate intervals.

Thus dosage schedules entail three variables: the size of the priming dose, the size of the maintenance dose and the dosage interval. The size of the priming dose (mg/kg) is calculated by multiplying the experimentally determined effective plasma concentration (mg/l) by the 'apparent' volume of distribution and adding to this value the maintenance dose. The apparent volume of distribution is a measure of the relative tissue to plasma concentration of the drug after equilibration. The maintenance dose and the dosage interval depend on the permissible degree that the plasma level can oscillate and still produce a therapeutic effect without evoking toxicity. The appropriate dosage regimen can be readily calculated from the biological half-life of the drug. Since these kinetics are discussed in detail by other authors, we need not discuss them further.

For certain drugs, the time is approaching when a different dosage schedule for each individual will be needed. Drugs are becoming more effective but also more toxic, and it is often difficult to take advantage of these agents unless dosage schedules are tailored based on the optimal plasma concentration. It must be emphasized, however, that such individualized regimens will be important mainly for drugs with a highly variable person-to-person rate of metabolism. Furthermore, they would be valid only for drugs whose therapeutic effects depend on the steady-state plasma level and would not apply to non-reversibly acting drugs, such as reserpine, alkylating agents and monoamine oxidase inhibitors.

**Elucidation of Mechanisms of Drug Interactions**

In recent years much concern over drug interactions has evolved because doctors frequently prescribe more than one drug or are unaware that the patient is taking drugs prescribed by other physicians. An important type of drug interaction occurs when one drug alters the plasma concentration of another. For example, a number of drugs in therapeutic doses can stimulate the activity of a wide diversity of microsomal drug-metabolizing enzymes. An especially difficult therapeutic situation can arise when a patient is treated at the same time with a coumarin anticoagulant and a variety of other drugs. For example, various barbiturates accelerate the metabolism of the coumarin drugs (O'Reilly & Aggeler, 1970). If the administration of the barbiturate is discontinued, the coumarin levels rise and can lead to internal bleeding.

These studies also demonstrate, incidentally, that cross-over studies using subjects as their own controls must now be carefully scrutinized, since a first drug may stimulate the metabolism of a second drug, thereby increasing its metabolic rate and invalidating the comparison.

One drug can also interact with another by inhibiting its metabolism. Thus, phenyramidol administered to a subject already on anticoagulant therapy with bishydroxycoumarin raises the plasma levels of the anticoagulant which may result in bleeding (Solomon & Schrogie, 1966). To complicate matters, a number of drugs first inhibit drug-metabolizing enzymes and later stimulate them, the net result depending on the timing of the dosage schedule. Perhaps an argument in favour of more potent drugs is that inhibition or stimulation of drug metabolism is not related to pharmacological potency but to the plasma level of the therapeutic agent. Thus drug interactions involving metabolism are less likely with more potent drugs.

In another type of interaction, changes in urinary pH may have a profound influence on the elimination of certain drugs. Acidic drugs, such as salicylate, are excreted more rapidly if the urine is made alkaline, while basic drugs, such as quinidine and amphetamine, are excreted more quickly if the urine is acidified (Hollister & Levy, 1965; Gerhardt, Knouss, Thyrum, Luchi & Morris, 1969; Davis, Kopin, Lemberger & Axelrod, 1971). This becomes clinically relevant when renal excretion is a major pathway of drug elimination. Thus, when the urine is made acidic by the ingestion of ammonium chloride or large amounts of vitamin C, the response to a standard dose of quinidine may be inadequate. In contrast, if the urine is made more alkaline by the ingestion of sodium bicarbonate, amphetamine may become toxic.

One drug may be eliminated in the urine by active tubular secretion; another drug, similarly secreted, may interfere with the elimination of the first drug. For example, phenylbutazone potentiates the hypoglycaemic effect of acetohexamide by interfering with the urinary excretion of its active metabolite (Field, Ohta, Boyle & Remer, 1967).

A drug may inhibit the absorption of another to such an extent that drug concentrations in plasma may be too low to be effective. For example, both plain sodium bicarbonate and most commercial antacids decrease the absorption of tetracyclines and pentobarbitone (Barr, Adir & Garrettson, 1971; Hurwitz & Sheehan, 1971). Substances such as desipramine that decrease the motility of the gut also decrease the absorption rate of phenylbutazone through delayed gastric emptying (Consolo, Morselli, Zaccala & Garattini, 1970).

The antagonism of guanethidine's antihypertensive action by desipramine (Mitchell, Cavanaugh, Arias & Oates, 1970) and by amphetamine (Chang, Costa & Brodie, 1965) also can be evaluated by measuring guanethidine concentrations in patients' plasma and urine. In this way, desipramine was shown to antagonize the effect of guanethidine by preventing its uptake by adrenergic nerve endings, whereas amphetamine counteracted guanethidine's action by releasing guanethidine from nerve endings (Oates, Mitchell, Feagin, Kaufmann & Shand, 1971).

**Value of Measuring Drug Concentrations in Studies of Drug-Induced Tissue Lesions**

We have been studying the possibility that the occasional cellular damage caused by many drugs is mediated through chemically reactive biotransformation products. This would imply that organic compounds are not always converted to less toxic substances but may also be transformed in part to chemically highly reactive compounds which can then react with various tissue macromolecules to cause tissue damage or to form antigens.

To test this hypothesis, we first used rats to study a number of industrial organic compounds that are remarkably inert chemically, yet reproducibly cause necrosis in that part of the liver which contains the highest activity of drug-metabolizing enzymes, the centrilobular region. Key parameters used in these studies were the relationships between plasma levels of the toxic agents and the degree of liver damage when the drug-metabolizing enzymes were induced or inhibited by appropriate compounds. Biochemical evidence indicates that the centrilobular necrosis produced in rats by bromobenzene, and a number of other halogenated hydrocarbons, is mediated through a chemically active metabolite formed by oxidation by liver microsomes (Brodie *et al.*, 1971; Reid *et al.*, 1971; Mitchell *et al.*, 1971). Phenobarbitone pretreatment stimulates the disappearance of bromobenzene from plasma and tissues but markedly potentiates the liver necrosis. In contrast, SKF 525-A ($\beta$-diethylaminoethyl diphenylpropylacetate), or piperonyl butoxide, inhibits the disappearance of bromobenzene yet prevents the liver necrosis.

These studies led us to investigate the nature of the active metabolite. By using $^{14}C$-labelled bromobenzene we have been able to demonstrate that the hydrocarbon bonds covalently with liver protein *in vivo* and that *in vitro* a covalent complex of bromobenzene and glutathione is formed (Krishna, Eichelbaum & Reid, 1971). From these data and the pattern of metabolites found in bile and urine, it is evident that the sequence of events is as follows: P-450 enzymes first convert bromobenzene to an epoxide, which then reacts along several pathways. Part of the epoxide rearranges to form a phenol; part is inactivated by reacting with water to form the dihydrodiol (by action of a hydrase); part is inactivated by reaction with glutathione (by the action of a glutathione transferase); and part reacts with tissue macromolecules to cause liver necrosis.

A hint of possible environmental and genetic factors in the hepatotoxicity produced by an agent that forms an active intermediate is disclosed by the *in vivo* actions of methylcholanthrene and glutathione (formed by pretreatment with cysteine), both of which prevent the bromobenzene-induced lesions without affecting plasma levels. Methylcholanthrene appears to act by increasing the activity of the epoxide hydrase, thereby diverting the epoxide along a harmless pathway; glutathione appears to act directly to form a harmless complex (Jollow, Zampaglione & Gillette, 1971).

Our conclusions for the halogenated aromatic hydrocarbons are similar to those of McLean and co-workers using carbon tetrachloride. On the basis of increased liver toxicity after pretreatment of animals with phenobarbital and of decreased toxicity after SKF 525-A, these workers concluded that the toxicity of carbon tetrachloride was mediated by an active intermediate formed by microsomal enzymes (Garner & McLean, 1969).

Having established the concept of drug metabolism as a cause of drug toxicity for appropriate model compounds, we have begun to investigate therapeutic agents.

We first turned our attention to paracetamol, a drug which, in large doses, produces acute centrilobular hepatic necrosis and renal tubular necrosis in man (Prescott, Roscoe, Wright & Brown, 1971) and in rats (Boyd & Bereczky, 1966). As the major metabolite of phenacetin, it also has been implicated in the 'analgesic nephropathy' syndrome currently prevalent in many European countries and in Australia.

Again, by studying the relation between plasma concentrations and the extent of liver damage after stimulation and inhibition of paracetamol's metabolism, we have established that the hepatic necrosis produced by paracetamol and its analogues in rats and mice is also mediated through a chemically reactive metabolite, possibly a hydroxamic acid (Mitchell *et al.*, 1972). Covalent bonding with tissue macromolecules in animals has been shown *in vivo* and *in vitro* and, in the latter case, a carbon monoxide-sensitive, mixed-function oxidase from liver was required to be present for bonding to occur. Interactions, of paracetamol with hepatic stores of glutathione, similar to those described above for bromobenzene have also been demonstrated.

## Conclusion

Several contributors discuss in detail the theoretical considerations and restrictions underlying the use and measurement of drug plasma levels and present extensive data for particular drugs from their own studies. For this reason, we have chosen to summarize the many areas where measurement of drug concentrations in plasma has been found to be helpful. Drug plasma levels have been used to explain biological variability in drug response, to distinguish reversibly acting from non-reversibly acting drugs, to define drugs acting through an active metabolite, and to screen drugs more efficiently. Special emphasis was given to the value of plasma level measurements in the development of optimal dosage regimens and in the elucidation of mechanisms underlying drug interactions and adverse drug reactions.

## REFERENCES


Barr, W. H., Adir, J. & Garrettson, L. (1971). Decrease of tetracycline absorption in man by sodium bicarbonate. *Clin. Pharmac. Ther.*, **12**, 779–784.

Boyd, E. M. & Bereczky, G. M. (1966). Liver necrosis from paracetamol. *Br. Pharmac. Chemother.*, **26**, 606–614.

Brodie, B. B. (1964). In: *Absorption and Distribution of Drugs*, ed. Binns, T. B., p. 199. Baltimore: Williams & Wilkins.

Brodie, B. B., Reid, W. D., Cho, A. K., Sipes, G., Krishna, G. & Gillette, J. R. (1971). Possible mechanism of liver necrosis caused by aromatic organic compounds. *Proc. natn. Acad. Sci. U.S.A.*, **68,** 160–164.

Burns, J. J. (1962). In: *Proceedings of the First International Pharmacological Meeting*, vol. **6,** ed. Brodie, B. B. & Erdos, E. G., p. 277. Oxford: Pergamon Press.

Burns, J. J. (1965). In: *Evaluation of New Drugs in Man*, ed. Eaimis, E., p. 21. Oxford: Pergamon Press.

Burns, J. J., Berger, B. L., Lief, P. A., Woolack, A., Papper, E. M. & Brodie, B. B. (1955). The physiological disposition and fate of meperidine (Demerol) in man and a method for its estimation in plasma. *J. Pharmac. exp. Ther.*, **114,** 289–298.

Chang, C. C., Costa, E. & Brodie, B. B. (1965). Interaction of guanethidine with adrenergic neurons. *J. Pharmac. exp. Ther.*, **147**, 303–312.

Consolo, S., Morselli, P. L., Zaccala, M. & Garattini, S. (1970). Delayed absorption of phenylbutazone caused by desmethylimipramine in humans. *Eur. J. Pharmac.*, **10**, 239–242.

Davis, J. M., Kopin, I. J., Lemberger, L. & Axelrod, J. (1971). Effects of urinary pH on amphetamine metabolism. *Ann. N.Y. Acad. Sci.*, **179,** 493–501.

Dingell, J. V., Sulser, F. & Gillette, J. R. (1964). Species differences in the metabolism of imipramine and desmethylimipramine (DMI). *J. Pharmac. exp. Ther.*, **143**, 14–22.

Duncan, W. A. M. (1963). The importance of metabolism studies in relation to drug toxicity. A general review. *Proc. Eur. Soc. Study Drug Toxicity*, **2**, 67–72.

Field, J. B., Ohta, M., Boyle, C. & Remer, A. (1967). Potentiation of acetohexamide hypoglycemia by phenylbutazone. *New Engl. J. Med.*, **277**, 889–894.

GARNER, R. C. & MCLEAN, A. E. M. (1969). Increased susceptibility to carbon tetrachloride poisoning in the rat after treatment with oral phenobarbitone. *Biochem. Pharmac.*, **18**, 645–650.

GERHARDT, R. E., KNOUSS, R. P., THYRUM, P. T., LUCHI, R. J. & MORRIS, J. J. (1969). Quinidine excretion in aciduria and alkaluria. *Ann. intern. Med.*, **71**, 927–933.

GILLETTE, J. R. (1965). Drug toxicity as a result of interference with physiological control mechanisms. *Ann. N.Y. Acad. Sci.*, **123**, 42–54.

GSELL, O. & MULLER, W. (1950). Parentale pyramidon-pyrazolidin-therapie von rheumatismus und infekten mittels irgrapyrin. *Schweiz. med. Wschr.*, **80**, 310–316.

HOLLISTER, L. & LEVY, G. (1965). Some aspects of salicylate distribution and metabolism in man. *J. Pharm. Sci.*, **54**, 1126–1129.

HURWITZ, A. & SHEEHAN, M. B. (1971). The effects of antacids on the absorption of orally adminstered pentobarbitol in the rat. *J. Pharmac. exp. Ther.*, **179**, 124–131.

JOLLOW, D., ZAMPAGLIONE, N. & GILLETTE, J. R. (1971). Mechanism of protection from bromobenzene hepatotoxicity by 3-methylcholanthrene. *Pharmacologist*, **13**, 288.

KRISHNA, G., EICHELBAUM, M. & REID, W. D. (1971). Isolation and characterization of liver proteins containing covalently bound $^{14}$C-bromobenzene metabolites. *Pharmacologist*, **13**, 196.

MARSHALL, E. K. (1940). Experimental basis of chemotherapy in the treatment of bacterial infections. *Bull. N.Y. Acad. Med.*, **16**, 722–731.

MITCHELL, J. R., CAVANAUGH, J. H., ARIAS, L. & OATES, J. A. (1970). Guanethidine and related agents. III. Antagonism by drugs which inhibit the norepinephrine pump in man. *J. clin. Invest.*, **49**, 1596–1604.

MITCHELL, J. R., REID, W. D., CHRISTIE, B., MOSKOWITZ, J., KRISHNA, G. & BRODIE, B. B. (1971). Bromobenzene-induced hepatic necrosis: species differences and protection by SKF 525-A. *Res. Commun. Chem. Path. Pharmac.*, **2**, 877–888.

MITCHELL, J. R., POTTER, W. Z., JOLLOW, D., DAVIS, D. C., GILLETTE, J. R. & BRODIE, B. B. (1972). Acetaminophen-induced hepatic necrosis. I. Potentiation by inducers and protection by inhibitors of drug-metabolizing enzymes. *Fedn Proc. Fedn Am. Socs exp. Biol.* (in press).

OATES, J. A., MITCHELL, J. R., FEAGIN, O. T., KAUFMANN, J. S. & SHAND, D. G. (1971) Distribution of guanidinum antihypertensives—mechanism of their selective action. *Ann. N.Y. Acad. Sci.*, **179**, 302–309.

O'REILLY, R. A. & AGGELER, P. M. (1970). Determinants of the response to oral anticoagulants in man. *Pharmac. Rev.*, **22**, 35–96.

PRESCOTT, L. F., ROSCOE, P., WRIGHT, N. & BROWN, S. S. (1971). Plasma-paracetamol half-life and hepatic necrosis in patients with paracetamol overdosage. *Lancet*, **1**, 519–522.

QUINN, G. P., AXELROD, J. & BRODIE, B. B. (1958). Species, strain and sex differences in metabolism of hexobarbital, amidopyrine, antipyrine and aniline. *Biochem. Pharmac.*, **1**, 152–159.

REID, W. D., CHRISTIE, B., KRISHNA, G., MITCHELL, J. R., MOSKOWITZ, J. & BRODIE, B. B. (1971). Bromobenzene metabolism and hepatic necrosis. *Pharmacology* (in press).

SHANNON, J. A. (1946). The study of antimalarials and antimalarial activity in the human malarias. *Harvey Lect. Ser.*, **41**, 43–89.

SHANNON, J. A., EARLE, D. P., BRODIE, B. B., TAGGART, J. V. & BERLINER, R. W. (1944). The pharmacological basis for the rational use of atabrine in the treatment of malaria. *J. Pharmac. exp. Ther.*, **81**, 307–330.

SOLOMON, H. M. & SCHROGIE, J. J. (1966). The effect of phenyramidol on the metabolism of bishydroxycoumarin. *J. Pharmac. exp. Ther.*, **154**, 660–666.

WEISS, C. F., GLAZKO, A. J. & WESTON, J. K. (1960). Chloramphenicol in the newborn infant. A physiological explanation of its toxicity when given in excess doses. *New Engl. J. Med.*, **262**, 787–794.

TWO

# Plasma Concentrations and Pharmacological Response in Animals

H. KEBERLE, J. W. FAIGLE, P. HEDWALL, W. RIESS AND J. WAGNER

*Research Department, Pharmaceuticals Division, Ciba–Geigy Limited, Basle, Switzerland*

## Introduction

One particularly important aspect of pharmacokinetics is the search for correlations between drug concentrations and pharmacological activity. Studies of this kind can in principal be performed *in vitro*, in the animal or in man.

The importance of experiments *in vitro* and in the animal is:

1. they supplement the information gained from pharmacological experiments:
2. they ensure greater safety in human experiments in that they provide data on pharmacologically and toxicologically active concentrations.
3. they make it possible to choose experimental conditions that would not be permissible in investigations in human beings.

In this paper three different studies *in vitro* and on animals are discussed in which we attempt to establish relations between concentration and activity.

## Sulphonamides

The first example is taken from a study of antibacterially active sulphonamides. The object of this study was to find out why it is that many sulphonamides that are highly potent *in vitro* should be completely devoid of any activity *in vivo*.

Since we wanted to examine the pharmacokinetics and the chemotherapeutic effects of a whole series of sulphonamides we decided to label all the compounds with $S^{35}$. The experiments were carried out on mice because chemotherapeutic effects are easy to detect in this species and only small quantities of radioactively labelled substance are required for the metabolic and pharmacokinetic studies.

The structures, bacteriological activity and physical properties of the three sulphonamides are shown in Table 1. Considering first their bacteriological activity, it is evident that all three are roughly equally

TABLE 1

| Structure | Bacteriological activity (*S. aureus*) | | Solubility mg/100 ml | | | Free in plasma water at conc. of 100 $\mu$g/ml |
|---|---|---|---|---|---|---|
| 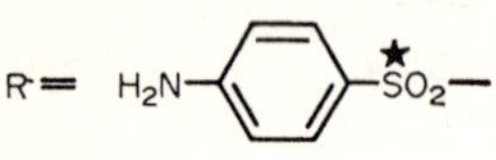 | *in vitro* M.I.C.* $\mu$g/ml | *in vivo* $ED_{50}$† mouse p.o. mg/kg | Water pH 7·4 | $CHCl_3$ | pKa | |
| 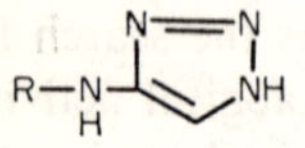 Hydrophile | 10 | >1000 | 3000 | 8 | 6·6 | 42 |
| 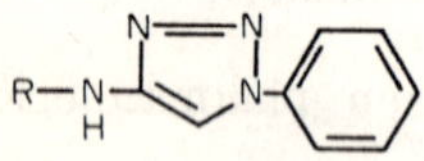 Semi-lipophile | 5 | 50 | 10 | 113 | 6·7 | 4 |
| 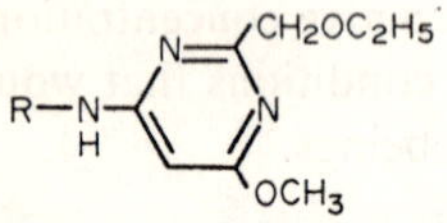 Lipophile | 5 | 250 | 260 | 2000 | 6·2 | 6 |

* M.I.C. = minimum inhibitory concentrations.
† $ED_{50}$ = estimated dose to protect 50% of infected mice.

active *in vitro*, at concentrations of 5–10 $\mu$g/ml; whereas *in vivo*, in the mouse, there are very appreciable differences between them. The first preparation remains completely inactive up to an oral dose of 1000 mg/kg, the second shows very good activity at 50 mg/kg and the third is only moderately effective at 250 mg/kg.

A comparison of the solubility of the three compounds in water at pH 7·4 and in chloroform shows that the first dissolves very well in water and the third very well in chloroform. The second preparation, on the other hand, which is the most active *in vivo*, is not readily soluble either in

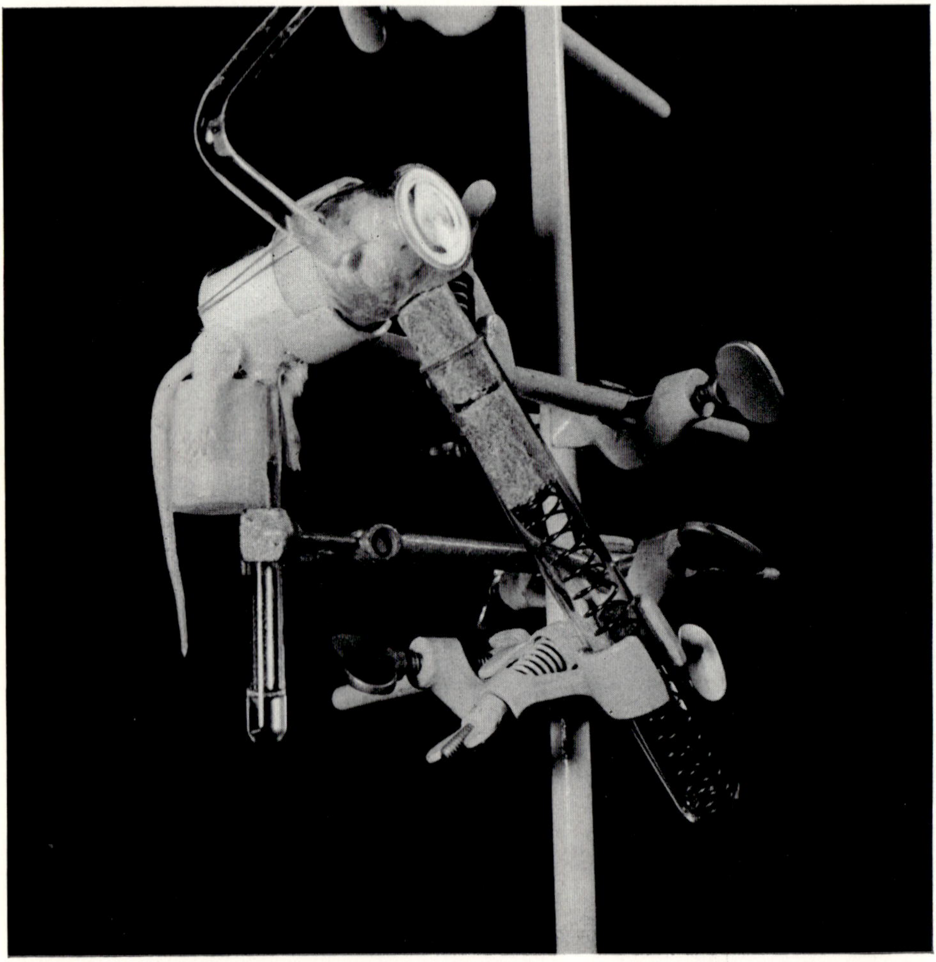

FIG. 1. Device for the efficient separation of urine and faeces in mice.

water or in chloroform. The penultimate column of Table 1 indicates that this difference is not due to the acid character of the sulphonamides, since all three have a similar pKa. The last column shows that the first sulphonamide, i.e. the hydrophilic one, which is inactive in the animal, is bound least of all to plasma proteins. At a total concentration of 100 $\mu$g/ml, the concentration of the unbound part is about ten times higher than in the case of the other two sulphonamides. Consequently, the inactivity of the

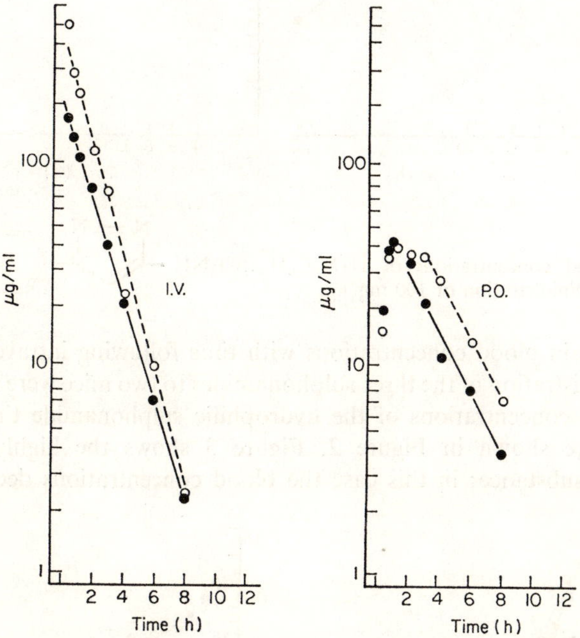


FIG. 2. Blood concentrations of $H_2N.C_6H_4.SO_2NH$ 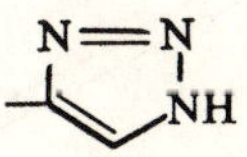 in two mice after administration of 100 mg/kg.

hydrophilic sulphonamide *in vivo* has certainly nothing to do with the extent to which it is ionized or bound to protein, but must be due to some other factor(s). To ascertain whether the metabolism and pharmacokinetics of the compounds could provide an explanation, experiments were carried out on individual mice. For these studies a new type of restriction cage was developed, which is shown in Figure 1. This cage separates the urine and faeces very efficiently. Blood samples were taken from the tail vein. Since samples of as little as 0·5 to 1 $\mu$l suffice for analysis, it was possible to study the pharmacokinetics of a substance after oral and intravenous administration to the same mouse.

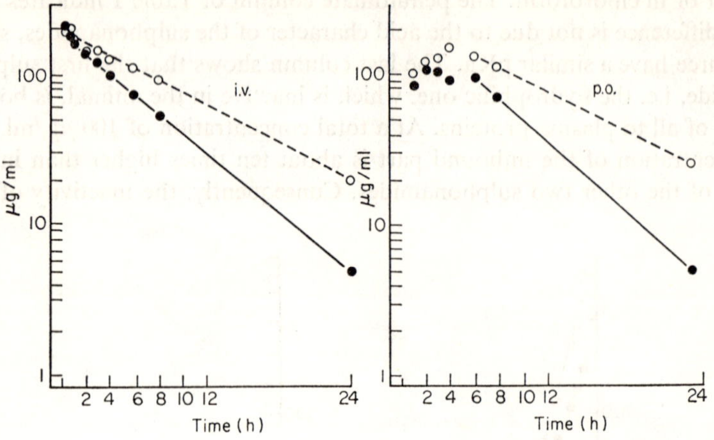


FIG. 3. Blood concentrations of $H_2N.C_6H_4.SO_2NH$— 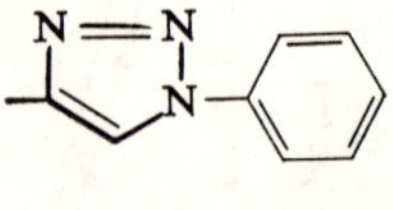 in two mice after administration of 100 mg/kg.

Changes in blood concentrations with time following intravenous and oral administration of the three sulphonamides to two mice were measured. The blood concentrations of the hydrophilic sulphonamide that proved inactive are shown in Figure 2. Figure 3 shows the highly effective lipophilic substance; in this case the blood concentrations decline more

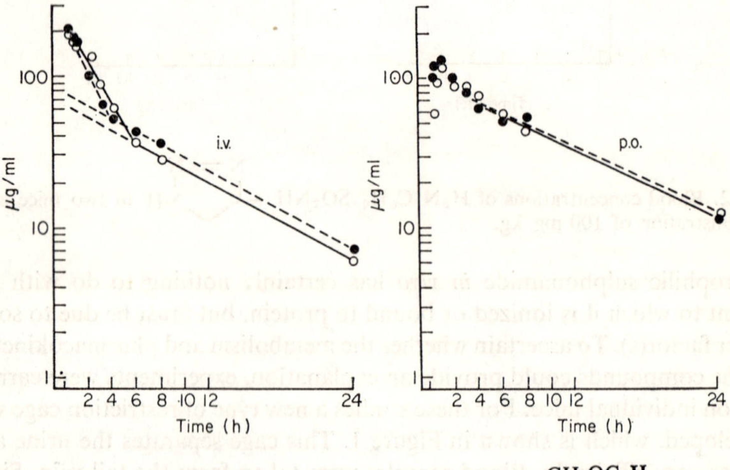


FIG. 4. Blood concentrations of $H_2N.C_6H_4.SO_2NH$— 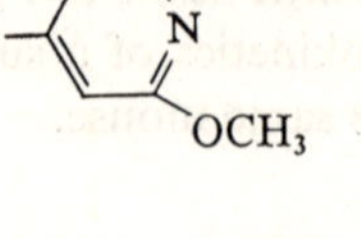 in two mice after administration of 100 mg/kg.

slowly. Blood concentrations of the lipophilic, moderately active preparation showing a pronounced biphasic decline are shown in Figure 4.

The data in Table 2 summarize the pharmacokinetic and metabolic

TABLE 2

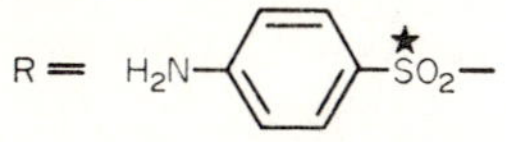

| Structure | t50% h i.v. | % of dose excreted within 24 h in: Urine i.v. | Urine p.o. | Faeces i.v. | Faeces p.o. | % of dose excreted in unchanged form in urine |
|---|---|---|---|---|---|---|
| 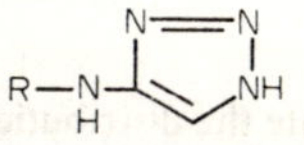 Hydrophile | 1·2 | 87 | 91 | 10 | 3 | 53 |
| 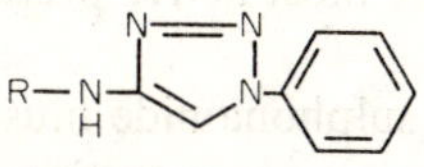 Semi-lipophile | 6·0 | 49 | 28 | 46 | 41 | 2 |
| 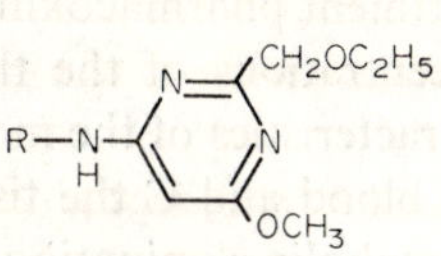 Lipophile | 7 | 89 | 93 | 7 | 13 | 3 |

results. The half-lives, calculated from the decline of the blood concentrations, are 1·2 h for the hydrophilic sulphonamide and 6 h for the semi-lipophilic compound; the 'half-life' of the lipophilic compound is 1·8 h for the first phase, and 7 h for the second phase. When the amounts of substance excreted in the urine and faeces after intravenous and oral administration are compared, it is apparent that all the preparations are totally absorbed from the gut.

The last column shows that 53% of the dose of the hydrophilic compound is recovered from the urine in the form of unchanged substance, as against 2% and 3% of the other two preparations.

The metabolic and pharmacokinetic data indicate that the inactivity of the hydrophilic sulphonamide *in vivo* cannot be explained in terms of either absorption or metabolism. Nor can the short half-life and the low blood concentrations of this preparation be the reason if the relevant concentrations, namely the concentrations of the free sulphonamide in plasma, are taken into consideration. The hydrophilic sulphonamide, being the least protein-bound, reaches during the first 6 h after the administration

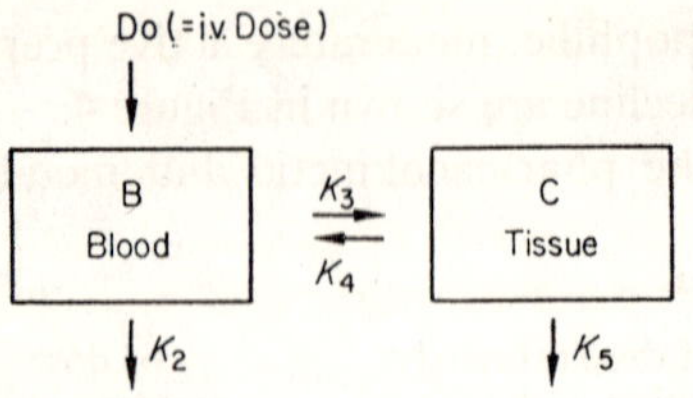


| Sulphonamide type | Rate constants $K_2$ | $K_3$ | $K_4$ | $K_5$ |
|---|---|---|---|---|
| hyrdrophile | 1·0 | 0·2 | 0·2 | 0·1 |
| semi-lipophile | 0·05 | 1·0 | 1·0 | 0·1 |
| lipophile | 0·01 | 1·0 | 0·2 | 0·1 |

Rate constants:

$K_2$ = Renal elimination
$K_3$ = Penetration into tissue compartment
$K_4$ = Back-flow from tissue compartment
$K_5$ = Metabolic elimination

FIG. 5. Characteristics of a two compartment model used to simulate the distribution of sulphonamides.

approximately the same level in plasma water as the most active preparation.

We think the lack of activity of the hydrophilic sulphonamide must be due to slow distribution, or in other words poor tissue penetration. To explain this we tried, with the aid of a two-compartment pharmacokinetic model, to simulate the course of the blood concentrations of the three sulphonamides on an analogue computer. The characteristics of the model used are shown in Figure 5, where B denotes the blood and C the tissue compartment. The rate constants for renal and metabolic elimination are

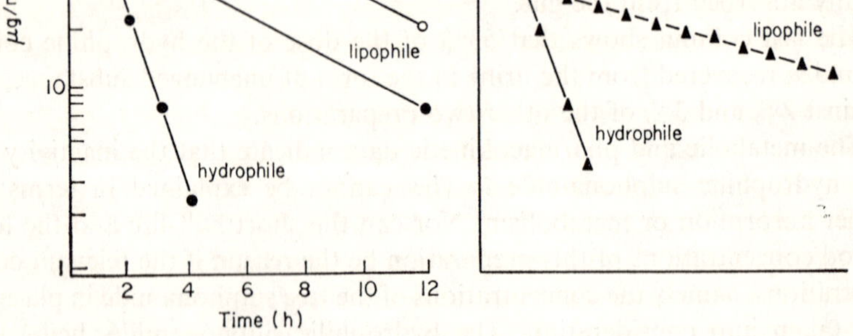


FIG. 6. Blood concentrations of three sulphonamides.

$k_2$ and $k_5$. Penetration into tissues and diffusion back into the blood are represented by $k_3$ and $k_4$ respectively. In Figure 6 experimentally determined curves and those derived from the analogue computer using the constants in Figure 5 are shown. On the basis of these data it can be inferred that the characteristic features of the hydrophilic inactive sulphonamide are rapid renal elimination, slow metabolism and slow penetration into and diffusion out of the tissue. The semilipophilic, i.e. the most active compound, undergoes slow renal and metabolic elimination and penetrates rapidly into tissue. The only difference between the semilipophilic and the lipophilic compound is that the latter diffuses more slowly out of the tissues, $k_4$ being smaller than $k_3$. Such a situation arises if a drug has a marked affinity for the tissues and consequently accumulates there.

In conclusion, it is not possible to predict the chemotherapeutic activity of a sulphonamide *in vivo* merely from the concentrations reached in blood or plasma water alone.

It appears that active sulphonamides undergo relatively slow renal and metabolic elimination and are rapidly and evenly distributed throughout the body. High tissue concentrations are not necessarily an advantage in the case of sulphonamides.

## Niridazole

The second study concerns the schistosomicide niridazole. The structure of niridazole is shown in Figure 7.

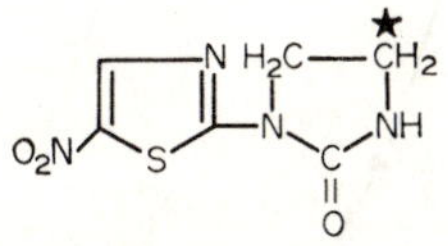


FIG. 7. Structure of niridazole (Ambilhar®), a schistosomicide.

The fate of niridazole in the organism was investigated in rats, rabbits, dogs and humans. It was found that an oral dose is slowly but well absorbed. As is shown in Figure 8, analysis of the blood revealed that the metabolites attain far higher concentrations in whole blood or plasma than does the unchanged drug itself (Faigle & Keberle, 1966). In the blood of the host the parasite is therefore exposed not only to niridazole, but also to high concentrations of metabolites. This raises the question whether the schistosomicidal activity is attributable to the drug or to its metabolites. Clearly, this question has a decisive bearing on the relation between the blood concentration and the chemotherapeutic effect, and consequently on the dosage of the drug. This question was answered by the results of the following experiments. After the administration of labelled niridazole to mice infected with *Schistosoma mansoni*, micro-autoradiographs revealed that radioactive substances had accumulated and become fixed in the worms. This accumulation must be correlated with the schistosomicidal effect, because the highest level of radioactivity was found in those areas of the parasite where the first morphological changes appear.

The autoradiographs, however, provided no information about the nature of the substance that had penetrated the parasite or of the substance that had become fixed in the parasite. This problem was clarified by the following *in vitro* experiment.

Live schistosomes were incubated in a solution consisting of $C^{14}$-niridazole and plasma from untreated animals. In a parallel experiment, the incubation was performed with plasma containing niridazole metabolites. A comparison of the results obtained in this experiment clearly revealed that accumulation of radioactive substances only occurred in the parasites exposed to niridazole, and not in those exposed to its metabolites. Accordingly, only the schistosomes in the niridazole solution sustained damage. On the other hand, when the niridazole-treated worms were analysed, it was found that the radioactivity accumulated in the tissues was accounted for not by niridazole, but by metabolites.

The processes taking place *in vivo* can be summed up as follows. Only the unchanged drug can penetrate from the blood of the host, into the

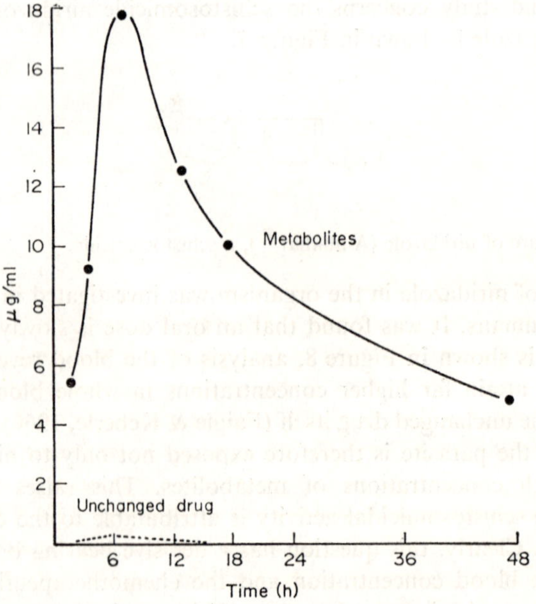


FIG. 8. Blood levels of niridazole and its metabolites in man, following a single dose of 25 mg/kg.

parasite. In the parasite, the drug is broken down into metabolites that are eliminated only very slowly, if at all. This leads, in the course of time, to accumulation of metabolites in the parasite (Faigle & Keberle, 1966).

Further confirmatory information was obtained when live schistosomes were incubated in calf serum in the presence of three different concentrations of $^{14}$C-niridazole, namely 10, 1·6 and 0·7 $\mu$g/ml. The incubation was continued until the parasites were killed. During incubation, the uptake of radioactive substances by the schistosomes was recorded.

The results of this experiment are outlined in Figure 9. This graph shows

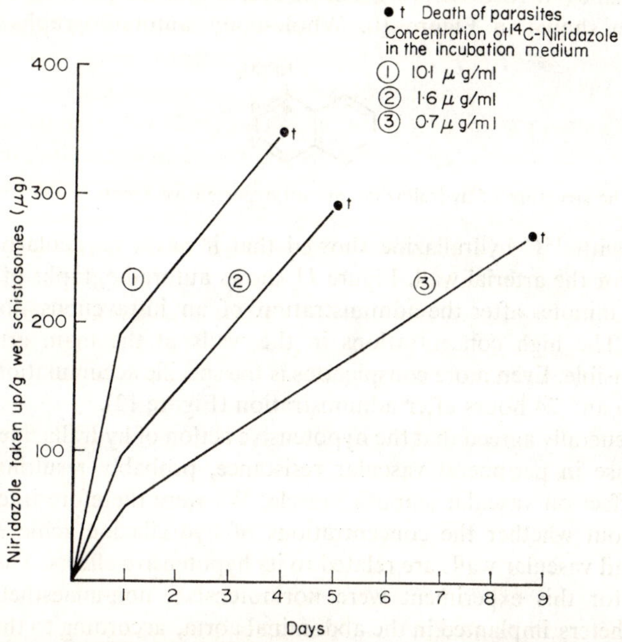


FIG. 9. Uptake of niridazole by *S. mansoni* during incubation in a medium containing various concentrations of the drug.*

that the schistosomes continue to take up niridazole until they die. When high concentrations of niridazole are present in the medium, the drug is taken up more rapidly than in the presence of low concentrations. The total quantity of radioactive metabolites accumulated in the parasite up to the time of their death is roughly the same at all serum concentrations of the drug (300 $\mu$g/g schistosomes). Apparently the parasite does not die until it has absorbed the requisite quantity of niridazole (Faigle & Keberle, 1969).

The time taken to achieve this lethal concentration is dependent on the concentration of niridazole in the medium. At the highest concentration death occurs after 3 days, and at the medium concentration after 5 days;

* Reproduced by permission of the *Annals of the New York Academy of Sciences.*

the lowest concentration employed is still capable of killing the schistosomes, but only after 9 days. This experiment demonstrates the interesting fact that to achieve a chemotherapeutic effect with niridazole time is at least as important as producing a definite concentration of the drug in the blood plasma of the host.

## Hydrallazine

The final example is from a study carried out with the hypotensive agent hydrallazine (APRESOLIN®). The structure and the position of the $^{14}C$ label are shown in Figure 10. Whole-body autoradiographs of mice

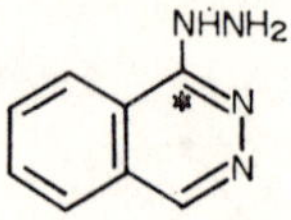


FIG. 10. The structure of hydrallazine, an antihypertensive agent.

treated with $^{14}C$ hydrallazine showed that it has a particularly marked affinity for the arterial wall. Figure 11 shows autoradiographs of a mouse 1 and 5 minutes after the administration of an intravenous dose of 10 mg/kg. The high concentrations in the walls of the main arteries are clearly visible. Even more conspicuous is the specific accumulation demonstrable 6 and 24 hours after administration (Figure 12).

It is generally agreed that the hypotensive action of hydrallazine is due to a decrease in peripheral vascular resistance, probably resulting from a direct effect on vascular smooth muscle. We were therefore interested in finding out whether the concentrations of hydrallazine achieved in the blood and vascular walls are related to its hypotensive effects. The animals chosen for this experiment were normotensive, non-anaesthetized rats with catheters implanted in the abdominal aorta, according to the method of Weeks & Jones (1960). In these rats we measured the decrease in blood pressure and the concentrations of hydrallazine in the blood, the aorta and the mesenteric artery after an intravenous dose of 5 mg/kg. The results are presented in Figure 13. The top curves show the blood pressure recorded in the controls and the reduction in blood pressure in the treated animals. It is evident that the hypotensive effects persists for at least 24 h. The middle curves illustrate the concentrations of hydrallazine in the aorta and mesenteric artery. The bottom curve indicates the course of the blood concentrations. Compared with the blood concentration, the concentrations in the aorta and mesenteric artery are very high, They also decline more slowly than the concentration in the blood. After 24 h 35 $\mu$g/g are still found in the aorta and 12 $\mu$g/g in the mesenteric artery, whereas the blood only contains 0·1 $\mu$g/ml.

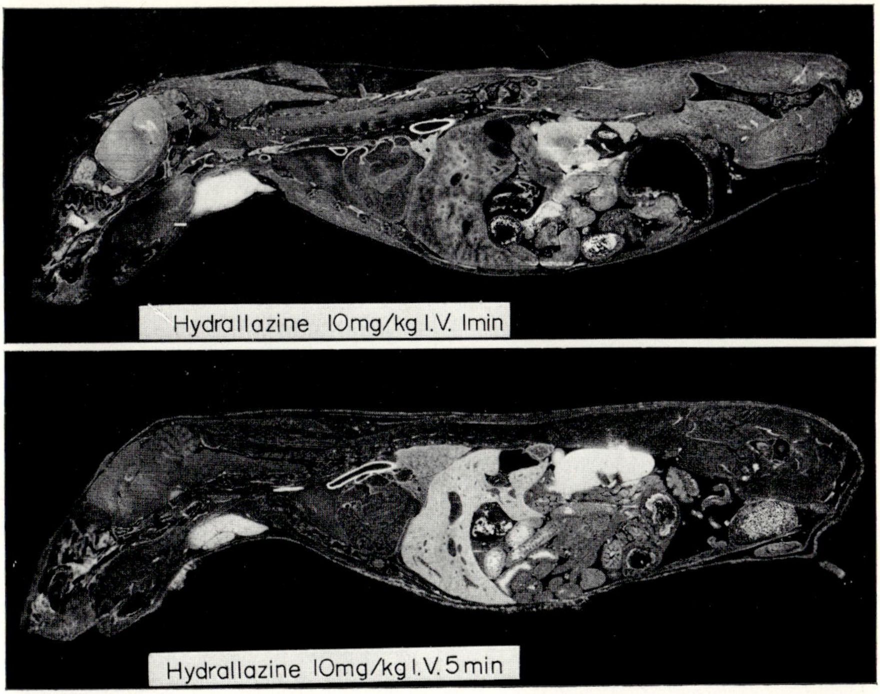


FIG. 11. Whole-body autoradiography of mice 1 min (upper) and 5 min (lower) after intravenous administration of $^{14}C$-hydrallazine (10 mg/kg).

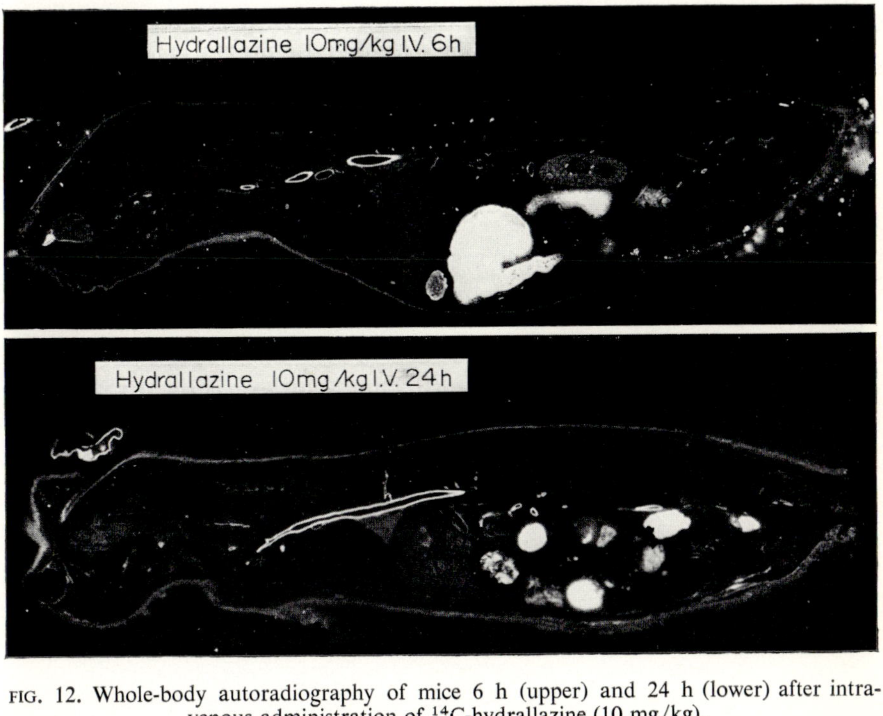


FIG. 12. Whole-body autoradiography of mice 6 h (upper) and 24 h (lower) after intravenous administration of $^{14}C$-hydrallazine (10 mg/kg).

Parallel to this experiment in intact rats, we also carried out an *in vitro* test on the isolated perfused mesenteric artery of the rat using the method of McGregor (1965). In this case the degree to which hydrallazine inhibited the pressor response, induced by electrical stimulation of the periarterial nerves, was measured. The inhibitory effect was determined at various concentrations of hydrallazine in the perfusion fluid. At the same time,

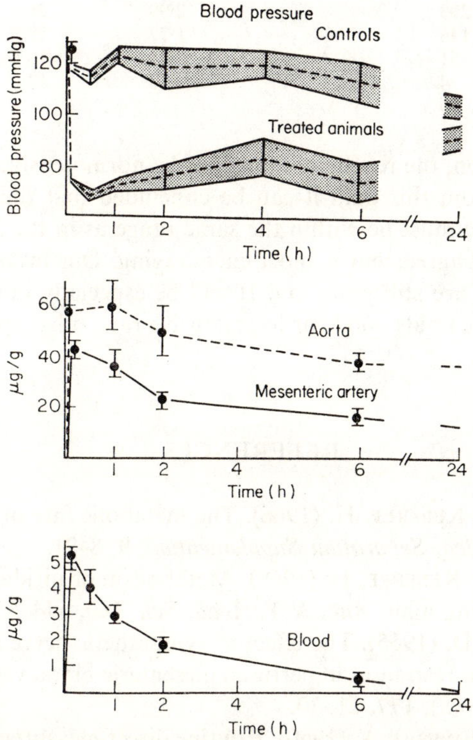


FIG. 13. Time course of changes in blood pressure (top graph); concentrations of hydrallazine in aorta and mesenteric artery (middle graph); and concentration of hydrallazine in blood (bottom graph). Following a dose of 5 mg/kg $^{14}C$-hydrallazine in normotensive rats.

the accumulation of the drug in the arterial wall was determined. The results obtained in this experiment are shown on the left-hand side of Table 3.

When the concentrations in the perfusion fluid are compared with those measured in the mesenteric artery, it is evident that the arterial concentrations are invariably much higher. The saturation concentration appears to be about 200 $\mu g/g$. The pharmacological effect is measurable at a concentration of as little as 0·1 $\mu g/ml$ in the perfusion fluid or 4 $\mu g/g$ in the artery.

TABLE 3

Concentration and activity of $^{14}C$-hydrallazine

| *in vitro* perfusion | | | *in vivo* normotensive rat | | |
|---|---|---|---|---|---|
| Perfusion fluid $\mu g \times 4/ml$ | Mesenteric Artery $\mu g \times 4/g$ | Effect | Blood $\mu g \times 4/ml$ | Mesenteric Artery $\mu g \times 4/g$ | Effect |
| 21 | 194 | + | 5·27 | 42·2 | + |
| 10 | 203 | + | 2·99 | 36·1 | + |
| 4 | 136 | + | 1·77 | 22·3 | + |
| 1 | 51 | + | 0·49 | 16·6 | + |
| 0·1 | 4 | + | 0·13 | 12·0 | (+) |
| 0·01 | 0·3 | 0 | | | |

For comparison, the results obtained in the normotensive rats are listed on the right. From this data it can be concluded that the effective concentration *in vivo* must lie within the same range as in the *in vitro* experiment. This good agreement is most encouraging. Our investigations with this preparation are still going on. It will be especially interesting to see whether the same holds good for hypertensive rats, other species and man also.

## REFERENCES


FAIGLE, J. W. & KEBERLE, H. (1966). The metabolic fate of CIBA 32,644-Ba. *Acta Tropica, Separatum Supplementum*, **9,** 8–21.

FAIGLE, J. W. & KEBERLE, H. (1969). Metabolism of niridazole in various species including man. *Ann. N.Y. Acad. Sci.*, **160,** 544–557.

MCGREGOR, D. D. (1965). The effect of sympathetic nerve stimulation on vasoconstrictor responses in perfused mesenteric blood vessels of the rat. *J. Physiol.* (*Lond.*), **177,** 21–30.

WEEKS, J. R. & JONES, J. A. (1960). Routine direct measurement of arterial blood pressure in unanesthetized rats. *Proc. Soc. Exp. Biol. Med.*, **104,** 646–648.

# THREE

# Plasma Concentrations of Drugs and Pharmacological Response in Man

FOLKE SJÖQVIST AND LEIF BERTILSSON

*Departments of Clinical Pharmacology, University of Linköping, and the Karolinska Institutet (Huddinge University Hospital), Stockholm, Sweden*

## Introduction

During recent years clinical pharmacologists and clinicians have realized the usefulness of monitoring plasma concentrations of certain drugs in patients. For example studies reported by Alexanderson and Lund in this symposium show that the effects of nortriptyline and diphenylhydantoin are much better correlated in patient populations to their steady-state plasma concentrations than to dosage. This also may be true for other drugs which are extensively metabolized in the body. A fixed dose (*X* mg per kg)

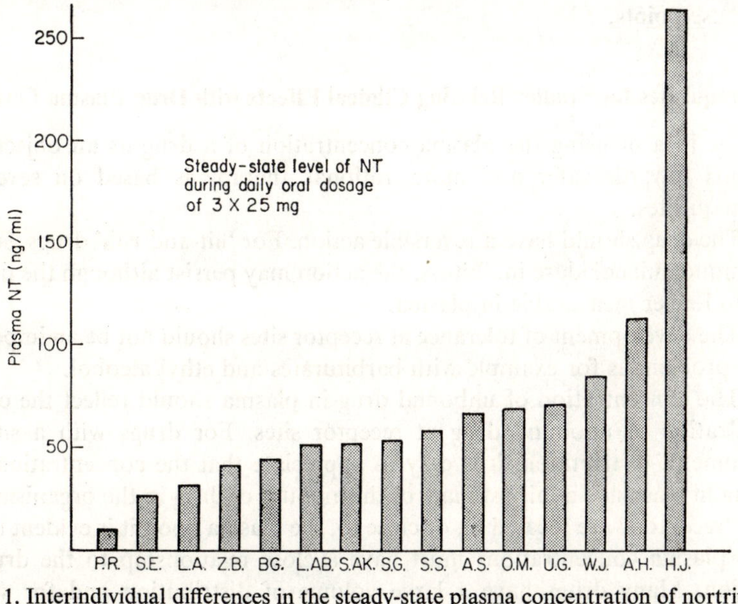


FIG. 1. Interindividual differences in the steady-state plasma concentration of nortriptyline in patients treated with 25 mg t.i.d. From Hammer & Sjöqvist (1967).

of such a drug may give a ten-fold interindividual range in the steady-state plasma concentrations (Figure 1) due to the combined influence of genetic and environmental factors on drug metabolism (Alexanderson *et al.*, 1969; Hammer & Sjöqvist, 1967).

It must be emphasized that there is no general biochemical test available to detect slow drug metabolizers. The clinically used laboratory procedures for liver function are of very little, if any, predictive value for an individual's ability to metabolize drugs. The position with drugs that are excreted unchanged by the kidney is much better because laboratory tests, such as serum creatinine or creatinine clearance, are useful guidelines for the reduction of the dosage, when there is impairment of renal function.

Why is it then that few doctors, even in university hospitals, ask for drug plasma levels as an objective means to maintaining an adequate dosage schedule? The truth is that even if physicians were to request such analyses, reliable data on the relationship between plasma levels and effects exist for very few drugs. This is in turn explained by the fact that few medical centres are equipped for this type of research which must be based on collaboration between clinicians, analytical chemists and pharmacologists.

Our paper attempts to review problems that may be encountered in this type of work. Our own studies of the relationship between plasma concentration and clinical effects of the tricyclic antidepressant drug nortriptyline (*cf.* Alexanderson *et al.* in this symposium) will serve to illustrate some of these points.

## Prerequisites for Studies Relating Clinical Effects with Drug Plasma Levels

The idea of using the plasma concentration of a drug as an objective means towards safer and more rational therapy is based on several prerequisites.

1. The drug should have a reversible action. For 'hit-and-run' drugs, such as monoamineoxidase inhibitors, the action may persist although the drug is no longer measurable in plasma.
2. The development of tolerance at receptor sites should not be an important problem as for example with barbiturates and ethyl alcohol.
3. The concentration of unbound drug in plasma should reflect the concentration of unbound drug at receptor sites. For drugs with a small volume of distribution, it is easy to appreciate that the concentration of drug in plasma is a fair estimate of the amount of drug in the organism. If the 'receptors' are located in, or close to, the plasma pool, it is evident that the plasma concentrations must have a close relationship to the drug's action. Many drugs have a large volume of distribution and for such compounds attempts to relate effects and plasma levels have been looked

upon with scepticism, because 'so little drug' is available in plasma compared with the tissues. The tissue level has been thought to be more important for the pharmacological effect than the plasma level. Besides there being few experimental studies on this point, and human studies are extremely difficult to perform, it can be appreciated that, independently of the volume of distribution of the drug, plasma and tissue levels should be in equilibrium after some period of chronic treatment. The length of this period will vary considerably between drugs. In our studies of nortriptyline, which has an apparent volume of distribution of 20–40 l/kg, the pharmacological effects were measured after three weeks' treatment, i.e. when the plasma and tissue compartments were in equilibrium. There is little reason to believe that the ratio between the concentrations of unbound nortriptyline in plasma and in the biophase surrounding hypothalamic monoaminergic receptor sites should differ markedly between patients as long as we consider distribution as a passive process depending upon the physico-chemical properties of the drug rather than upon the genetic constitution of the individual. The possible importance for drug response of minor interindividual differences in drug binding should nevertheless be explored in man.

4. It is essential in studies of this kind that the pharmacological effects of the drugs are recorded in an accurate way. For a few drugs such as tricyclic antidepressants (see below) and adrenergic beta blockers, it is possible to use their antagonism of other compounds (tyramine and isoprenaline, respectively) as a suitable pharmacodynamic variable. Yet, the crucial question about the relationship between drug plasma level and *clinical* effects has to be tackled using methods which give an index of the amelioration of the symptoms and degree of disease. For psychopharmacological agents we often have to rely upon rating procedures. The ratings should then be performed under blind conditions, i.e. the raters being unaware of the drug plasma levels in the patients. It is also an advantage to know that there is a high degree of correlation between two independent 'blind' raters since the subjective judgement of different observers may differ radically.

Even measuring such an apparently simple parameter as systemic arterial blood pressure imposes a number of questions: should we measure it continuously or at a few occasions every day, in the sitting, standing or lying position, at rest or after exercise or both, in the clinic or at home?

It is very important that the variable being measured is relevant for the pharmacological effect of the drug, otherwise no relationship to drug plasma levels can be expected.

It is our impression that the development of accurate methods for recording the effects of drugs in man and particularly in patients is the rate limiting step in this type of research. In the clinic the situation is often complicated by the fact that patients are given more than one drug at the same time.

5. There are a number of points to take into consideration regarding the drug and its chemical assay. For the convenience of the academic investigator we would like to select a drug which is only active *per se*. However, with the drugs used in practice the pharmacological effects of the metabolites are often unknown and the main metabolites may not even be identified. For drugs like imipramine, chlorpromazine and propranolol

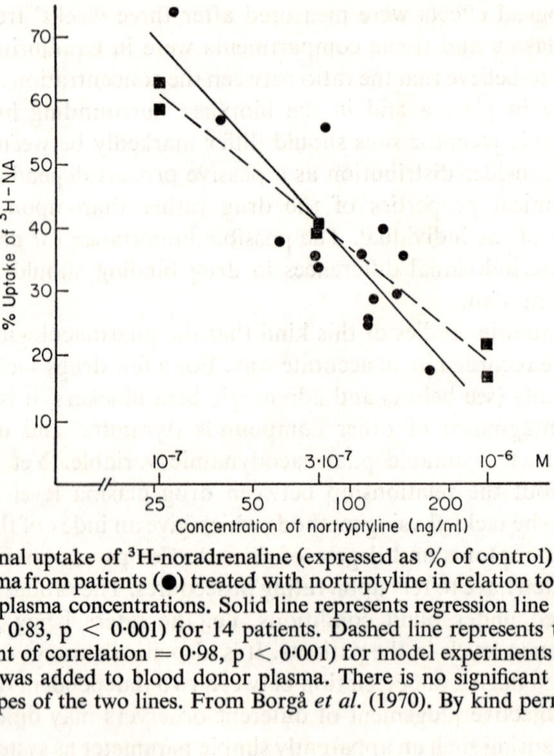


FIG. 2. Neuronal uptake of $^{3}$H-noradrenaline (expressed as % of control) in irises incubated in plasma from patients (●) treated with nortriptyline in relation to 'endogenous' nortriptyline plasma concentrations. Solid line represents regression line (coefficient of correlation = 0·83, $p < 0{\cdot}001$) for 14 patients. Dashed line represents the regression line (coefficient of correlation = 0·98, $p < 0{\cdot}001$) for model experiments (■) in which nortriptyline was added to blood donor plasma. There is no significant difference between the slopes of the two lines. From Borgå *et al.* (1970). By kind permission of the publisher.

active metabolites are known to be formed and then we may have to measure several compounds in plasma.

We would like to discuss briefly our approach when we were faced with the fact that the probable metabolites of nortriptyline could not be synthesized within reasonable time. We then turned to model experiments using the adrenergic nerve plexus of the rat's iris. Upon incubation under suitable conditions these neurons take up through their axonal membrane the noradrenaline which has been added to the test tube (Borgå *et al.*, 1970). This uptake is quantitatively inhibited by tricyclic antidepressants. The test can be performed with human plasma as incubation medium.

A comparison of the results obtained in patients undergoing treatment with nortriptyline with those obtained when nortriptyline was added to the incubation bath in concentrations corresponding to those occurring in plasma in these patients is shown in Figure 2. There is no significant difference in the degree of inhibition of noradrenaline uptake between the two experiments. This is strong evidence that active (in terms of the uptake mechanism) metabolites of nortriptyline play no major role in the action of this compound. Many polar metabolites are very rapidly cleared from plasma and therefore never reach particularly high concentrations compared to the parent compound. It may thus be possible to utilize *in vitro* experiments or to return to animal experiments (using e.g. inhibitors or

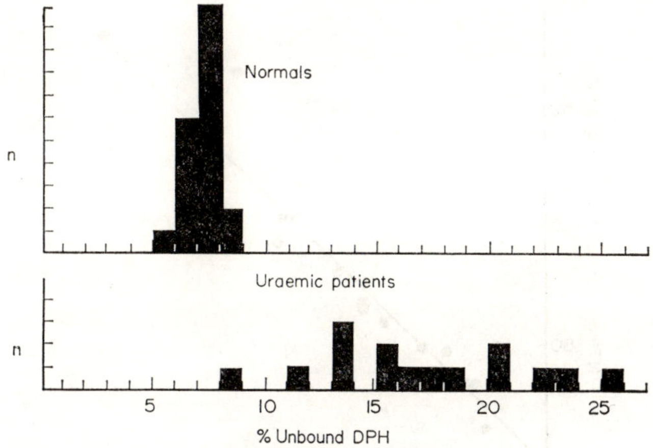


FIG. 3. Diagram of percentage unbound diphenylhydantoin in plasma of 20 normal volunteers (upper scale) and of 15 uraemic patients (lower scale). Modified from Reidenberg *et al.* (1971).

inducers of drug metabolism) when we wish to assess the effects of possible metabolites.

Another question is whether *total or unbound plasma levels* should be measured or both. It appears quite clear that usually it is enough to measure the total plasma concentration. Under normal conditions the interindividual differences in plasma protein binding seem to be small (*cf.* Borgå *et al.*, 1969; Lund *et al.*, 1971; Alexanderson & Borgå, 1972). When the patient is treated simultaneously with two or more acidic drugs like warfarin and phenylbutazone, it is known that the pharmacological action of the displaced drug (warfarin) will increase because the unbound pharmacologically active level is increased (O'Reilly & Levy, 1970). Since this fraction of the drug is available to the metabolic sites in the liver, the metabolism may be enhanced and the total level of drug in plasma decreased. We have recently shown that the unbound fraction of diphenylhydantion is increased markedly in patients with uremia (Reidenberg *et al.*, 1971). These patients can therefore be expected to respond therapeutically or with side-effects at much lower total plasma levels than normal epileptics (Figure 3).

Ideally the drug has *steady-state kinetics* with minor fluctuations of drug plasma levels during the day. In this case the time for sampling plasma may be of little importance. For other drugs very strict protocols have to be set up, the plasma level being measured at specific time points in relation to dosage.

Regarding the chemical *analytical methods* it appears obvious to the specialist that the assay must be both sensitive and selective. Much work

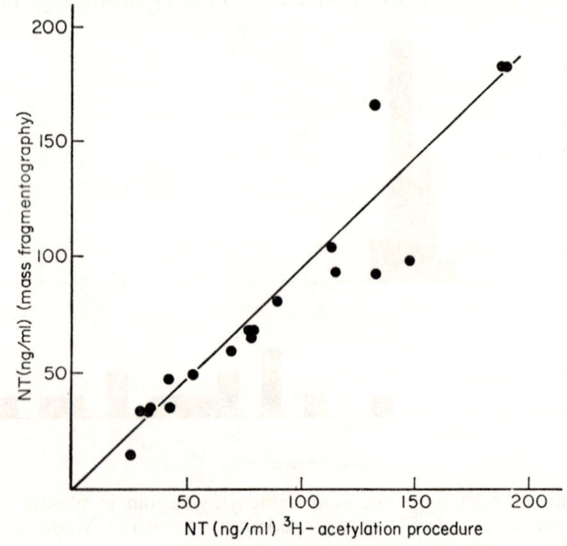


FIG. 4. Plasma samples from patients treated with NT were analysed by mass fragmentography and the *in vitro* $^3$H-acetylation procedure (Hammer & Brodie, 1967). In most of the cases a good agreement were found with the two methods. From Borgå *et al.* (1971). With kind permission of the publisher.

in this area has been performed with methods of equivocal specificity. One should try to attack the problem with the most accurate method available and to validate previous findings with new analytical methods as they become available. In our own work on nortriptyline, we have initially used the method of Hammer & Brodie (1967) for *in vitro* acetylation of the drug with $^3$H-labelled acetic anhydride. During the progress of the work, we have developed and adopted mass fragmentography (Hammar *et al.*, 1969) as an even more sensitive method with unequivocal specificity (Borgå *et al.*, 1971). The use of this latter method has essentially validated our previous results (Figure 4).

In many conventional analytical methods the drug history of the

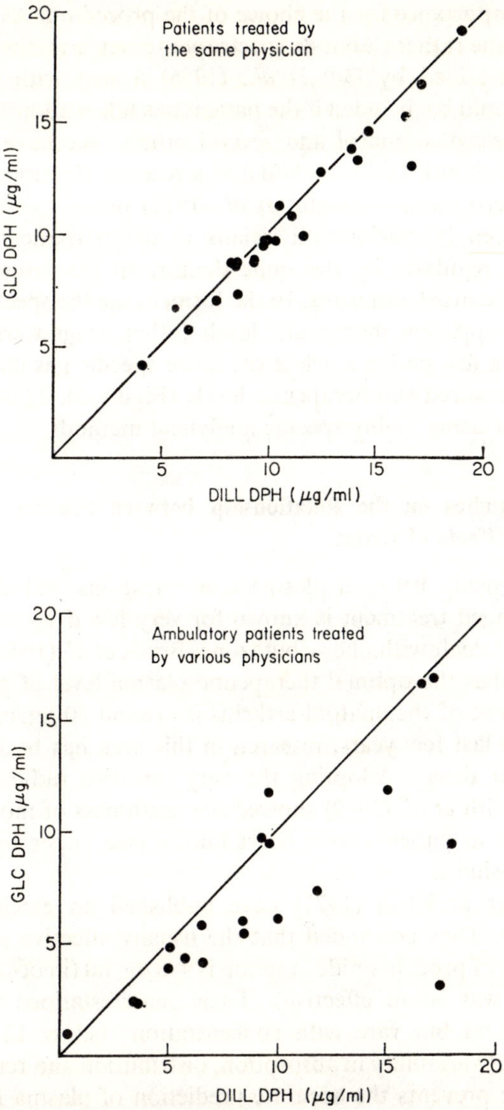


FIG. 5. Comparison of two methods for measuring diphenylhydantoin (DPH) in plasma: gas-chromatography according to Berlin *et al.* (1972) versus spectrophotometry according to Dill *et al.* (1956). The spectrophotometric method has been used with or without countercurrent extraction depending upon the drug history of the patient.
(a). The analyses have been performed in patients who have been seen by the same physician for about two years. Good agreement between the methods.
(b). The analyses have been performed in patients seen by various physicians. Discrepancies are found between the results of the two methods. Probably an incorrect drug history has been obtained whereby the spectrophotometric method has not been properly adjusted with counter current extraction.

patient has importance for the choice of the procedure. As an example of this point; in the rather elaborate spectrophotometric method for diphenylhydantoin described by Dill *et al.*, (1956) a step with countercurrent extraction should be included if the patient has taken additional drugs such as barbiturates, dicoumarol and several others. We have compared the results obtained with Dill's method and a recently developed gas chromatographic micro method (Berlin *et al.*, 1972) under two conditions, i.e. in patients seen by various physicians in the outpatient clinic and in patients seen regularly by the same doctor. In the latter case the two methods gave consistent results. In the former case the spectrophotometric method gave apparent therapeutic levels (other drugs were interfering in the assay) in a few patients, while the more specific gas chromatographic procedure measured subtherapeutic levels (Figure 5). This underlines the importance of using highly specific analytical methods.

## Controlled Studies on the Relationship between Plasma Concentrations and Clinical Effects of Drugs

The relationship between plasma concentrations and effects of drugs during prolonged treatment is known for very few drugs. An early study on this subject dealt with phenylbutazone. Bruck *et al.* (1954) showed quite conclusively that the optimal therapeutic plasma level of phenylbutazone in the treatment of rheumatoid arthritis is around 80 $\mu$g/ml.

During the last few years, research in this area has been published on cardiovascular drugs. Adopting the very sensitive radio-immunological technique, Smith *et al.* (1969) showed the usefulness of monitoring serum digoxin levels in patients with heart failure (see paper by Chamberlain in this symposium).

Koch-Weser & Klein (1971) have published an extensive study on procainamide. They concluded that the usually effective anti-arrhythmic concentration of procainamide in serum is 4–8 $\mu$g/ml (in occasional patients 8–16 $\mu$g/ml was more effective). Toxic manifestations were common above 16 $\mu$g/ml but rare with concentrations below 12 $\mu$g/ml. Large interindividual variability in absorption, distribution and renal excretion of procainamide prevents the accurate prediction of plasma levels from the dose administered.

A finding of great interest was that patients with low cardiac output and extrarenal azotemia had a decreased volume of distribution and elimination rate of procainamide which both tended to increase the plasma levels. It is now becoming widely recognized that the disease state often may modify the kinetics of the drug. It may be inappropriate to use kinetic data obtained in healthy volunteers to predict dosage schedules in ill patients (*cf.* Reidenberg *et al.*, 1971).

Of psychotropic drugs, lithium is unique by not being metabolized. The work of Schou *et al.* (1970) shows that toxic effects of lithium usually occur at serum concentrations above 2 meq/l. The monitoring of serum lithium concentrations has now become an accepted routine procedure partly due to the availability of a relatively simple analytical method. For other psychoactive drugs there is little information on this point; exceptions being diphenylhydantoin (Lund *et al.*, 1971; Lund, this symposium) and nortriptyline (Åsberg *et al.*, 1970, 1971; Alexanderson *et al.*, this symposium).

*Clinical Implications*

At our hospital we are now monitoring plasma concentrations of phenylbutazone, digoxin, diphenylhydantoin, procainamide, lithium and nortriptyline (serum levels of certain antibiotics are run by the Clinical Bacteriology Department). We are prepared to increase this service when controlled trials prove the value of monitoring plasma levels of other drugs.

It is important that these measurements be performed on sound clinical indications to avoid an overwhelming burden on the laboratory. A rough guess is that such measurements would be helpful for the therapist in about 10% of patients treated with the drugs listed above. Our policy requires that the clinicians specify the indications for the measurements (poor therapeutic response, suspicion of side-effects, etc.). They also have to submit a complete drug history, since this will influence the assay methods and the interpretation of data. We, on our side, provide the clinician with a kinetic and clinical interpretation of the analytical data and try to follow up the analyses at the bedside. Thus therapeutic wardrounds are organized during which the pharmacokinetic and pharmacodynamic basis of interindividual differences in drug response are discussed. This organization permits a most rewarding feed-back between our department and different clinical departments such as Internal Medicine, Neurology and Psychiatry.

It is intended to keep this rather strict policy since it is a common experience that insufficient dialogue between the laboratory and clinical staffs will ultimately reduce the intellectual content of the work. We thus try to discourage an abuse of drug determinations in plasma but encourage an intelligent use of this service. Under these conditions the costs of the laboratory work will be small compared with the therapeutic gains. As an example, during two years' monitoring of diphenylhydantoin plasma levels (around 1000 analyses) we have found about 20 undiagnosed intoxications. One of these patients was receiving state pension and one was already in an institution for the chronically ill. All could return to work after reduction of the dose to the lower end of the recommended range.

These patients had been previously seen by academic neurologists but their symptoms had not been thought to be due to diphenylhydantoin intoxication.

## Discussion

This paper tries to make the point that carefully controlled studies on the relationship between drug plasma levels and clinical effects may provide a clue to safer and more effective therapy. This research must be properly designed, otherwise we will end up no more enlightened than we were before. A stereotyped approach to the use of plasma levels in 'therapy control' will not suffice. The investigator should be prepared to find no relationship between plasma level and his pharmacodynamic parameter and then ask the questions: is the drug activated in the body? did we measure it specifically? and did we record the relevant pharmacodynamic variable? The investigator should be prepared to find the unexpected as e.g. the curved relationship between antidepressant effect of nortriptyline and steady state plasma concentration described by Åsberg *et al.* (1971). A correct interpretation of such data may unravel novel pharmacodynamic knowledge. It is becoming increasingly obvious that there may be inter-individual variability in receptor site sensitivity to drugs, the best example being the hereditary resistance to coumarin anticoagulant drugs (O'Reilly *et al.*, 1968). The only way to discover such findings is to measure drug plasma levels in relation to response.

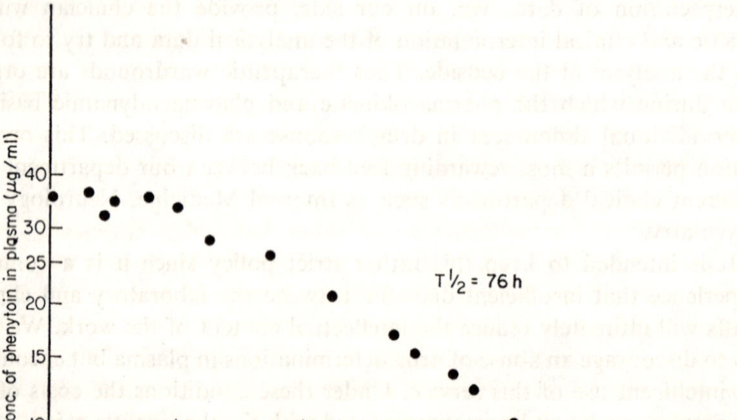


FIG. 6. Example of a 'therapeutic' intoxication with phenytoin. The plasma level stays constant for about 50 h after stopping the drug intake in a patient showing clinical signs of intoxication. It takes about a week before the plasma concentration has declined to the therapeutic range.

In addition to ensuring that dosage is appropriate, there are other obvious indications for measuring drug plasma levels in the clinic such as diagnosing and treating attempted suicide (e.g. phenobarbital and salicylates) and treatment of patients with poor kidney function (e.g. with ototoxic antibiotics). Another area of investigation involves inadvertent intoxication produced by a therapeutic regime. Repeated plasma sampling, with studies of the disappearance of drug in relation to symptoms, may be rewarding. Many neurologists seem to be unaware of the very slow decline of toxic diphenylhydantoin (DPH) plasma levels to the therapeutic range. In the case described in Figure 6 there was a clear tendency for the side-effects to vanish before the plasma concentrations started to decline significantly.

Finally, another aspect of the usefulness of monitoring plasma concentrations of drugs should be pointed out. As mentioned previously, a rigid approach to the clinical use of plasma concentrations should be discouraged. There are other reasons, besides pharmacokinetic explanations, why a drug may be ineffective. For example, the diagnosis may be wrong or the drug has not been properly selected. We would again like to exemplify with antidepressants. It is now thought that at least two distinct subtypes of endogenous depression may occur, hypothetically called noradrenaline- and serotonin-depressions. The former are characterized by motor retardation and are said on empirical grounds to respond preferentially to drugs such as desmethylimipramine which block the amine uptake in noradrenaline neurons. Consequently it may be assumed that in this group of patients biochemical changes occur in noradrenergic neurons. As support for this Bunney and his colleagues at the National Institute of Health, USA, (personal communication) have found low levels of the main noradrenaline metabolite 3-methoxy-4-hydroxyphenylglycol (MHPG) in body fluids of certain patients with depression. Furthermore, selected cases with retarded depression respond to DOPA, while this is not true for the majority of patients (Bunney *et al.*, 1971).

In serotonin depressions, on the other hand, the depressed mood dominates the clinical picture and some of these patients may even show hyperactivity. It has been reported that in depressed patients as a whole (without subdivision of the patients) the levels of the acid metabolite of serotonin, 5-hydroxyindole-3-acetic acid (5-HIAA), in CSF are low compared with controls (Ashcroft & Sharman, 1960; Dencker *et al.*, 1966). This finding could not be confirmed in another series (Roos & Sjöström, 1969), but it was shown that depressed patients have lower 5-HIAA levels in CSF than controls after blocking the transport of the acid from CSF with probenecid, indicating a slower turn-over of the amine. Presumably such patients should be treated with a blocker of serotonin uptake such as chlorimipramine.

In clinical trials of antidepressants very little consideration has been paid to the possibility that the patients have different types of diseases and therefore would require different drugs. In fact most trials of new antidepressants tend to show improvement figures comparable to those reported for older drugs such as imipramine, which in turn performs slightly better than placebo. This could be explained by the fact that a considerable proportion of patients in the respective trials is given the wrong drug.

Other therapeutic failures may be explained by the findings reviewed in

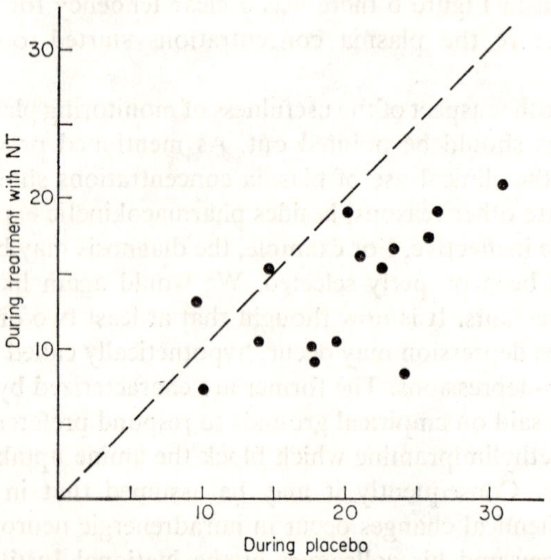


FIG. 7. Concentration of 5-HIAA in CSF in ng/ml before and during treatment with nortriptyline. A dotted line has been drawn at 45° and if nortriptyline had no effect on 5-HIAA all the observational points would be distributed along this line. Data to the right of the dotted line thus indicate that the levels have declined during treatment with nortriptyline compared to the preceding placebo period ($p < 0{\cdot}01$).

this symposium by Alexanderson *et al.*, i.e. that there seems to be a critical range of plasma concentrations of nortriptyline (rather than a fixed level) which gives an antidepressant effect. A considerable proportion of patients never reaches this range on usual clinical doses.

There are also therapeutic failures even within this optimal therapeutic range. We have become interested in the question: are there any clinical or biochemical differences between patients who respond and those who do not respond at this apparently optimal range of nortriptyline plasma levels?

In other words, by controlling the kinetics of the drug it may be possible to get a new dimension for studies of the pathophysiology of disease. A specific mass fragmentographic method for 5-HIAA has been developed (Bertilsson *et al.*, 1972). Using this method it has been found that nortriptyline itself lowered the 5-HIAA level in CSF (Figure 7). Even more interestingly, a subgroup of patients with endogenous depression ('serotonin depressions') has particularly low levels of 5-HIAA in CSF (Åsberg *et al.*, 1973). These data suggest that it is not possible to decide whether a low CSF level of 5-HIAA is due to drug therapy or to the disease *unless* actual

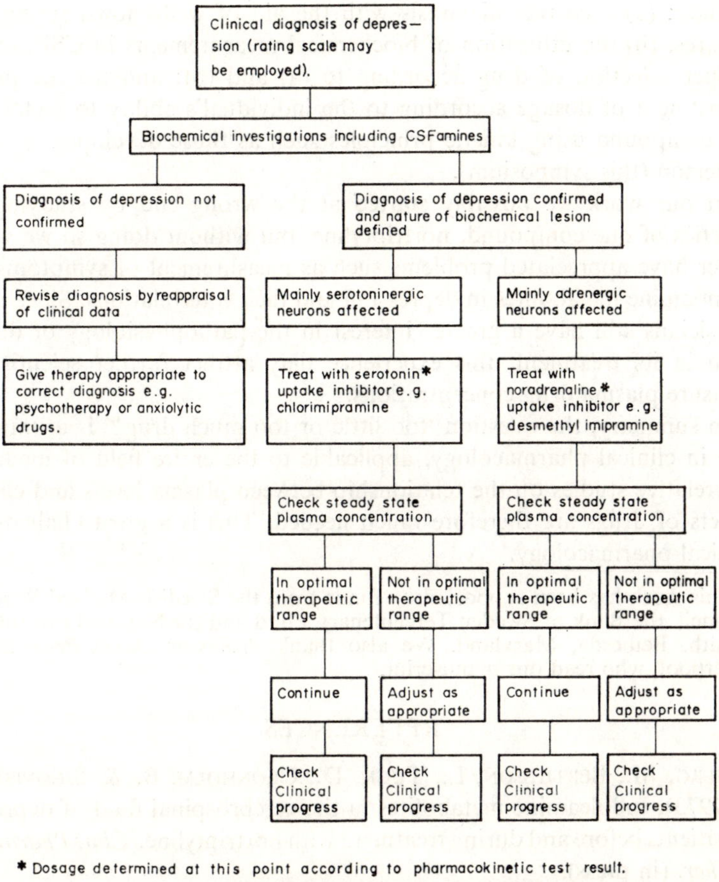


FIG. 8. Flow chart showing decision-making in the management of depression. *N.B.* This figure is meant to stimulate rather than provoke or depress the reader.

measurements ascertain that no drug can be detected in the patient. This may explain some discrepancies in the literature regarding 5-HIAA levels in CSF in depressed patients. As a rule the investigators have not kept drug therapy under strict control and none has measured drug levels.

It thus becomes apparent that, under pharmacokinetically controlled conditions, certain biochemical changes in CSF may turn out to be very useful in studies relating plasma levels of psychotropic drugs to pharmacodynamic action. Such studies may throw light on interindividual variability in turn-over rates of monoamines in the neuron systems affected in depression.

Figure 8 is not representative of the decision-making in today's psychiatry but may provide a glimpse of future treatment of depression. The decisions include: (a) a correct diagnosis with the aid of well-known rating procedures, (b) the utilization of biochemical measurements in CSF, (c) the proper selection of drug according to (a) and (b); and (d) the proper adjustment of dosage according to the individual's ability to metabolize the compound using kinetic principles such as those developed by Alexanderson (this symposium).

In our work we possibly started at the wrong end by studying the kinetics of one compound, nortriptyline, but without doing so we would never have appreciated problems such as measurement of symptoms and monoamine metabolites in depression and their interrelations. Since many physicians still have a greater interest in the pathophysiology of disease than in its treatment, this experience may attract further scientists to measure plasma drug concentrations.

In summary, the question 'too little or too much drug?' is a universal one in clinical pharmacology, applicable to the entire field of medicine. Correlative studies on the relationship between plasma levels and clinical effects of drugs are therefore much needed. This is a great challenge to clinical pharmacology.

This work has been supported by funds from the Swedish Medical Research Council, the Bank of Sweden Tercentenary Fund and the National Institutes of Health, Bethesda, Maryland. We also thank Professor David Price Evans, Liverpool, who read our manuscript.

## REFERENCES

ÅSBERG, M., BERTILSSON, L., TUCK, D., CRONHOLM, B. & SJÖQVIST, F. (1973). Indoleamine metabolites in the cerebrospinal fluid of depressed patients before and during treatment with nortriptyline. *Clin. Pharmacol. Ther.* (in press).

ÅSBERG, M., CRONHOLM, B., SJÖQVIST, F. & TUCK, D. (1970). The correlation of subjective side effects with plasma concentrations of nortriptyline. *Brit. Med. J.*, **4**, 18–21.

ÅSBERG, M., CRONHOLM, B., SJÖQVIST, F. & TUCK, D. (1971). Relationship between plasma level and therapeutic effect of nortriptyline. *Brit. Med. J.*, **3**, 331–334.

ALEXANDERSON, B., SJÖQVIST, F., & PRICE EVANS, D. A. (1969). Steady-state plasma levels of nortriptyline in twins: Influence of genetic factors and drug therapy. *Brit. Med. J.*, **4**, 764–768.

ALEXANDERSON, B. & BORGÅ, O. (1972). Interindividual differences in plasma protein binding of nortriptyline in man—a twin study. *Europ. J. Clin. Pharmacol*, **4,** 196–200.

ASHCROFT, G. W. & SHARMAN, D. F. (1960). 5-Hydroxyindoles in human cerebrospinal fluids. *Nature.* **186,** 1050–1051.

BERLIN, A., AGURELL, S., BORGÅ, O., LUND, L. & SJÖQVIST, F. (1972). Micromethod for the determination of diphenylhydantoin in plasma and cerebrospinal fluid—a comparison between a gas chromatographic and a spectrophotometric method. *Scand. J. Lab. Clin. Invest.*, **29,** 281–287.

BERTILSSON, L., ATKINSON, JR, A., ALTHOUS, J. R., HÄRFAST, Å., LINDGREN, J. E. & HOLMSTEDT, B. (1972). Quantitative determination of 5-hydroxyindole-3-acetic acid in cerebrospinal fluid by gas chromatography—mass spectrometry. *Anal. Chem.*, **44,** 1434–1438.

BORGÅ, O., AZARNOFF, D. L., PLYM FORSHELL, G. & SJÖQVIST, F. (1969). Plasma protein binding of tricyclic antidepressants in man. *Biochem. Pharmacol.*, **18,** 2135–2143.

BORGÅ, O., HAMBERGER, B., MALMFORS, T. & SJÖQVIST, F. (1970). The role of plasma protein binding in the inhibitory effect of nortriptyline on the neuronal uptake of norepinephrine. *Clin. Pharmacol. & Ther.*, **11,** 581–588.

BORGÅ, O., PALMER, L., LINNARSON, A. & HOLMSTEDT, B. (1971). Measurement of nortriptyline in body fluids of man with mass fragmentography. *Anal. Letters*, **4,** 837–844.

BRUCK, E., FEARNLEY, M., MEANOCK, I. & PATLEY, H. (1954). Phenylbutazone therapy. Relation between the toxic and therapeutic effects and the blood level. *Lancet*, **1:** 225–229.

BUNNEY, JR., W. E., BRODIE, H. K. H., MURPHY, D. L. & GOODWIN, F. K. (1971). Studies of Alpha-methyl-para-tyrosine, L-dopa and L-tryptophan in Depression and Mania. *Am. J. Psychiat.*, **127,** 872–881.

DENCKER, S. J., MALM, U., ROOS, B.-E. & WERDINIUS, B. (1966). Acid monoamine metabolites of cerebrospinal fluid in mental depression and mania. *J. Neurochem.*, **13,** 1545–1548.

DILL, W. A., KAZENKO, A., WOLF, L. M. & GLAZKO, A. J. (1956). Studies on 5, 5-diphenylhydantoin in animals and man. *J. Pharmacol. Exper. Therap.*, **118,** 270–279.

HAMMAR, C-G., HOLMSTEDT, B., LINDGREN, J. E. & THAM, R. (1969). The combination of gas chromatography and mass spectrometry in the identification of drugs and metabolites. *Adv. in Pharmacol. and Chemother.*, **7,** 53–89.

HAMMER, W. & BRODIE, B. B. (1967). Application of isotope derivative technique to assay of secondary amines: Estimation of desipramine by acetylation with $H^3$-acetic anhydride. *J. Pharmacol. Exp. Therap.*, **157,** 503–507.

HAMMER, W. & SJÖQVIST, F. (1967). Plasma levels of monomethylated tricyclic antidepressants during treatment with imipramine-like compounds. *Life Sci.*, **6**, 1895–1903.

KOCH-WESER, J. & KLEIN, S. W. (1971). Procainamide dosage schedules, plasma concentrations and clinical effects, *J.A.M.A.*, **215**, 1454–1460.

LUND, L., LUNDE, P. K. M., RANE, A., BORGÅ, O. & SJÖQVIST, F. (1971). Plasma protein binding, plasma concentrations and effects of diphenylhydantoin in man. *Ann. N.Y. Acad. Sci.*, **179**, 723–728.

O'REILLY, R. A. & LEVY, G. (1970). Pharmacokinetic analysis of potentiating effect of phenylbutazone on anticoagulant action of warfarin in man. *J. Pharm. Sci.*, **59**, 1258–1262.

O'REILLY, R. A., POOL, J. G. & AGGELER, P. M. (1968). Hereditary resistance to coumarin anticoagulant drugs in man and rat. *Ann. N.Y. Acad. Sci.*, **151**, 913–931.

REIDENBERG, M. M., ODAR-CEDERLÖF, I., VON BAHR, C., BORGÅ, O. & SJÖQVIST, F. (1971). Protein binding of diphenylhydantoin and desmethylimipramine in plasma from patients with poor renal function. *New Engl. J. Med.*, **285**, 264–267.

ROOS, B-E. & SJÖSTRÖM, R. (1969). 5-Hydroxyindoleacetic acid (and homovanillic acid) levels in the cerebrospinal fluid after probenecid application in patients with manic-depressive psychosis. *Pharmacol. Clin.*, **1**, 153–155.

SCHOU, M., BAASTRUP P. C., GROF, P., WEIS, P. & ANGST, J. (1970). Pharmacological and clinical problems of lithium prophylaxis. *Brit. J. Psychiat.*, **116**, 615–619.

SMITH, T. W., BUTLER, V. P. & HABER, E. (1969). Determination of therapeutic and toxic serum digoxin concentrations by radioimmunoassay. *New Engl. J. Med.*, **281**, 1212–1216.

# FOUR

# Blood Concentrations of Compounds in Animal Toxicity Tests

S. B. DE C. BAKER[1] AND D. M. FOULKES

*Imperial Chemical Industries, Pharmaceuticals Division, Macclesfield, Cheshire*

## Introduction

The purpose of animal toxicity studies is to assess the safety of a potential drug for man. The studies can be divided into three parts:

1. The definition of the nature of the toxicity in the animal.
2. The determination of the relevance of this toxicity to man.
3. Work designed to assist in the early detection and interpretation of changes in the clinical trial.

In animal tests it is necessary to establish what changes can be induced by the compound; these may be morphological, biochemical or behavioural. Before such a test one has no idea of the results and one therefore monitors as many parameters as possible, selecting these carefully to give the maximum information. To reduce the chances of missing something, 'excessive' amounts of test compound are sometimes administered, but this in turn creates its own problems of accumulation of drug or its metabolites, or of altered metabolism. Once the changes in animals have been defined their significance has to be assessed. Unless we know how much of the compound reaches the tissue, sensible interpretation is impossible, and it is important that blood levels of compounds are checked during a toxicological test. This is not always possible, often because a suitable method has not been developed or the amounts of the circulating drug are too small to detect. When this occurs one is forced to use a radio-tracer technique and the significance of the toxicological findings have to be interpreted retrospectively from labelling studies usually performed on completion of the tests. Both the pharmacological and toxicological effects should be related to the blood levels to obtain a comprehensive picture of the test from which some idea of the significance of the results can be deduced.

The relevance of a toxic change, observed in a test species, for man cannot be determined unless the mechanism of the effect is understood in the animal, as illustrated in the following example. A compound is

[1] Present address: Noble's Hospital, Douglas, Isle of Man.

tolerated by rats at the level of 500 mg/kg for three months when it is administered as a single daily oral dose. In the rat it is rapidly absorbed, has a short half-life of 2 to 3 h with 90% of the excretion occurring through the kidney, and the peak concentration in the urine is thus very high. This concentration produces a hyperplastic change in the bladder epithelium. If twice the dose, 1000 mg/kg, is given in the diet so that the absorption takes place over a longer period, the urinary concentrations never reach the high levels and the bladder epithelial change is avoided. The dose, and the spread of the doses if applied to man, preclude such changes occurring in clinical use of this drug. This example highlights a practical problem posed by the results of toxicity tests. A single dose of a drug with a short half-life means that the blood levels swing widely from excessive to nil over 24 h. The very high blood levels may produce an exaggerated expression of some aspects of the toxicity. Multiple doses daily can be given to a limited number of animals, but this is simply not practicable for large numbers. Administering the drug in the subject's diet is at best erratic, and blood levels throughout the ensuing 24 h in individual animals cannot be accurately gauged. Careful thought, therefore, has to be given to the method and timing of the dosing, and in most cases a compromise and an understanding of the implications is needed in order to make the best choice of dosage regimen.

The study of blood levels in animals presents problems, besides the chemical one of devising a sensitive technique, early in the life of an experimental drug. One must know exactly what the method measures; does it measure only the drug itself? does it include conjugates and simple metabolites? or is it even less specific? It is not known at the time of the study whether the whole molecule, or part of it, is responsible for the observed toxicity and activity. For example, quindoxin (Grofas)[1] a growth promoter for chickens, is estimated in the blood by a method which converts the drug to quinoxaline which is then measured by a gas chromatographic method. As it happens, the chicken's gut flora also rapidly converts the compound to quinoxaline, the active compound. Had the chemical method measured unchanged drug only, little or none would ever have been found in the blood by chemical means.

[1] The word 'Grofas' is a trade mark, the property of Imperial Chemical Industries Ltd. Chemical formula:

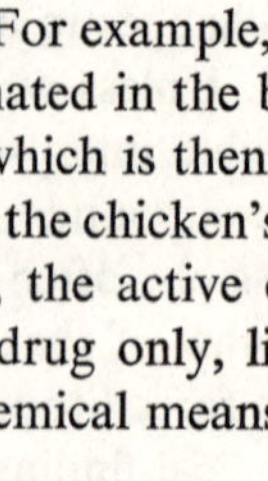

A necessary adjunct to the chemical methods is the use of radiolabelled compounds. If a comparison is made between the levels of total radioactivity in the blood and the levels of compound by chemical assay any substantial discrepancy can be ascribed to the drug's metabolites which may have to be identified and tested for pharmacological and toxicological activity separately.

**Factors Affecting Drug Assessment**

The study of blood levels during a toxicity test is not just a simple 'one off' measurement; the levels should be monitored throughout the test as so many factors can cause variations which could radically alter our judgement of the safety of a compound. Some of these factors are listed below:

species difference
sex difference
pregnancy
alteration in absorption
enzyme induction or inhibition
overloading of metabolic pathways and/or
accumulation of compound in certain tissues.

*Species Differences*

Species differences in the relation between dose and subsequent blood levels is well known, yet the disturbing fact is how frequently we extrapolate

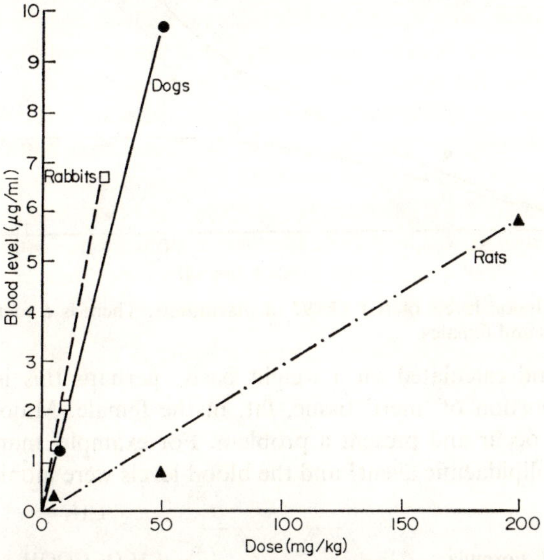


FIG. 1. Species difference in relationship of dose to blood levels. Difficulties arise if rat doses are given blindly to rabbits.

results obtained from one species to another without giving sufficient thought to the implications. One of the commonest examples is the choice of species for teratogenic studies when governmental guide lines demand work in a species sensitive to thalidomide, recommending rabbits. The doses used are commonly based on those employed in chronic toxicity tests in a different species, the rat. The graph (Figure 1) shows what may happen under such conditions. The rabbit blood levels are far higher at lower doses of compound than those of the rats. This particular problem came to light because the rat doses were also given to rabbits, resulting in a high incidence of foetal resorptions. One wonders how many drugs are abandoned due to failure to appreciate problems of this sort, or conversely how many teratogenic studies with negligible blood levels of drug are passed by regulatory bodies.

*Sex Differences*

A small sex difference is common; usually females have a slightly higher blood level of administered drug than males for a given dose when

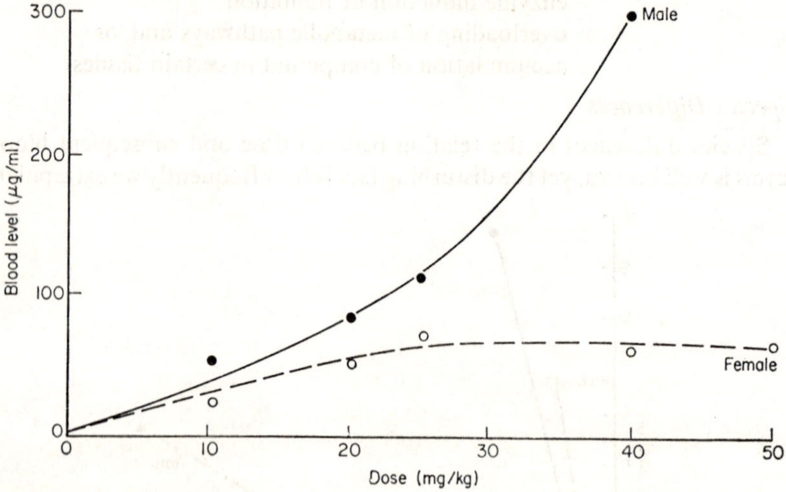


FIG. 2. Mean blood levels of ICI 55,897 in marmosets. There is a marked difference between males and females.

measured and calculated on a weight basis; perhaps this is due to the higher proportion of 'inert' tissue, fat, in the female. Major differences can and do occur and present a problem. For example, marmosets were given a hypolipidaemic agent[1] and the blood levels were monitored. Apart

[1] ICI 55,897. Formula:

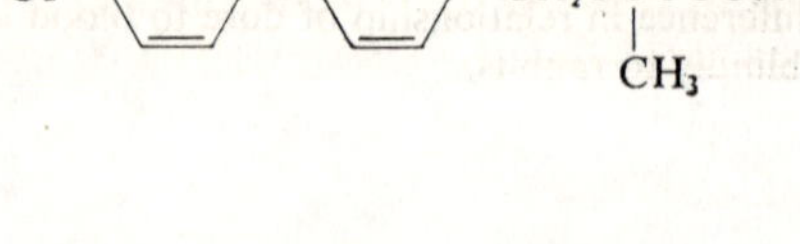

from an unusual variability, we found that the females had markedly lower blood levels than the males. The graph (Figure 2) shows the mean levels achieved by males and females given the compound daily on a weight basis. The reason for this difference has not yet been elucidated, but many of the females were pregnant and this could be part of the explanation. During teratogenic studies with this compound the effect of pregnancy on

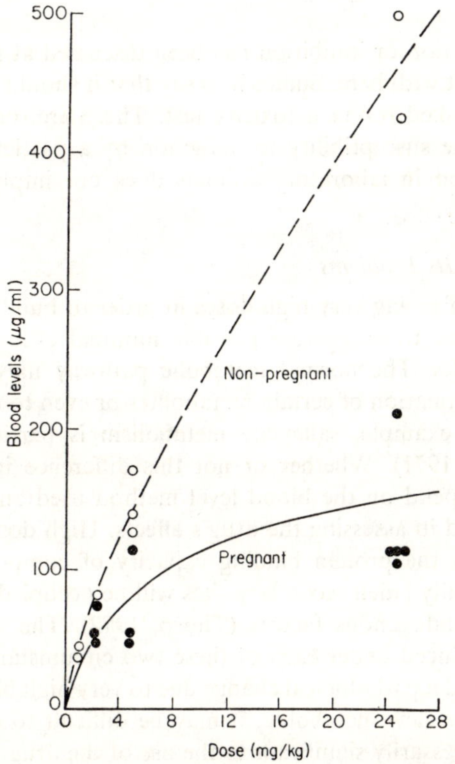


FIG. 3. Relationship of dose to blood levels in pregnant and non-pregnant rats.

the blood levels was demonstrated clearly. Non-pregnant females receiving standard doses on a weight basis showed levels three times those of their pregnant counterparts (Figure 3). So in carrying out teratogenic studies one should not only concern oneself with inter-species blood levels but also consider possible changes within a species due to pregnancy, and other conditions.

*Altered Absorption and Clearance*

The time of day in relation to food can influence the rate of absorption from an oral dose and thus the toxicity. This is clearly demonstrated in acute studies. It may not be very important in the assessment of safety but may present problems in the interpretation of the blood level data. The drug itself may cause lesions which then alter absorption. This is commonly seen in toxicity studies of anti-inflammatory compounds in dogs in which ulceration of the small intestine is common. The usual picture is one of blood levels falling off towards the end of a test, an observation most often made in tests using higher dose levels, or in any animal which is particularly ill.

Enzyme induction or inhibition has been discussed at great length and need not be dealt with here. Suffice it to say that it should always be borne in mind and looked for in a toxicity test. There are, of course, species differences in the susceptibility to induction by a particular compound; enzyme induction in laboratory animals does not imply that man will respond similarly.

*Overdosage and Its Problems*

The custom of giving very high doses in order to build a safety margin into the test, and to exaggerate possible minimal effects, may produce misleading results. The normal metabolic pathway may be overloaded leading to accumulation of certain metabolites or even to the formation of new ones. For example, salicylate metabolism is particularly dose-dependent (Levy, 1971). Whether or not this difference in metabolism is detected will depend on the blood level method used and the metabolic studies employed in assessing the drug's effects. High doses can also produce changes in the protein binding capacity of compounds; once the primary site is fully laden secondary sites will be occupied which can then displace other endogenous factors (Thorp, 1972). The significance of a toxic effect produced under each of these two circumstances is in doubt. Having produced a pathological change due to very high blood levels, or to the presence of a new metabolite, it may be difficult to persuade people that it is not necessarily significant to the use of the drug in treating man; especially if the lesions so produced are such emotive ones as cataracts or tumours.

*Blood Levels and Tissue Levels*

We have discussed blood levels as if they were synonymous with tissue concentrations. This is obviously not true, and any marked localization of a compound in an organ or a particular tissue, e.g. fat, could make nonsense of an interpretation of a change in that organ based on blood levels of the compound. Accumulation may also give rise to an apparent prolonged half-life of the compound after chronic dosing; the tissue may be acting as a store from which the compound is only slowly released. A dose calculated from the blood half-life of a compound based on an acute study

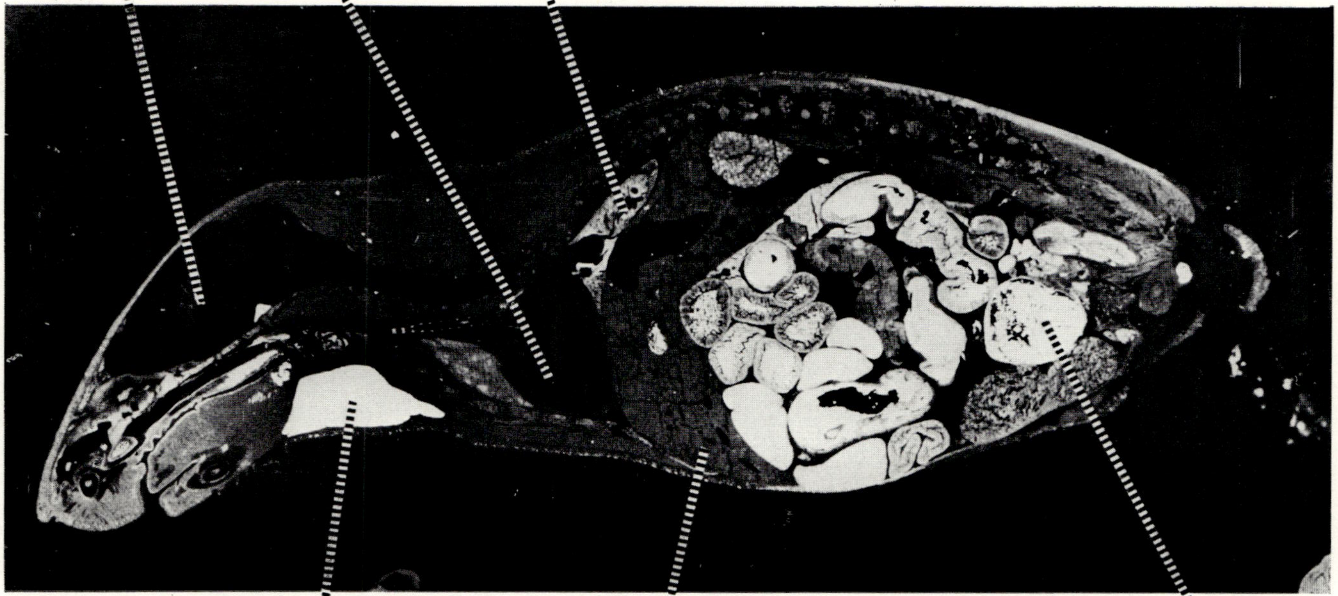


FIG. 4. Autoradiograph showing the distribution of practolol in mice one hour after dose.

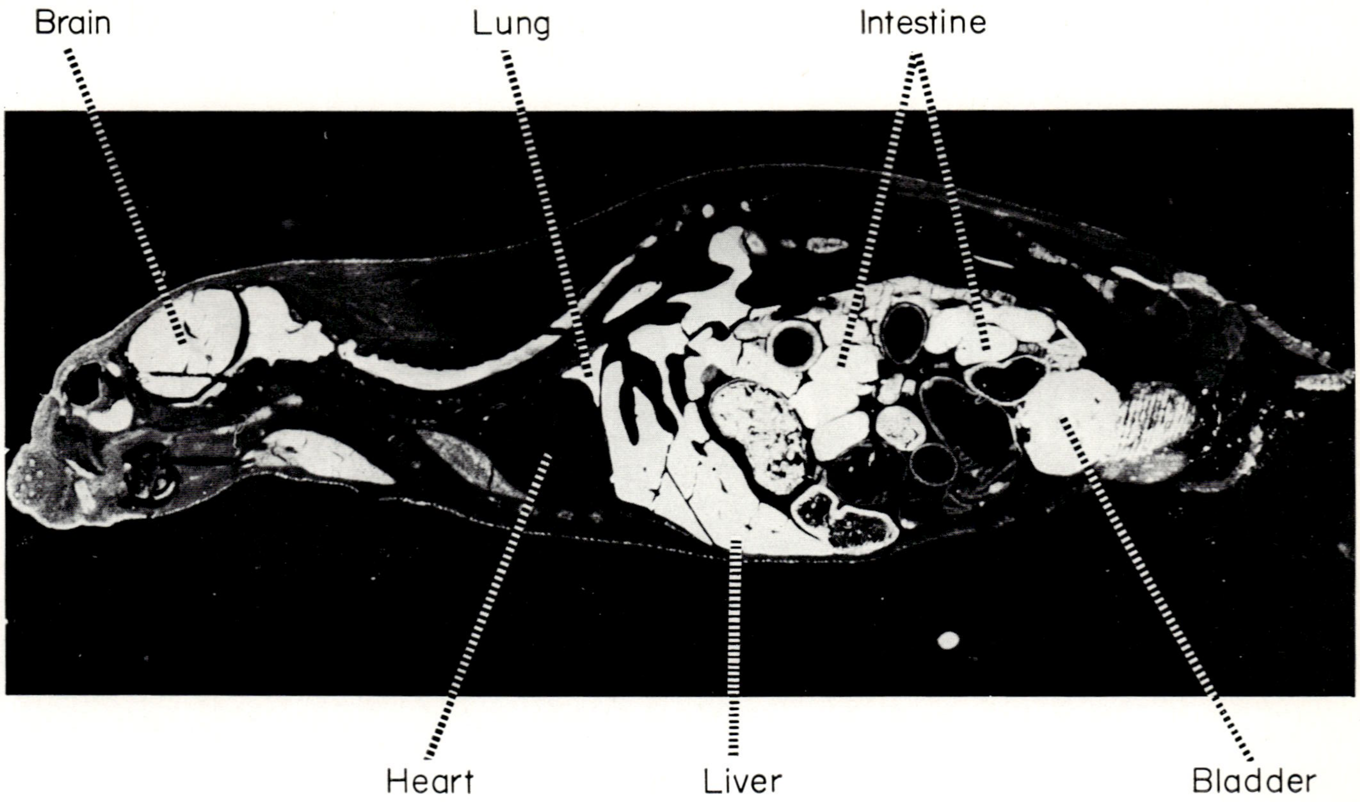


FIG. 5. Autoradiograph showing the distribution of propranolol in mice one hour after dose.

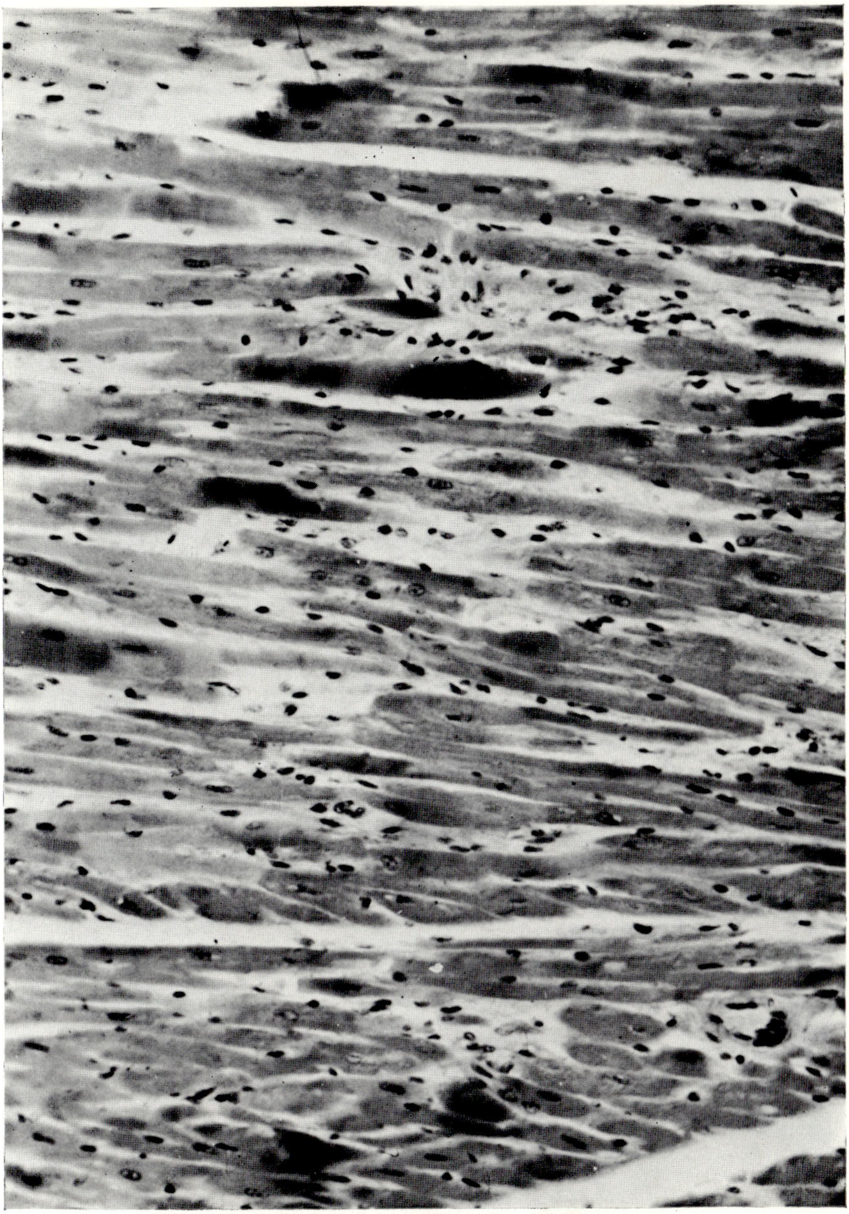

FIG. 7. Myocardial changes secondary to ICI 55,695 in dogs.

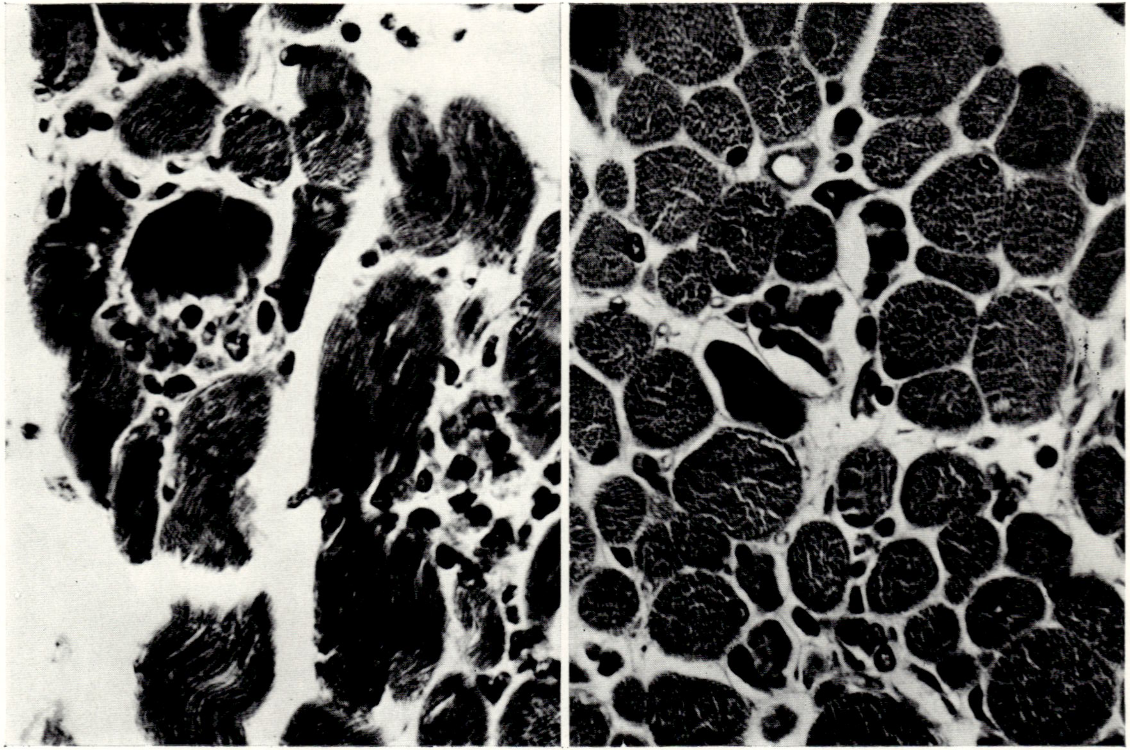

FIG. 8. Changes in skeletal muscles of lambs given ICI 55,695 (left), and cod liver oil (right). The changes are typical of vitamin E deficiency.

could be sadly wrong for chronic dosing, the blood levels could rise unexpectedly once the storage capacity is full. The best way of detecting a possible tissue accumulation of drug is whole body autoradiography followed by a more detailed radio-tracer study of the particular tissues involved. Figures 4 and 5 show a comparison between the distribution of labelled propranolol and practolol. This is very useful at times as it may indicate the likely mechanism of a different toxicological or pharmacological effect.

## The Relationship between Toxicity and Blood Levels

It is often assumed that there is a direct relationship between toxicity and blood levels of a drug. This is more likely to be true for the pharmacological effect than for the toxicity since the compound has usually been carefully selected for its therapeutic effect and probably has a direct action. The toxicological effect is unwanted and its pathogenesis is likely to be complex and indirect. We can appreciate that there may be a relationship between blood levels and acute toxic effects; for example, tubular necrosis secondary to mercuric chloride (but even in this case some measure of protection can be given). The liver changes caused by carbon tetrachloride depend on the hepatic enzyme complement as well as on the dose received. The two examples cited above are very simple, compared with many cases of drug toxicity, but even here we cannot always expect a close blood level–effect relationship. In the chronic situation there are many opportunities for indirect mechanisms to operate. Anti-inflammatory drugs produce peptic ulceration in many species, but the incidence is very erratic. A clear-cut $L.D._{50}$ is very difficult to obtain since death occurs from perforation of an ulcer and there is marked individual variation in susceptibility to this lesion. Figure 6 shows the lethality of an anti-inflammatory

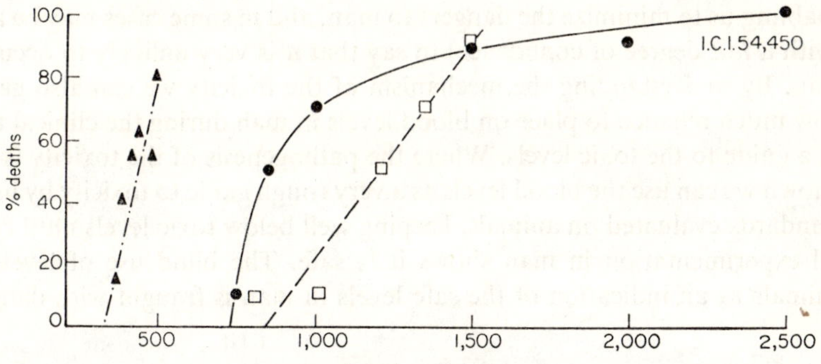


FIG. 6. Lethality of doses of an anti-inflammatory drug ICI 54,450 compared with two compounds showing a more usual pattern.

drug compared with the more common findings in acute tests. The $L.D._{50}$ of ICI 54,450 is about 850 mg/kg, but there are still some animals resistant to ulceration at 2000 mg/kg. The mechanism of ulceration is probably related to the pharmacological action of the compound preventing the healing of minor traumatic injuries. This explanation is supported by the observation that rats develop skin lesions on the back of the neck where they are picked up daily for dosing, and dogs show sores over the pressure areas. Whether or not the animal develops an ulcer depends on the chance of acquiring a primary traumatic lesion. Thus the incidence, although to some extent dose-related at low levels when the anti-inflammatory action is incomplete, will be erratic at high levels when the dose giving maximal anti-inflammatory action has been exceeded.

The situation becomes more complicated when the toxic action is produced by interference with vitamins or hormonal function. A hypolipidaemic agent[1] was found to produce myocardial necrosis in dogs (Figure 7) which was thought to be related to a vitamin E deficiency. This idea was supported by comparing the effects of the compound and cod liver oil in lambs which are very susceptible to vitamin E deficiency. The lesions produced were identical in both treatments and were typical of 'white muscle' disease (Figure 8). Man is relatively resistant to vitamin E deficiency and could receive this compound; in this respect it is no more toxic than cod liver oil. The correlation between blood levels and toxicity is not necessarily close within a species and is even less so between species.

## The Relevance of Animal Toxicity to Man

Having defined what the toxic changes are in animals one has the very difficult problem of assessing the safety for man. By knowing the pathogenesis of a lesion in laboratory animals we have at least some knowledge enabling us to minimize the dangers to man, and in some cases may be able (with a fair degree of confidence) to say that it is very unlikely to occur in man. By understanding the mechanism of the toxicity we can also gauge how much reliance to place on blood levels in man during the clinical trial as a guide to the toxic levels. Where the pathogenesis of the toxicity is not known we can use the blood levels as a very rough guide to toxicity by using standards evaluated on animals, keeping well below toxic levels until careful experimentation in man shows it is safe. The blind use of levels in animals as an indication of the safe levels in man is fraught with danger.

[1] ICI 55,695. Formula:
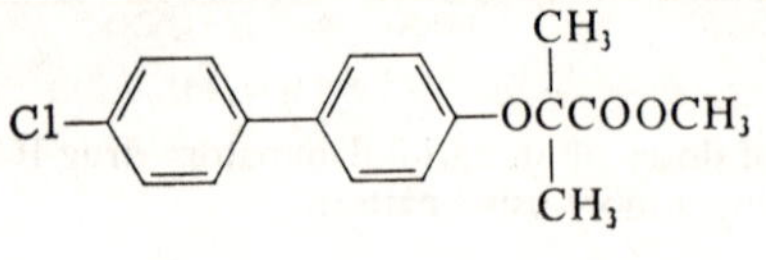

The difficulties inherent in the interpretation of animal data make it more sensible to do further clinical studies on man, only using animals to solve specific problems as they arise.

ICI 54,450[1] (Alcock, 1971) produced no adverse effects in animals other than ulceration of the alimentary tract (typical of anti-inflammatory

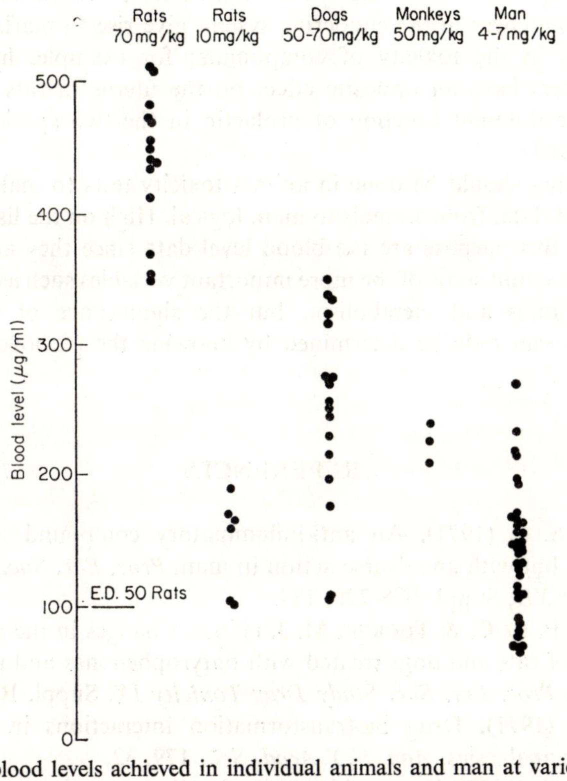


FIG. 9. The blood levels achieved in individual animals and man at various doses of ICI 54,450.

compounds), but in man it caused jaundice. A comparison of the blood levels in animals and man (Figure 9) showed that those of the animals were sufficient to have a reasonable safety margin. After jaundice had been observed in man, a large number of animal species were screened in an attempt to find one susceptible to jaundice with 54,450, but none was found.

It is fashionable to blame metabolism for the species differences and common sense indicates that the test species should be selected on the basis

[1] ICI 54,450. Formula:

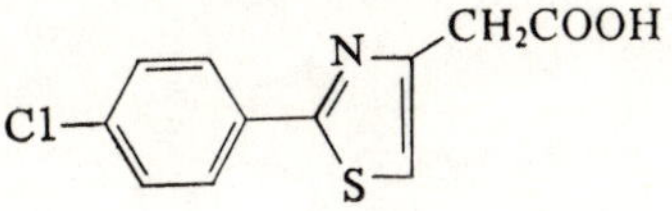

of their similarity to man in this respect. This is undoubtedly very important and must be borne in mind in any toxicity test, but there are species differences, other than strictly metabolic, which can influence the toxicity. In the example given earlier, of vitamin E deficiency induced by a test-compound, the species difference is in no way related to the metabolism of the compound but to the species sensitivity to vitamin E deficiency. Species differences in the endocrine system give rise to marked apparent differences in the toxicity of compounds; for example, hypothalamic tranquillizers have an opposite effect on the uterus in rats and dogs—due to the different function of prolactin in the two species (Baker & Tucker, 1967).

Everything should be done in animal toxicity tests to make the extrapolation of data, from animals to man, logical. High on the list of requirements for this purpose are the blood level data since they automatically take into account some of the more important variables such as absorption, excretion rates and metabolism, but the significance of many other differences can only be determined by knowing the pathogenesis of the effects.

## REFERENCES

ALCOCK, S. J. (1971). An anti-inflammatory compound non-toxic to animals but with an adverse action in man. *Proc. Eur. Soc. Study Drug Toxicity XII*, Suppl. ICS **220,** 184.

BAKER, S. B. DE C. & TUCKER, M. J. (1967). Changes in the reproductive organs of rats and dogs treated with butyrophenones and related compounds. *Proc. Eur. Soc. Study Drug Toxicity IX*, Suppl. ICS **145**, 113.

LEVY, G. (1971). Drug biotransformation interactions in man: non-narcotic analgesics. *Ann. N.Y Acad. Sci.*, **179**, 32.

THORP, J. M. (1972). Inter and intra-species differences in protein binding. *Proc. Eur. Soc. Study Drug Toxicity XIII* (in press).

# FIVE

# Plasma Concentrations and Drug Toxicity in Man

L. F. PRESCOTT, P. ROSCOE AND J. A. H. FORREST

*The Regional Poisoning Treatment Centre and University Department of Therapeutics, The Royal Infirmary, Edinburgh, Scotland*

**Introduction**

Although at first glance it might appear self-evident that drug toxicity and plasma concentrations should be closely related, it is often difficult or impossible to demonstrate a close correlation under clinical conditions. In this paper we discuss some of the possible reasons for the failure to relate plasma concentrations to toxicity, and the principles involved are illustrated with examples of toxicity associated with both the therapeutic use and overdosage of drugs.

On theoretical grounds a good correlation with plasma concentrations is unlikely unless toxic effects are directly related to the amount of active drug in the affected tissue at a given time. The different 'mechanisms' of drug toxicity must therefore be considered, and it is obvious that many types of drug reaction have to be excluded (Table 1). For example, in allergic and hypersensitivity reactions the immunological state of the individual rather than the amount of drug determines the response, and in

TABLE 1. *Drug toxicity—a classification*

| |
|---|
| Exaggerated therapeutic effect |
| Secondary pharmacological actions |
| Idiosyncrasy |
| Allergic and hypersensitivity reactions |
| Drug-specific organ toxicity |
| Local tissue irritation |
| Change in drug effects due to disease |
| Interference with natural defence mechanisms |
| Interference with nutrient absorption, protein synthesis and growth |
| Teratogenesis and carcinogenesis |
| Genetically controlled abnormalities in response |
| Pharmacokinetic abnormalities |
| Drug interactions |
| Errors of drug formulation or administration |

a previously sensitized person minute quantities may cause fatal anaphylaxis. Alkylating agents, monoamine oxidase inhibitors and organophosphorus insecticides combine irreversibly with cell constituents, and their effects persist long after the drugs have disappeared from the circulation, while in the special case of drug withdrawal reactions, 'toxicity' occurs only after the drug has been discontinued. In addition, the incidence and severity of drug toxicity reactions are influenced by many factors: age, the disease itself, complications such as abnormal electrolyte, acid-base or hormonal balance, hypoxia, cardiac or peripheral circulatory failure, malnutrition, uraemia and previous or concurrent drug therapy may all predispose to toxicity in certain circumstances. Toxicity is often attributed to just one of several drugs being taken at the same time, and the contribution of the other drugs is ignored, even though they may act on the same tissues.

**The Time Factor**

Failure to appreciate the kinetics of drug distribution is a constant source of confusion, and it is often taken for granted that the plasma and tissue concentrations of a drug are directly related. This assumption is valid only when the drug in the plasma has reached distribution equilibrium with the drug in the tissues, and the time taken to reach equilibrium varies from one tissue to another depending on the blood supply and the physicochemical properties of the drug. Major discrepancies must be expected between drug effects and plasma concentrations immediately after *i.v.* injections and in other situations where there are rapid shifts of drug from plasma to tissues or vice versa. This effect may contribute to the extreme range in 'blood' thiopentone concentrations (1 to 22 $\mu$g/ml) observed in patients regaining consciousness after thiopentone-nitrous oxide anaesthesia (Dundee, 1956). The time at which blood samples are taken in relation to the time and route of drug administration is obviously of crucial importance, and plasma concentrations are most likely to accurately reflect tissue concentrations during chronic administration of drugs with a long biological half-life. With some drugs (*e.g.*, lithium and nicotinic acid) toxic reactions seem to be related more to the rate of increase of the plasma concentrations rather than to the maximum concentration (Svedmyr, Harthon & Lundholm, 1969; Gershon, 1970).

The time factor is important for other reasons. Often, toxicity depends on the duration of drug therapy, and there may be a closer correlation between toxicity and the variation in average plasma concentration with time. For example, methotrexate can be given intermittently (i.v.) in large doses with little risk of toxicity, whereas chronic oral therapy with much smaller doses may cause progressive hepatic lesions (Dahl, Gregory, &

Scheuer, 1971; Price, 1971). The route of administration may be an important factor here however. The duration of exposure to the drug is also a major factor in the pathogenesis of conditions such as analgesic nephropathy, haemolytic anaemia associated with a direct antiglobulin (Coombs) test in patients receiving α-methyldopa, and chloroquin retinopathy. On the other hand, tolerance to the side-effects of drugs may develop rapidly. The drowsiness observed when treatment is begun with α-methyldopa is usually short-lived unless the dose is increased, and Åsberg, Cronholm, Sjöqvist & Tuck (1970) were able to correlate plasma concentrations of nortriptyline with side effects during the first three weeks of therapy, but not during the fourth week.

## Methodology

The recognition and recording of clinical drug toxicity is notoriously unreliable. There is a difficulty in deciding what constitutes a genuine toxic reaction and in making a quantitative assessment. Hypotension, depression of respiration, altered consciousness, tachycardia or fever present little difficulty, but subjective complaints such as pruritis, headache, dizziness, anxiety or nausea are not so easy to assess. There is also difficulty in dissociating these manifestations from the effects of the underlying disease and the inevitable polypharmacy. Incidental observations made during the course of another investigation are rarely satisfactory, and there is no substitute for a well-designed prospective double-blind study (e.g. Åsberg *et al.*, 1970). Apparent lack of correlation may be due to indirect drug action and measurement of an inappropriate biological function. For example, there is no direct relationship between the plasma concentration of coumarin anticoagulants and prothrombin-complex activity at any time, but a close correlation can be demonstrated with the rate of synthesis of clotting factors (O'Reilly & Levy, 1970).

There are also major problems in the estimation of drug concentrations in plasma. The ideal sample for analysis is probably plasma water from arterial blood, but this cannot be obtained as a routine practice. Data are often presented simply as 'blood levels', presumably derived from analysis of whole blood samples. Drugs are generally taken up by red cells according to their lipid solubility, and highly ionized compounds such as quaternary ammonium bases scarcely enter red cells at all (Schanker, Nafpliotis & Johnson, 1961). 'Blood levels' may have to be corrected for haematocrit, and often cannot be compared directly with plasma concentrations. The concentration of 6-mercaptopurine in human red cells, for example, is less than 1% of that in plasma (Loo, Luce & Sullivan, 1968), while desmethylimipramine is concentrated about ten-fold in red blood cells (Von Bahr & Borgå, 1971). The corresponding red cell concentration factor for alkyl mercury compounds is about 100! In an attempt to avoid confusion, 'blood', serum and plasma concentrations of drugs will be quoted as cited in the original literature reports.

With drugs which are highly bound to plasma proteins, the extent of binding should also be taken into account since effects are thought to be related only to the concentration of unbound drug. The binding of diphenylhydantoin is decreased by a factor of from 2 to 3 in patients with uraemia (Reidenberg, Odar-Cederlöf, Von Bahr, Borgå & Sjöqvist, 1971), and reduced binding of sulphonamides has been noted in other disease states. Of particular importance is the fact that binding may be reduced disproportionately in patients receiving multiple drug therapy (Anton, 1968). The increased sensitivity to thiopentone observed in patients with impaired renal function may perhaps be explained on the basis of decreased binding of the drug to plasma proteins (Dundee & Richards, 1954).

A further cause of confusion is the use of non-specific analytical methods which may not only measure inactive metabolites but may also be subject to interference from other drugs taken at the same time. This is a major problem with self-poisoning, where ingestion of several drugs at once is common (Cameron & Wright, unpublished results; Brown, 1971). The use of non-specific methods which also measure inactive metabolites led to the widely accepted, but quite mistaken, belief that forced alkaline diuresis is effective therapy for overdosage with short- and medium-acting barbiturates. More recently, a similar myth was perpetuated concerning the value of peritoneal dialysis and forced diuresis for the 'treatment' of tricyclic antidepressant intoxication (Royds & Knight, 1970). In this case, the extremely non-specific methyl orange method was used and this would have measured not only inactive tricyclic metabolites but also the chlorpromazine, diazepam and lignocaine which had been given to the patients for therapeutic reasons. Most hospital laboratories still rely on ultraviolet spectrophotometric methods for the estimation of barbiturates, and many commonly used drugs can cause gross interference (Tompsett, 1969). This is much less of a problem with gas-liquid chromatography.

It is essential to know whether toxicity is due to the parent drug or to metabolites. Unfortunately, such information is often not available, and there are exceptions to the general rule that drug metabolites are pharmacologically inactive. Toxicity can be attributed to metabolites of many compounds, including sulphonamides, phenacetin, methoxyflurane, carbon tetrachloride and bromobenzene. Highly active metabolites may be formed in very small amounts within the target cells, and there may be little point in trying to relate toxicity to the plasma concentrations of unchanged drug. Indeed, there may even be an inverse relationship. Pretreatment with phenobarbitone increases experimental hepatotoxicity induced by carbon tetrachloride or bromobenzene, while the severity of the lesion is decreased by treatment with SKF 525A. If these effects are due to changes in microsomal enzyme activity, lower concentrations of the parent drug due to rapid metabolism would be associated with more marked toxicity rather than higher concentrations of drug resulting from inhibition of metabolism (Brodie *et al.*, 1971).

## Toxicity and the Therapeutic Use of Drugs

Toxicity has been related to the plasma concentrations of a number of drugs, and the central nervous system effects of phenacetin, pentazocine and nortriptyline may be cited as examples (Prescott, Steel & Ferrier, 1970; Berkowitz, Asling, Schider & Way, 1969; Åsberg *et al.*, 1970). Failure to demonstrate a correlation is mentioned less often, perhaps because a lack of correlation has not been expected. In one controlled study, volunteers were given 200 mg of pentobarbitone (Hollister & Clyde, 1969). Surprisingly, there was a significant correlation between aggressiveness and the serum concentrations of barbiturate at 8 h and a paradoxical tendency for low sleepiness scores to be associated with high drug concentrations. Social and personal factors rather than the serum barbiturate concentrations were thought to have determined the response. In another study neither hypotensive action nor central nervous system depression could be related to the plasma concentrations of α-methyldopa measured either as the 2-$^{14}C$ labelled drug or by a spectrophotofluorometric method (Prescott *et al.*, 1966). The probable explanation in this case is that α-methyldopa acts indirectly through metabolites and measurements of total plasma radioactivity would have included both unchanged drug and metabolites.

### *Cardiac Glycosides*

Plasma concentrations of digoxin during chronic oral therapy have been related to toxicity in numerous recent reports (Grahame-Smith & Everest, 1969; Smith & Haber, 1970, 1971; Smith & Willerson, 1971; Oliver, Parker & Parker, 1971; and others). With the radioimmunoassay method a fairly consistent picture has emerged, and the dividing line between therapeutic and toxic concentrations seems to be 1·5 to 2 ng/ml. Oliver *et al.*, (1971) reported average digoxin concentrations of 0·5, 1·6 and 3 ng/ml respectively in inadequately digitalized and adequately digitalized patients and those with toxicity (Figure 1). Smith & Haber (1970) observed concentrations of less than 2 ng/ml in 90% of 131 patients without toxicity, whereas this value was exceeded in 87% of those with unequivocal evidence of digitalis intoxication. There was considerable overlap, however, between the plasma digoxin concentrations in patients with and without toxicity (Table 2). The plasma concentrations of digitoxin were about ten times higher, presumably due to extensive plasma protein binding and there was a greater overlap between the groups. With the $^{86}$rubidium-red-cell-uptake-inhibition method, plasma digoxin concentrations in patients

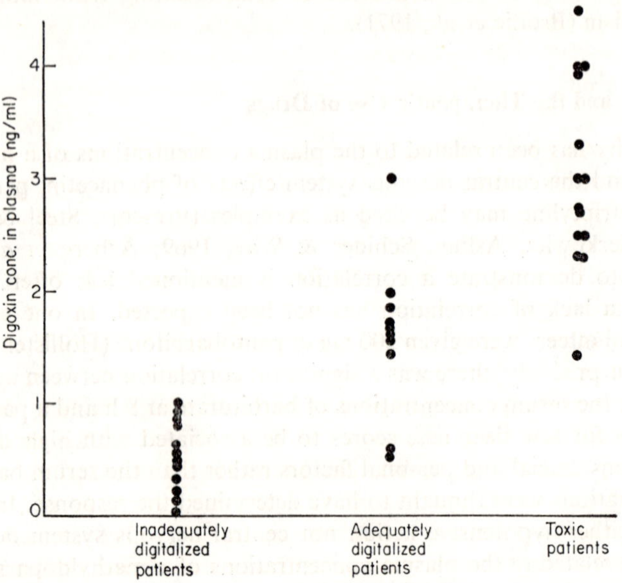


FIG. 1. Plasma digoxin concentrations in patients judged to be inadequately digitalized, adequately digitalized and toxic (Oliver *et al.*, 1971).*

with and without toxicity ranged from 4 to 8 and 0·8 to 4·5 ng/ml respectively (Grahame-Smith & Everest, 1969).

The current wave of enthusiasm for the estimation of digoxin concentrations as an aid to the diagnosis of digitalis toxicity must be tempered by recent reports which have failed to confirm earlier observations. Fogelman, LaMont, Finkelstein, Rado & Pearce (1971) found no correlation between plasma digoxin concentrations (radioimmunoassay) and electrocardiographic evidence of toxicity in 101 patients. The mean values for toxic,

TABLE 2. *Serum concentrations of digoxin and digitoxin (radioimmunoassay)*

| | serum concentrations (ng/ml) | | | |
|---|---|---|---|---|
| | Patients without toxicity | | Patients with toxicity | |
| Drug | Mean ± S.D. | Range | Mean ± S.D. | Range |
| Digoxin | 1·4 ± 0·7 | 0·3–3·0 | 3·7 ± 1·0 | 1·6–13·7 |
| Digitoxin | 17 ± 8 | 3–39 | 34 ± 6 | 26–43 |

From Smith & Haber (1971).

* Reproduced by permission of the *American Journal of Medicine*.

possibly toxic and non-toxic patients were 1·69 ± 1·29, 1·61 ± 0·79 and 1·41 ± 1·09 ng/ml respectively, and 7 of 18 definitely toxic patients had plasma digoxin concentrations of less than 1·0 ng/ml. In one woman with nausea, vomiting, diarrhoea, chromatopsia, paroxysmal atrial tachycardia with block and frequent premature ventricular beats, the digoxin concentration was only 0·41 ng/ml and symptoms cleared when the drug was discontinued. This lack of correlation could not be explained on the basis of hypokalaemia or renal failure, and is of particular significance since estimations were requested specifically by clinicians because of suspected digitalis intoxication.

Very high plasma concentrations have been observed following deliberate or accidental overdosage with digoxin, and in five such cases the concentrations ranged from 11·1 to 42 ng/ml (Smith & Willerson, 1971). The patient with the highest value died with refractory hyperkalaemia, and the others (mean maximum concentration 15·1 ng/ml) all developed arrhythmias, but survived.

The response to cardiac glycosides is influenced by $K^+$, $Na^+$, $Ca^{++}$, $Mg^{++}$ and acid-base balance, hypoxia, thyroid state, autonomic activity and the underlying myocardial pathology. Furthermore, changes in electrolyte balance and thyroid function may alter the ratio of plasma to myocardial concentration of digoxin (Smith, 1971). Under the circumstances it is hardly surprising that toxicity and plasma concentrations are not always closely related, and a clinical 'bioassay' such as estimation of salivary $K^+$ and $Ca^{++}$ concentrations might yet prove more useful in practice (Wotman, Bigger, Mandel & Barkelstone, 1971).

*Chloramphenicol*

This drug produces direct reversible depression of erythropoiesis which tends to be related to dose and duration of therapy. Patients with and without renal or hepatic disease were given 2 g of chloramphenicol daily for up to 4 weeks, and toxicity was assessed by measurement of haematocrit, reticulocyte count, serum iron concentration and total iron-binding capacity. Erythropoietic depression occurred only in patients with hepatic or renal disease, and was associated with high serum concentrations of unchanged chloramphenicol (Figure 2). There was no such correlation with chloramphenicol metabolites (Suhrland & Weisberger, 1963). In another study, patients received either 4 g or 6 g of chloramphenicol daily and bone-marrow depression was observed in patients with plasma concentrations exceeding 25 μg/ml following the initial dose (Scott *et al.*, 1965). The high correlations in these reports can probably be explained by a direct effect of the unchanged drug on the bone marrow and the fact that a rise in the serum iron concentration is a relatively sensitive and easily measured index of erthyroid depression. Very young infants seem to be

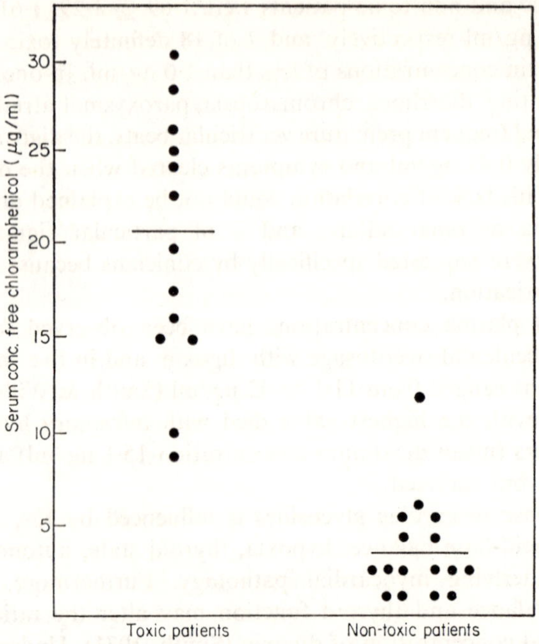


FIG. 2. Maximum serum concentrations of free chloramphenicol in patients with and without depression of erythropoiesis (redrawn from Suhrland & Weisberger, 1963). The horizontal lines represent mean values for each group.

uniquely sensitive to the toxic effects of chloramphenicol since the 'gray baby syndrome' apparently has no counterpart in adults.

*Diphenylhydantoin*

The central nervous system manifestations of diphenylhydantoin intoxication in epileptic patients correlate reasonably well with plasma concentrations (Kutt *et al.*, 1964; Stensrud & Palmer, 1964; Kutt, 1971; Lund, *et al.*, 1971, and others). Nystagmus on lateral gaze appears with concentrations of 15 to 25 µg/ml, ataxia occurs at about 30 µg/ml, and mental changes are seen with concentrations exceeding 40 µg/ml. According to Kutt *et al.*, (1964), it is frequently possible to estimate the plasma concentrations of diphenylhydantoin to within 5% merely by determining the severity of the nystagmus. Our own limited experience is in close agreement with the above classification. The initial plasma concentration of diphenylhydantoin was 44 µg/ml in one patient who was severely obtunded with such gross truncal ataxia that she was unable to sit up unaided, and in another patient admitted for investigation of 'posterior fossa tumour' the concentration was 54 µg/ml. In another study, however, toxicity was noted in only 9 of 18 patients with plasma diphenylhydantoin concentrations above 20 μg/ml, and in 7 of 10 patients with values above 30 μg/ml (Lund *et al.*, 1971). In further studies, Lund observed neurotoxicity in only 6 of 35 patients with concentrations above 20 μg/ml (this symposium, p. 227).

The relationship between plasma concentrations and toxicity of diphenylhydantoin is not clear cut in patients receiving large doses i.v. for the treatment of cardiac arrhythmias. Bigger, Schmidt & Kutt (1968) found that vertigo, nystagmus and drowsiness were invariably associated with plasma concentrations above 20 μg/ml, but that not all patients developed toxicity above this level. The plasma concentration was only 10·5 μg/ml in one patient who became hypotensive, while complete atrio-ventricular (A-V) block occurred in another acutely ill patient with a peak concentration of 22 μg/ml. Furthermore, Stone, Klein & Lown (1971) noted nystagmus and neurotoxicity with plasma diphenylhydantoin concentrations ranging from 8·6 to 35 μg/ml in patients with recurrent ventricular tachycardia.

Chronic administration and the rather slow elimination kinetics of diphenylhydantoin probably contribute to the generally good correlations observed by some investigators in epileptic patients. It is not clear why others have failed to confirm these findings. The less satisfactory correlations in patients with cardiac arrhythmias could be due to failure to reach equilibrium between drug in plasma and brain following i.v. injection and increased susceptibility to the toxic effects of the drug in severely ill patients. In adults with normal renal function there is little individual variation in the extent of binding of diphenylhydantoin to plasma proteins (Lund *et al.*, 1971; Reidenberg *et al.*, 1971). Salicylate and phenylbutazone, however, can cause significant displacement, even at therapeutic concentrations (Lunde, Rane, Yaffe, Lund & Sjöqvist, 1970), and the effects of diphenylhydantoin might be potentiated by these commonly used drugs. We have recently seen two patients who developed frank diphenylhydantoin intoxication following heavy consumption of aspirin in one case, and therapeutic doses of oxyphenbutazone in the other. The total plasma diphenylhydantoin concentrations were in the lower toxic range (20 and 23 μg/ml).

*Lignocaine and Other Local Anaesthetics*

Plasma or 'blood' concentrations of lignocaine have been measured by many investigators, and although it is often asserted that toxicity is related to concentration, the position is hopelessly confused. Bromage & Robson (1961) infused large amounts of lignocaine during and after general anaesthesia and did not observe toxic effects until 'blood' concentrations exceeded 10 μg/ml. The nonspecific methyl orange method was used, and no details were given of other drugs administered. Foldes, Molloy, McNall

& Koukal (1960), using the same analytical method, noted neurotoxicity at a mean plasma concentration of 5·3 μg/ml after an average dose of 6·4 mg/kg had been infused over 18 min in 12 normal volunteers. In another study in normal volunteers, 200 mg of lignocaine was given i.v. over 20 min 20 s, and 3 min after the start of injection the mean plasma concentration was 4 μg/ml. Subjective central nervous system effects and mild electroencephalographic abnormalities occurred in some individuals, but these were not related in any way to the plasma concentrations. Similar results were obtained with prilocaine (Eriksson, 1966).

Central nervous system toxicity has been associated with an even greater range of plasma or 'blood' concentrations of lignocaine in patients with myocardial infarction and cardiac arrhythmias. Jewitt, Kishon & Thomas (1968) observed twitching, confusion and disorientation with 'blood' concentrations of lignocaine of only 2·7 and 3·0 μg/ml in patients receiving infusions at the rate of 1 to 2 mg/min. On the other hand, no comparable side-effects were noted in a 31-year-old woman who was given 5·5 g of the drug in 20 h. At the end of this period the serum lignocaine concentration was said to be 21 μg/ml, but the method of assay was not stated and the patient had received innumerable other drugs (Bedynek, *et al.*, 1966). In another report, stupor and focal convulsions occurred in three patients given very large doses of lignocaine when the 'blood' concentrations were 22·8, 10·9 and 6·8 μg/ml (Gianelly, Von der Groeben, Spivak & Harrison, 1967).

Dr. J. Nimmo has recently studied plasma lignocaine concentrations in patients with myocardial infarction given 100 mg of the drug i.v. over 2 min. There was roughly a ten-fold range in the initial plasma concentrations, and transient neurotoxicity was observed in three patients with concentrations at 3 min of 8·3, 4·9 and 1·8 μg/ml (Figure 3). Interestingly, the patient with the highest concentration (19 μg/ml) was quite unaffected, while a patient with one of the lowest values became quite dizzy and lightheaded. None of these patients had severe cardiac failure or hypotension, and lignocaine was estimated in plasma by gas-liquid chromatography (Prescott & Nimmo, 1971). Obviously, there is an initial inverse relationship between plasma and tissue concentrations. If distribution is slow and the drug is confined mainly to the circulation it cannot do any harm, but if the concentration is low in plasma due to rapid tissue uptake then toxicity may be anticipated. It was formerly believed that lignocaine was rapidly metabolized by the liver, with a plasma half-life of about 20 min, and that toxic effects would always be short lived. However, the rapid disappearance of the drug from plasma following bolus i.v. injections is due largely to distribution rather than metabolism. When equilibration between drug in plasma and tissues had been reached after chronic infusions of 24 to 48 h, the plasma half-life is 3 to 4 h because of slow release of drug from peripheral tissue stores. Under these conditions, toxicity associated with high plasma lignocaine concentrations is likely to be prolonged (Prescott & Nimmo, 1971).

Central nervous system toxicity may therefore occur under different conditions with plasma or 'blood' concentrations of lignocaine ranging from 1·8 to more than 21 μg/ml. It is impossible to relate plasma concentrations to toxicity without taking into account at least the amount of drug given,

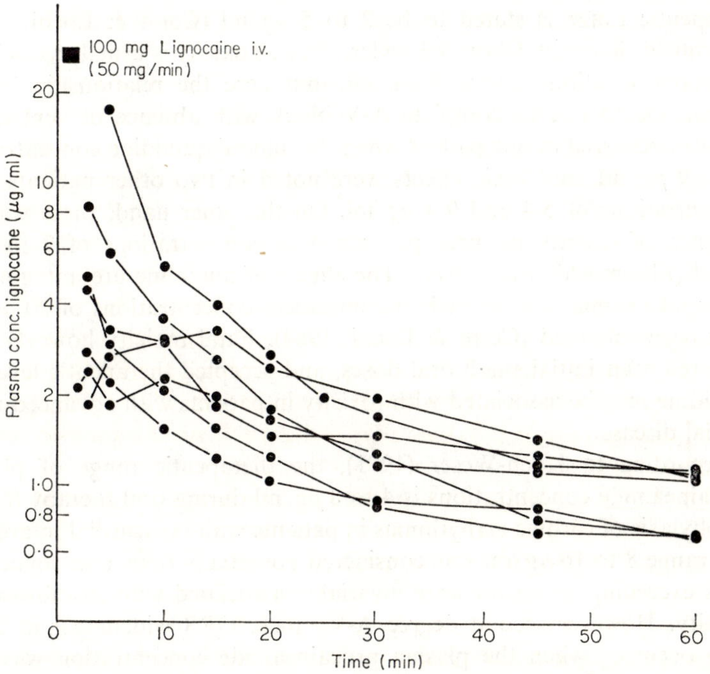


FIG. 3. Plasma concentrations of lignocaine following i.v. injection of 100 mg over 2 min in patients with myocardial infarction. Central nervous system toxicity was observed in three patients with lignocaine concentrations of 8·3, 4·9 and 1·8 μg/ml at 3 min.

the route and rate of administration, the specificity of the analytical methods, the time interval between administration and sampling, whether concentrations are rising or falling, the duration of therapy, administration of other drugs, the condition of the patient and the underlying pathology. Furthermore, lignocaine concentrations in whole blood and plasma are not equivalent.

Similar problems are likely to be encountered with other local anaesthetics. Thus the plasma concentrations varied from 20 to 80 μg/ml in volunteers infused with procaine to the point when convulsions occurred (Wikinski, Usubiaga & Wikinski, 1970). These authors also described the case of a

39-year-old man who was inadvertently given 4 g of procaine i.v. over 2 min. The plasma concentration of procaine rose to 96 μg/ml, there was tachycardia, hypertension, maximal dilatation of the pupils and widening of the QRS complex but the patient miraculously survived.

*Quinidine and Procaineamide*

The antiarrhythmic effects of quinidine correlate fairly well with plasma or 'blood' concentrations, especially during oral administration, and the therapeutic range is stated to be 2 to 5 μg/ml (Conn & Luchi, 1964; Bloomfield, Romhilt, Chou & Fowler, 1971). Toxicity is usually associated with concentrations above 8 μg/ml, but here the relationship is less certain. Death due to complete A-V block with absence of ventricular complex occurred in one patient when the 'blood' quinidine concentration was 6.9 μg/ml, and toxic effects were noted in two other patients with concentrations of 5·4 and 9·4 μg/ml. On the other hand, there was no evidence of toxicity in three patients with concentrations of 9 to 11·2 μg/ml (Bloomfield *et al.*, 1971). The effects of quinidine are antagonized by hypokalaemia, and in such circumstances concentrations of 20 μg/ml have been tolerated (Conn & Luchi, 1964). Fatal toxicity however, has occurred after initial small oral doses, and accepted therapeutic levels of quinidine may be associated with toxicity in patients with advanced myocardial disease.

According to Koch-Weser (1971), the therapeutic range of plasma procaineamide concentrations is 4 to 8 μg/ml during oral therapy for the prophylaxis of cardiac arrhythmias in patients with myocardial infarction. The range 8 to 16 μg/ml was considered potentially toxic and concentrations exceeding 16 μg/ml were invariably associated with cardiovascular toxicity. However second degree A-V block, QRS widening and death have occurred when the plasma procaineamide concentration was 10·2 μg/ml (Koch-Weser, Klein, Foo-Canto, Kastor & DeSanctis, 1970). With these drugs, toxicity is greatly influenced by the underlying myocardial pathology, and in the case of quinidine, by the electrolyte balance.

**Drug Overdosage**

Until fairly recently, the only information concerning plasma concentrations of drugs taken in overdosage and poisons was that obtained by forensic pathologists. Clinical toxicology is still a neglected speciality and there are very few centres with the clinical experience and laboratory facilities necessary to obtain adequate data from sufficiently large numbers of patients. Nevertheless, the literature is replete with case reports and accounts of survival after dialysis or forced diuresis following drug overdosage. Often there is no chemical evidence that the drug in question was indeed ever taken, the dose and time of ingestion can rarely be established with certainty, ingestion of several different drugs is commonplace and response may be influenced by age, underlying pathology or tolerance. Furthermore, the specificity of methods used for drug assay is often in doubt and determinations are usually carried out in an emergency situation. Under the circumstances, it is often not possible to make a meaningful analysis of toxicity in relation to plasma concentrations of drugs taken in overdosage.

Further complications are caused by the efforts of 'non-clinical' toxicologists who seldom deal with live patients but who still describe the clinical features and management of poisoned patients with an air of authority (Matthew, 1971). Impressive tabulations of 'therapeutic', 'toxic' and 'lethal' values for 'blood levels' of drugs appear from time to time (Parker et al., 1970; Wert, 1970; Winek, 1971). Not only is the concept of a 'lethal blood level' quite meaningless in practice, but such compilations often contain gross errors and obvious discrepancies. For example, Winek (1971) lists the following 'lethal blood levels': salicylate 500 μg/ml; amitriptyline 10 to 20 μg/ml; short-acting barbiturates 10 μg/ml, intermediate-acting barbiturates 30 μg/ml; phenobarbitone 80 to 150 μg/ml, and methaqualone 30 μg/ml. According to Wert (1970), 'lethal blood levels' of barbiturates are 10 to 50 μg/ml, and 'low values are significant in the slower-acting forms while higher values are significant in more rapid acting drugs'. These figures simply do not make sense and bear no relation to modern clinical experience.

*Barbiturates*

It is widely believed that 'blood' or plasma barbiturate concentrations are a reliable guide to the severity of intoxication. This is a fallacy (Matthew & Lawson, 1966). We recently observed a five-fold range in the plasma concentrations of short- to medium-acting barbiturates in 10 patients admitted with Grade IV coma (no response to maximal painful stimulation). Consumption of other drugs or alcohol was excluded, none of the patients had significant underlying medical disease and barbiturate in plasma was estimated using a gas-liquid chromatographic method. There was no clear correlation between the maximum barbiturate concentration and the duration of coma or depth of coma as judged by the need for assisted ventilation (Table 3). Of even greater significance was the wide range in plasma concentrations on regaining consciousness to the point of response to verbal commands. There was evidence of marked tolerance to the central nervous system effects of barbiturate in patient No. 1. This 44-year-old barbiturate addict was twice admitted following overdosage of butobarbitone with maximum plasma concentrations of 100 and 118 μg/ml (Figure 4). On each occasion coma was of short duration, assisted

TABLE 3. *Plasma barbiturate concentrations and half-lives in 10 patients admitted in Grade IV coma following uncomplicated barbiturate overdosage*

| Patient | Age & sex | Barbiturate | Maximum plasma level (μg/ml) | Duration of coma (h) | Plasma level on regaining consciousness (μg/ml) | Plasma drug half-life* (h) |
|---|---|---|---|---|---|---|
| 1A | 44M | buto | 118 | 16 | 61 | 12 |
| 1A | 44M | buto | 100 | 24 | 52 | 12 |
| 2R | 74F | amylo | 55 | 13V | 32 | 13→6 |
| 3R | 47F | quinal | 67 | 42V | 8 | 14→7 |
| 4 | 52F | amylo | 66 | 40V | 22 | 56→13 |
| 5 | 27F | amylo + | 76 | 76V | 11 | 46→12 |
| | | quinal | 52 | | 3.7 | 33→11 |
| 6 | 23F | amylo | 47 | 30 | 26 | 15 |
| 7 | 33F | amylo | 43 | 36V | 14 | 13 |
| 8 | 24M | amylo + | 17 | 38 | 5.2 | 32→12 |
| | | quinal | 15 | | 1.7 | 18→7 |
| 9 | 22F | amylo + | 16 | 24 | 8.2 | 30→8 |
| | | quinal | 13 | | 4.9 | 35→8 |
| 10 | 27M | pento | 28 | 24 | 13 | 26→17 |

A = Addicted to barbiturates, R = barbiturates used regularly as hypnotics, V = assisted ventilation. * The first and second figures represent initial and terminal plasma barbiturate half-life values respectively. There was no change in half-life in patients 1, 6 & 7.

ventilation was not required and the patient was soon walking about with plasma concentrations of butobarbitone far in excess of those stated to be lethal or indications for immediate haemodialysis (Schreiner, 1970; Henderson & Merrill, 1966; Winek, 1971 and others). The clinical course in relation to plasma barbiturate concentrations in the case of a young

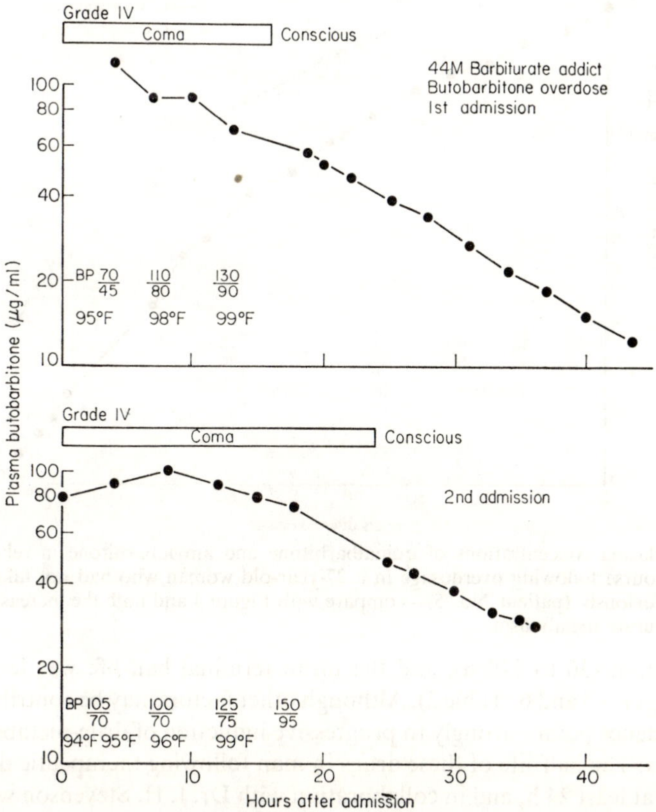


FIG. 4. Plasma butobarbitone concentrations in a 44-year-old barbiturate addict (patient No. 1) in relation to clinical course following butobarbitone overdosage on two separate occasions.

woman who denied previous consumption of hypnotics is shown in Figure 5 for comparison. Consciousness was not regained until the barbiturate concentration fell to 14·7 μg/ml. In this context it is interesting to note that Haider (1971) documented a completely flat (isoelectric) electroencephalogram in a patient when the 'blood' quinalbarbitone concentration was only 19 μg/ml.

We observed another interesting phenomenon which does not seem to have been described previously. The rate of fall of the plasma barbiturate concentrations increased markedly in most patients during the period of

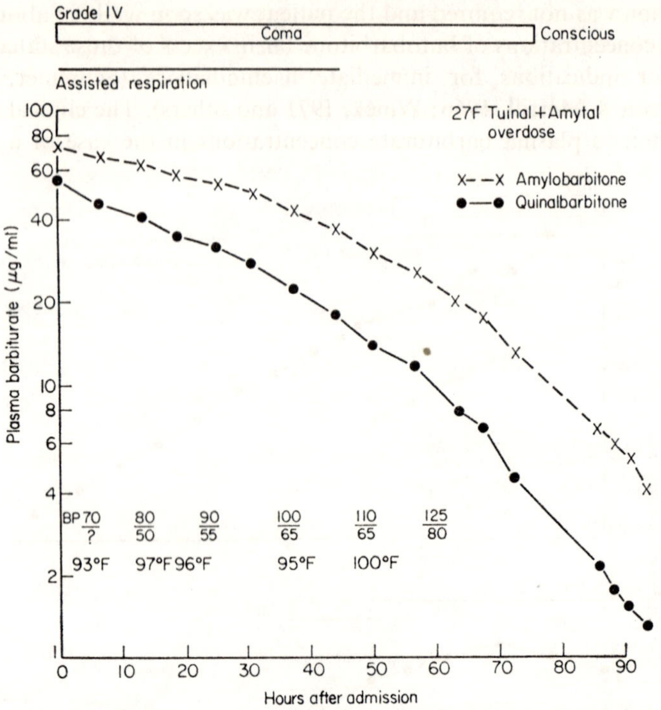


FIG. 5. Plasma concentrations of quinalbarbitone and amylobarbitone in relation to clinical course following overdosage in a 27-year-old woman who had not taken hypnotics previously (patient No. 5)—compare with Figure 4 and note the increasing rate of barbiturate metabolism.

observation (36 to 110 h), and the mean terminal half-life was less than 11 h (Figures 5 and 6; Table 3). Although other factors may be contributory, the evidence points strongly to progressive induction of drug-metabolizing enzymes. The half-life of these drugs in man following therapeutic doses is usually at least 24 h, and in collaboration with Dr. I. H. Stevenson we have found that the plasma antipyrine half-life is unusually short in these patients when they regain consciousness. There was no shortening of the plasma barbiturate half-life in the barbiturate addict and in two other patients.

Other investigators have observed a lack of correlation between barbiturate concentrations and depth or duration of coma (Matthew & Lawson, 1966; Henderson & Merrill, 1966; Setter, Maher & Schreiner, 1966; Hadden, Johnson, Smith, Price & Giardina, 1969; Hathway, 1971). In a minority of reports statistically significant correlations have been claimed, but these have been of a very low order, and in the individual case, the barbiturate concentration is of little if any prognostic value. The only exception seems to be in the case of intoxication with phenobarbitone (Setter *et al.*, 1966). Increased tolerance to hypnotics in persons previously taking large amounts of central nervous system depressant drugs has often been suggested as a possible explanation for the lack of correlation (Matthew & Lawson, 1966; Setter *et al.*, 1966; Hadden *et al.*, 1969). While this may account for disproportionately high plasma concentrations or rapid recovery in some patients, this is not always the answer. For instance, Brown & Proudfoot observed Grade IV coma in three barbiturate addicts

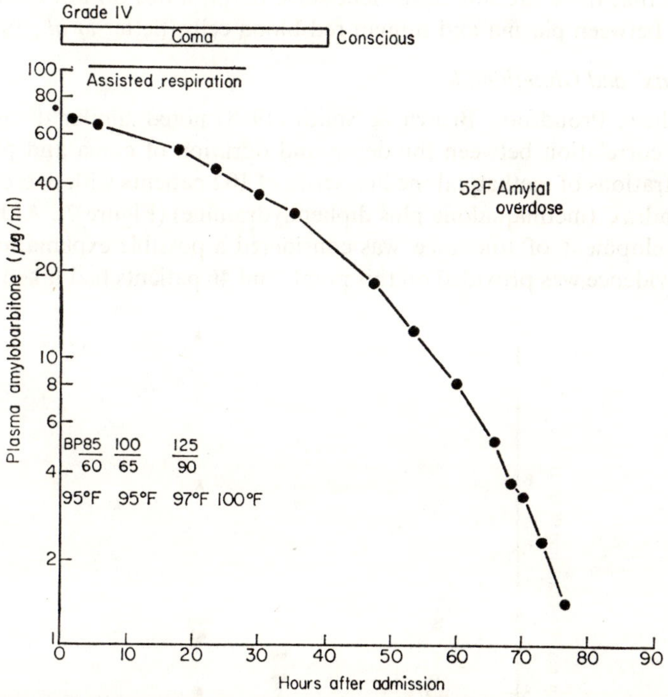


FIG. 6. Plasma concentrations of amylobarbitone following overdosage in patient No. 4. The rate of amylobarbitone metabolism increased steadily during the period of observation.

with medium-acting blood barbiturate concentrations of only 11, 22 and 13 μg/ml (see Hathway, 1971). Failure to relate duration of coma to maximum barbiturate concentration is due to the wide range in concentrations at which consciousness is regained and individual variation in the rate and extent of induction of barbiturate metabolism (Table 3).

Determination of drug concentrations in plasma is therefore of very limited value in the management of uncomplicated barbiturate intoxication, except for confirmation of the diagnosis should this be in doubt. It is much more important to know which drug is involved, since intoxication with phenobarbitone or barbitone results in prolonged coma and, if necessary, can be treated by forced alkaline diuresis. This technique is of no value in the case of short- and medium-acting drugs. Furthermore, for a given degree of intoxication the plasma concentrations of long-acting barbiturates are likely to be several times higher than the concentrations of short- to medium-acting drugs. Gas-liquid chromatography is particularly useful in this situation since the barbiturate can be quickly identified and its concentration measured at the same time. Often, no distinction is made between 'blood levels' and plasma concentrations, and again it must be stressed that these are not equivalent since barbiturates do not distribute equally between plasma and human red blood cells (Setter *et al.*, 1966).

### '*Mandrax*' *and Glutethimide*

Matthew, Proudfoot, Brown & Smith (1968) noted similar disturbing lack of correlation between the depth and duration of coma and plasma concentrations of methaqualone in a series of 102 patients with overdosage of 'Mandrax' (methaqualone plus diphenhydramine) (Figure 7). Although the development of tolerance was considered a possible explanation, no direct evidence was provided on this point, and 46 patients had taken other

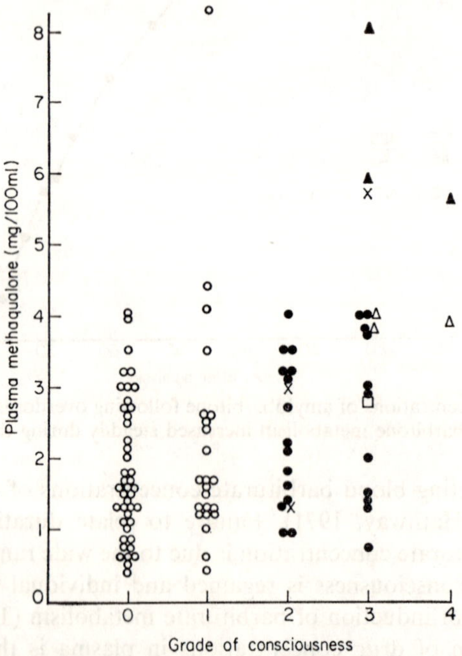


FIG. 7. Plasma concentrations of methaqualone and grades of consciousness in 102 patients following overdosage with 'Mandrax' (methaqualone plus diphenhydramine). Grades 0 to 4 represent level of consciousness as follows: 1—response to verbal commands, 2—response to mild painful stimulation, 3—minimum response to maximum painful stimulation, 4—no response to maximum painful stimulation. The duration of coma is indicated by the symbols: ○—conscious, ●—0 to 6 h, ×—7 to 12 h, △—13 to 18 h, ▲—19 to 24 h, □—37 to 48 h (Matthew *et al.*, 1968). Reproduced by permission of the Editor of the *British Medical Journal*.

drugs or alcohol. The contribution of the diphenhydramine to the intoxication cannot be assessed since it was not measured in plasma, and the assay for methaqualone may have included inactive metabolites (Brown, 1971).

The picture is similar with glutethimide intoxication. Wright & Roscoe (1970) found no useful correlation between plasma concentrations of glutethimide and depth and duration of coma or complications such as

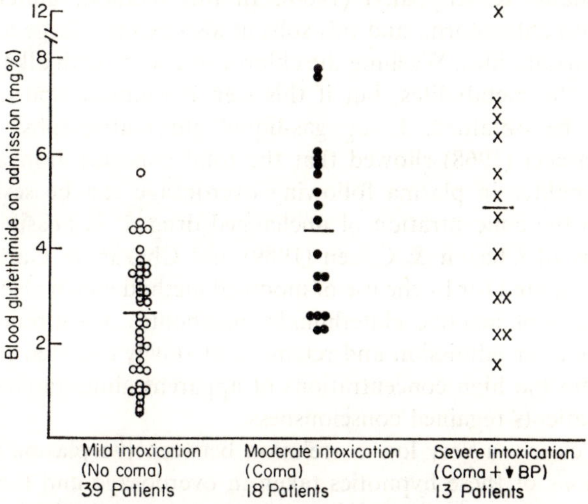


FIG. 8. Blood glutethimide concentrations in 70 patients on admission in relation to severity of intoxication. The horizontal lines represent mean values for eadh group and there is no statistically significant difference between the means of the moderately and severely intoxicated patients (Chazan & Garella, 1971).*

apnoea, papilleodema, hypotension and pulmonary oedema. It was impossible to give a prognosis or predict the likelihood of complications from the plasma glutethimide concentrations. Chazan & Cohen (1969) and Chazan & Garella (1971) also observed a lack of correlation between 'blood' glutethimide concentrations and the state of consciousness. In the latter report, there was marked overlap in the 'blood' glutethimide concentrations in 70 patients with mild, moderate and severe intoxication, but values above 50 $\mu$g/ml were seen almost exclusively in moderate and severe poisoning (Figure 8). Not only was there no relationship between the concentrations on admission and the duration of coma, but in 10 of 31 patients with moderate or severe intoxication *consciousness was regained with 'blood' glutethimide concentrations equal to or greater than the admission values*! Identical findings were described in the earlier report. Glutethimide concentrations in cerebrospinal fluid (CSF) were measured in 24 patients on admission and at 24-h intervals during coma. The CSF :

*Reproduced by permission of the *Archives of Internal Medicine*.

blood concentration ratio was 0·6 and there was a high correlation between 'blood' and CSF concentrations. As expected, there was no greater correlation between CSF concentrations of glutethimide and the clinical course.

These observations are very puzzling, and the increase in glutethimide concentrations between the time of admission and return of consciousness is particularly difficult to understand. In all the reports cited, glutethimide was estimated using the ultraviolet spectrophotometric method of Goldbaum, Williams & Koppanyi (1960). In this method, glutethimide is extracted into chloroform, and this solvent also extracts large amounts of interfering metabolites. Washing the chloroform twice with alkali removes 80–90% of the metabolites, but if this step is omitted, spuriously high values will be obtained. Using gas-liquid chromatography, Sunshine, Maes & Faracci (1968) showed that the total concentration of glutethimide metabolites in plasma following overdosage can be several times higher than the concentration of unchanged drug. It is possible that the observations of Chazan & Cohen (1969) and Chazan & Garella (1971) could be accounted for by the use of modified method which also measured large amounts of inactive glutethimide metabolites. Continuing absorption of drug after admission and retention of slowly excreted metabolites could explain the high concentrations of apparent glutethimide observed when the patients regained consciousness.

There is clearly a very low correlation between the plasma or 'blood' concentrations of these hypnotics taken in overdosage and the extent of central nervous system depression. This cannot be wholly explained by variation in response due to acquired or acute tolerance, age, underlying cardiac, renal or hepatic disease, consumption of other drugs or alcohol, hypoxia, increase in the relative concentration of acidic drugs in the brain as a result of respiratory acidosis, or the use of non-specific analytical methods. Alternative explanations are that plasma and brain concentrations are not related, or more likely, that there is enormous individual variation in the response to these drugs.

Assessment of the severity of intoxication can therefore be based only on the clinical condition of the patient. Nevertheless, the champions of haemodialysis and forced diuresis advocate the use of these relatively ineffective measures according to plasma drug concentrations (Berman, Jeghers, Schreiner, & Pallotta, 1956; Lee & Ames, 1965; Setter *et al.*, 1966 and others). Schreiner (1970), for instance, repeatedly cites concentrations of 35 μg/ml for short-acting barbiturates and 80 μg/ml for long-acting barbiturates as potentially lethal and indications for haemodialysis. Again, identification of the drug is important because unless the concentration is very high, haemodialysis does not remove biologically significant amounts of short-medium acting barbiturates, glutethimide or methaqualone. It must be stressed that reduction in the plasma concentration or 'half-life' of a drug during dialysis means nothing more than that drug has been removed from plasma. It tells us nothing about removal of drug from the tissues, which is what matters, and in practice this may amount to very little. Setter *et al.* (1966), for example, mention a patient with quinalbarbitone intoxication who was haemodialysed for 12 h. During this time the serum barbiturate concentration fell from 72 to 22 $\mu$g/ml, but the concentration in subcutaneous fat only decreased from 72 to 55 $\mu$g/ml. The proponents of haemodialysis do not like to discuss 'rebound intoxication' or the increase in plasma concentration which may occur when haemodialysis is discontinued, and this is often attributed to the 'narcotized gut syndrome' rather than to re-equilibration of drug between tissues and plasma (Kennedy *et al.*, 1969; Setter *et al.*, 1966). Little is known of the dialysance of drug metabolites, and recovery studies may be misleadingly optimistic unless the analytical methods are absolutely specific for the drug in its active form.

*Salicylates*

Although the clinical manifestations of uncomplicated salicylate intoxications are quite unmistakable, it is by no means simple to assess

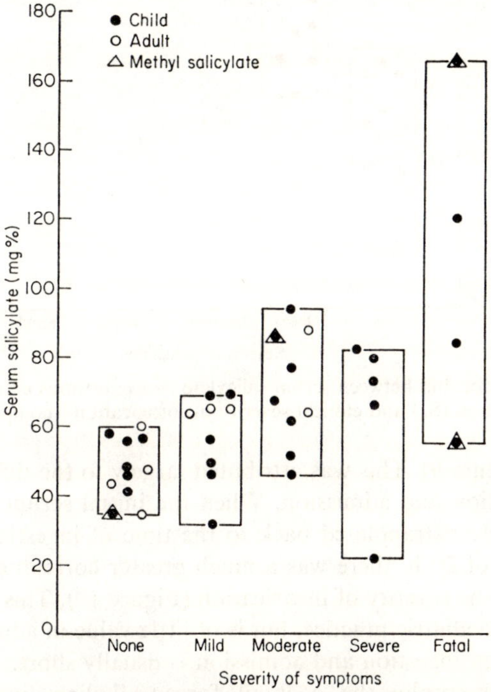


FIG. 9. The relationship between serum salicylate concentrations at the time of admission and clinical severity of salicylate intoxication (redrawn from Done, 1960).

the severity of the intoxication by clinical signs alone. For this reason we always use a simple and rapid side-room method for the estimation of salicylate in plasma (Brown, Cameron & Matthew, 1967). Mild salicylism is seen with concentrations of 250 to 350 $\mu$g/ml, but is said to occur at lower levels in children and 'sensitive' individuals. Done (1960) observed a very poor correlation between the clinical signs of intoxication in a mixed group of children and adults and serum salicylate concentration on

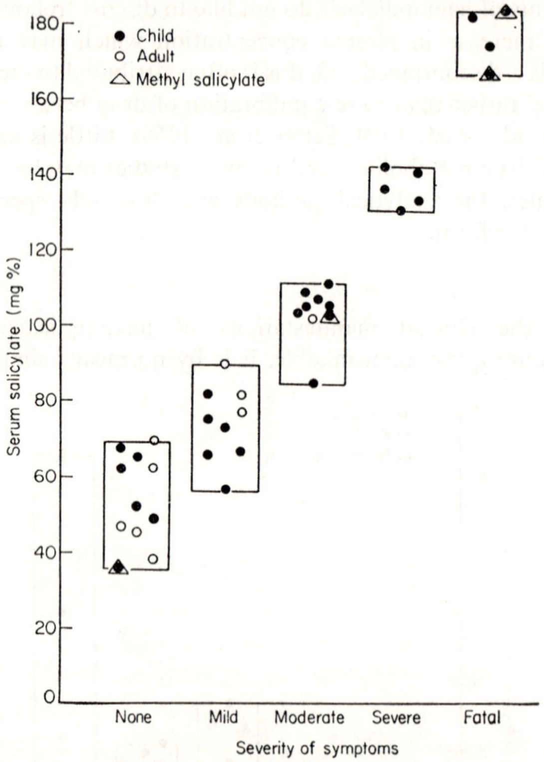


FIG. 10. The relationship between serum salicylate concentrations extrapolated back to the time of ingestion ($S_0$) and clinical severity of intoxication—compare with Figure 9 (Done, 1960).

admission (Figure 9). This was attributed largely to the different intervals between ingestion and admission. When the initial serum salicylate concentrations were extrapolated back to the time of ingestion ($S_0$) using a half-life value of 20 h, there was a much greater correlation between the $S_0$ values and the severity of intoxication (Figure 10). This approach may be helpful in paediatric practice, but is of little value in adults because the interval between ingestion and admission is usually short.

We routinely employ the 'cocktail' forced alkaline diuresis regime of Lawson *et al.*, (1969) in patients with plasma salicylate concentrations above 500 μg/ml. Although this is invariably followed by a striking relief of symptoms, in the patients studied by Lawson *et al.* (1969) there was only a modest fall in plasma salicylate concentrations and the urinary recovery of total salicylate during the diuresis was only about 1·8 g. Alkalosis causes a reduction in the brain salicylate concentrations (Davison,

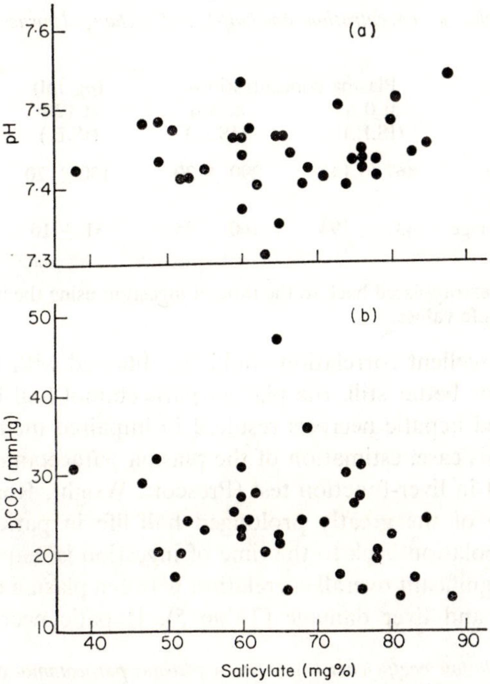


FIG. 11. The lack of correlation between (a) arterial pH and (b) arterial $pCO_2$ and peak plasma salicylate concentrations in 36 patients (Lawson *et al.*, 1969).*

1971), and the disproportionate amelioration of symptoms is presumably due largely to redistribution and haemodilution rather than elimination of salicylate. Some toxic effects of salicylate do not correlate at all with plasma concentrations. Hyperventilation often persists for 24 to 48 h, long after plasma salicylate concentrations have fallen to very low levels and other signs of intoxication have disappeared. In addition, there is no significant correlation between peak plasma salicylate concentrations in adults and abnormalities of acid-base equilibrium as measured by arterial blood pH and $pCO_2$ (Figure 11) (Lawson *et al.*, 1969).

*Paracetamol*

In contrast to the relationship between the corrected plasma salicylate concentrations ($S_0$) and toxicity observed by Done (1960), we found a

* Reproduced by permission of the *Quarterly Journal of Medicine*,

relatively low correlation between plasma concentrations of unchanged paracetamol during the first few hours after overdosage and subsequent hepatotoxicity. Indeed, the mean plasma paracetamol concentrations extrapolated back to 'zero time' using the individual half-life values were virtually identical in patients with or without hepatic necrosis (Table 4).

TABLE 4. *Mean plasma concentrations and half-life of unchanged paracetamol in poisoned patients*

| Patients | Plasma concentrations at 0 h* (IS.E.) | at 4 h (IS.E.) | (μg/ml) at 12 h (IS.E.) | Half-life (h) |
|---|---|---|---|---|
| With liver damage (17 patients) | 467 ± 143 | 290 ± 20 | 130 ± 20 | 7·6 ± 0·8 |
| Without liver damage (13 patients) | 437 ± 194 | 160 ± 25 | 31 ± 10 | 2·9 ± 0·3 |

* Concentrations extrapolated back to the time of ingestion using the individual plasma paracetamol half-life values.

However, an excellent correlation could be obtained with the concentrations at 12 h, or better still, the plasma paracetamol half-life. The paracetamol-induced hepatic necrosis resulted in impaired metabolism of the drug, and in this case, estimation of the plasma paracetamol half-life was in effect a built-in liver-function test (Prescott, Wright, Roscoe & Brown 1971). Because of the greatly prolonged half-life in patients with liver damage, extrapolation back to the time of ingestion is inappropriate, and there was no significant overall correlation between plasma concentrations at 'zero time' and liver damage (Table 5). Hepatic necrosis is almost

TABLE 5. *Correlation coefficients* (*r*) *between plasma paracetamol concentration and half-life and biochemical evidence of hepatic necrosis in* 30 *poisoned patients.*

| | r for plasma level at 0 h* | r for plasma level at 4 h | r for plasma half-life |
|---|---|---|---|
| Log. max GOT | 0·39 | 0·69 | 0·70 |
| Log. max HBD | 0·09 | 0·62 | 0·79 |
| Log max LDH | 0·05 | 0·59 | 0·75 |
| Max bilirubin | 0·16 | 0·24 | 0·64 |
| Max prothrombin | 0·31 | 0·35 | 0·71 |
| Min bicarbonate | −0·46 | −0·31 | −0·45 |

* Concentrations extrapolated back to the time of ingestion as in Table 4. For statistically significant correlations ($P < 0{\cdot}05$) with $N = 30$, r must exceed 0·36.

inevitable if the plasma paracetamol half-life exceeds 4 h (normal range 1·5 to 2·5 h), and the outcome is likely to be fatal if the half-life is more than 10 to 12 h. The plasma concentration curves have separated sufficiently by 12 h to enable a reasonably accurate prognosis to be given from the assay of a single plasma sample (Prescott *et al.*, 1971).

As with other drugs, the use of non-specific methods for the estimation of paracetamol has caused confusion. Contrary to popular belief, *p*-aminophenol cannot be detected in blood or urine as a metabolite of paracetamol, and it is hardly surprising that conflicting results are obtained when both unchanged drug and its inactive conjugates are hydrolysed to *p*-aminophenol and expressed as 'blood *p*-aminophenol levels'. In fact, there is an inverse relationship between plasma concentrations of paracetamol conjugates and liver damage, and the most sensitive prognostic index is the ratio of unchanged to conjugated paracetamol measured in plasma 12 h after overdosage. It is of course possible that minor unidentified metabolites of paracetamol cause the hepatic necrosis, but the severity of the lesion determines the plasma paracetamol half-life, and this explains the excellent clinical correlation.

**Summary**

Contrary to expectations, a high correlation between drug toxicity and plasma concentrations has been observed with relatively few drugs in clinical practice.

The different mechanisms involved in drug toxicity, individual variation in response, the route and rates of administration, drug distribution, physiological factors, age, underlying pathology and its complications, changes in drug binding to plasma proteins, tolerance and the effects of other drugs taken previously or concurrently must all be taken into account.

Clinically useful correlations have been demonstrated with diphenylhydantoin, chloramphenicol and cardiac glycosides, but there is usually considerable overlap in the concentrations reported in patients with and without toxicity. Even with digoxin, for which a strong case has been made, the mean values in toxic, possibly toxic and non-toxic levels did not differ significantly in one study.

There is an unexplained and most disturbing lack of correlation between plasma concentrations of barbiturates, methaqualone and glutethimide following overdosage, and both depth and duration of coma. This cannot be explained solely on the basis of acquired tolerance to hypnotics. Failure to relate duration of coma to plasma barbiturate concentration is due to the wide range in concentrations at which consciousness is regained and individual variation in the rate and extent of induction of barbiturate metabolism. In adults, salicylate concentrations correlate poorly with the clinical severity of intoxication, but a better correlation was observed in one study involving children when concentrations were extrapolated back to the time of ingestion. The extent of hepatic necrosis following paracetamol overdosage is closely related to the plasma paracetamol half-life.

In practice, major problems arise through failure to recognize the importance of drug distribution kinetics, lack of information concerning the activity of drug metabolites and the use of non-specific analytical methods for drug assay. At present relatively few clinical problems can be resolved merely by requesting a 'blood level'.

We are indebted to Dr. H. Matthew for support and encouragement, and we gratefully acknowledge assistance rendered by Dr. S. S. Brown of the Department of Clinical Chemistry and the Nursing Staff of the Regional Poisoning Treatment Centre, Edinburgh. We also thank Mrs. I. Mann and Mrs. J. Roberts for technical assistance. This work was supported by a grant from the Scottish Hospitals Endowment Research Trust.

## REFERENCES

ANTON, A. H. (1968). The effects of disease, drugs and dilution on the binding of sulphonamides in human plasma. *Clin. Pharmacol. Therap.*, **9**, 561–567.

ÅSBERG, M., CRONHOLM. B., SJÖQVIST, F. & TUCK. D. (1970). The correlation of subjective side effects with plasma concentrations of nortriptyline. *Brit. med. J.* **4**, 18–21.

BEDYNEK, J. L., WEINSTEIN, K. N., KAH, R. E. & MINTON, P. R. (1966). Ventricular tachycardia controlled by intermittent intravenous administration of lidocaine hydrochloride. *J. Amer. Med. Ass.* ,**198**, 553–555.

BERKOWITZ, B. A., ASLING, J. H., SCHNIDER, S. M. & WAY, E. L. (1969). Relationship of pentazocine plasma levels to pharmacological activity in man. *Clin. Pharmacol. Therap.*, **10**, 320–328.

BERMAN, L. B., JEGHERS, H. J., SCHREINER, G. E. & PALLOTTA, A. J. (1956). Haemodialysis, an effective therapy for acute barbiturate poisoning. *J. Amer. Med. Ass.*, **161**, 820–827.

BIGGER, J. T., Schmidt, D. H. & KUTT, H. (1968). Relationship between the plasma level of diphenylhydantoin sodium and its cardiac antiarrhythmic effects. *Circulation*, **38**, 363–374.

BLOOMFIELD, S. S., ROMHILT, D. W., CHOU, T. & FOWLER, N. O. (1971). Quinidine for prophylaxis of arrhythmias in acute myocardial infarction. *New Eng. J. Med.*, **285**, 979–986.

BRODIE, B. B., REID, W. D., CHO, A. K., SIPES, G., KRISHNA, G. & GILLETTE, J. R. (1971). Possible mechanism of liver necrosis caused by aromatic organic compounds. *Proc. Nat. Acad. Sci.* **68**, 160–164.

BROMAGE, P. R., & ROBSON, J. G. (1961). Concentration of lignocaine in the blood after intravenous, intramuscular, epidural and endotracheal administration. *Anaesthesia*, **16**, 461–478.

BROWN, S. S. (1971). Poisoning: clinical chemistry or chemical toxicity? *Ann. clin. Biochem.*, **8**, 98–104.

BROWN, S. S., CAMERON, J. C. & MATTHEW, H. (1967). Plasma salicylate levels in acute poisoning in adults. *Brit. med. J.*, **2,** 738–739.

CAMERON, J. C. & WRIGHT, N. A comparison of drug histories and results of urine screening in poisoned patients (to be published)

CHAZAN, J. A. & COHEN, J. J. (1969). Clinical spectrum of glutethimide intoxication. *J. Amer. Med. Ass.*, **208,** 837–839.

CHAZAN, J. A. & GARELLA, S. (1971). Glutethimide intoxication. A prospective study of 70 patients treated conservatively without hemodialysis. *Arch. intern. Med.*, **128,** 215–219.

CONN, H. L. & LUCHI, R. L. (1964). Quinidine as an antiarrhythmic agent. *Amer. J. Med.*, **37,** 685–699.

DAHL, M. G. C., GREGORY, M. M. & SCHEUER, P. J. (1971). Liver damage due to methotrexate in patients with psoriasis. *Brit. med. J.*, **1,** 625–629.

DAVISON, C. (1971). Salicylate metabolism in man. *Ann. N. Y. Acad. Sci.*, **179,** 249–268.

DONE, A. K. (1960). Salicylate intoxication. Significance of measurements of salicylate in blood in cases of acute ingestion. *Pediatrics*, **26,** 800–807.

DUNDEE, J. W. (1956). In: *Thiopentone and Other Thiobarbiturates*, pp. 119-121. Edinburgh: Livingstone.

DUNDEE, J. W. & RICHARDS, R. K. (1954). Effects of azotemia on the action of intravenous barbiturate anaesthesia. *Anaesthesiology*, **15,** 333–346.

ERIKSSON, E. (1966). Prilocaine. An experimental study in man of a new local anaesthetic with special regards to efficacy, toxicity and excretion. *Acta. Chir. Scand. Suppl.*, **358,** 25–36 and 37–46.

FOGELMAN, A. M., LA MONT, J. T., FINKELSTEIN, S., RADO, E. & PEARCE, M. L. (1971). Fallibility of plasma-digoxin in differentiating toxic from non-toxic patients. *Lancet*, **2,** 727–729.

FOLDES, F. F., MOLLOY, R., MCNALL, P. G. & KOUKAL, L. R. (1960). Comparison of toxicity of intravenously given local anaesthetic agents in man. *J. Amer. Med. Ass.*, **172,** 1493–1498.

GERSHON, S. (1970). Lithium in mania. *Clin. Pharmacol. Therap.*, **11,** 168–187.

GIANELLY, R., VON DER GROEBEN, J. O., SPIVACK, A. P. & HARRISON, D. C, (1967). Effect of lidocaine on ventricular arrhythmias in patients with coronary heart disease. *New Eng. J. Med.*, **277,** 1215–1219.

GOLDBAUM, L. R., WILLIAMS, M. A. & KOPPANYI, T. (1960). Determination of glutethimide in biological fluids. *Anal. Chem.*, **32,** 81–84.

GRAHAME-SMITH, D. G. & EVEREST, M. S. (1969). Measurement of digoxin in plasma and its use in the diagnosis of digoxin intoxication. *Brit. med. J.*, **1,** 286–289.

HADDEN, J., JOHNSON, K., SMITH, S., PRICE, L. & GIARDINA, E. (1969). Acute barbiturate intoxication, *J. Amer. Med. Ass.*, **209,** 893–900.

HAIDER, I. (1971). The electroencephalogram in acute barbiturate poisoning. In: *Acute Barbiturate Poisoning*, ed. by Matthew, H., pp. 147–174. Amsterdam: Excerpta Medica.

HATHWAY, D. E. (1971). Methods of chemical analysis for the barbiturates. In *Acute Barbiturate Poisoning*, pp. 55–73. Ed. by Matthew, H. Amsterdam: Excerpta Medica.

HENDERSON, L. W. & MERRILL, J. P. (1966). Treatment of barbiturate intoxication. *Ann Intern. Med.*, **64,** 876–891.

HOLLISTER, L. E. & CLYDE, D. J. (1968). Blood levels of pentobarbital sodium, meprobamate and tybamate in relation to clinical effects. *Clin. Pharmacol. Therap.*, **9,** 204–208.

JEWITT, D. E., KISHON, Y. & THOMAS, M. (1968). Lignocaine in the management of arrhythmias after acute myocardial infarction. *Lancet*, **1,** 266–270.

KENNEDY, A. C., LINDSAY, R. M., BRIGGS, J. D., LUKE, R. G., YOUNG, N. & CAMPBELL, D. (1969). Successful treatment of three cases of very severe barbiturate poisoning. *Lancet*, **1,** 995–998.

KOCH-WESER, J. (1971). Pharmacokinetics of procaineamide in man. *Ann. N.Y. Acad. Sci.*, **179,** 370–382.

KOCH-WESER, J., KLEIN, S. W., FOO-CANTO, L. L., KASTOR, J. A. & DESANCTIS, R. W. (1969). Antiarrhythmic prophylaxis with procaineamide in acute myocardial infarction. *New Eng. J. Med.*, **281,** 1253–1260.

KUTT, H. (1971). Biochemical and genetic factors regulating dilantin metabolism in man. *Ann. N.Y. Acad. Sci.*, **179,** 704–722.

KUTT, H., WINTERS, W. KOKENGE, R. & MCDOWELL, F. (1964). Diphenylhydantoin metabolism, blood levels and toxicity. *Arch. Neurol.*, **11,** 642–648.

LAWSON, A. A. H., PROUDFOOT, A. T., BROWN, S. S., MACDONALD, R. H., FRASER, A. G., CAMERON, J. C. & MATTHEW, H. (1969). Forced diuresis in the treatment of acute salicylate poisoning in adults. *Quart. J. Med.*, **38,** 31–48

LEE, H. A. & AMES, A. C. (1965). Haemodialysis in severe barbiturate poisoning. *Brit. med. J.*, **1,** 1217–1219.

LOO, T. L., LUCE, J. K., SULLIVAN, M. P. & FREI, E. (1968). Clinical pharmacologic observations on 6-mercaptopurine and 6-methylthiopurine mucleoside. *Clin. Pharmacol. Therap.*, **9,** 180–194.

LUND, L., LUNDE, P. K., RANE, A., BORGÅ, O. & SJÖQVIST, F. (1971). Plasma protein binding, plasma concentrations and effects of diphenylhydantoin in man. *Ann. N.Y. Acad. Sci.*, **179,** 723–728.

LUNDE, P. K. M., RANE, A., YAFFE, S. J., LUND, L. & SJÖQVIST, F. (1970). Plasma protein binding of diphenylhydantoin in man: interaction with other drugs and the effect of temperature and plasma dilution. *Clin. Pharmacol. Therap.*, **11,** 846–855.

MATTHEW, H. (1971). Acute poisoning. Some myths and misconceptions. *Brit. med. J.*, **1,** 519–522.

MATTHEW, H. & LAWSON, A. A. H. (1966). Acute barbiturate poisoning—a review of 2 years' experience. *Quart. J. Med.*, **35,** 539–552.

MATTHEW, H., PROUDFOOT, A. T., BROWN, S. S. & SMITH, A. C. A. (1968). Mandrax poisoning. Conservative management of 116 patients. *Brit. med. J.*, **2,** 101–102.

OLIVER, G. C., PARKER, B. M. & PARKER, C. W. (1971). Radioimmunoassay for digoxin. Technic and clinical application. *Amer. J. Med.*, **51,** 186–192.

O'REILLY, R. A. & LEVY, G. (1970). Kinetics of the anticoagulant effect of bishydroxycoumarin in man. *Clin. Pharmacol. Therap.*, **11,** 378–384.

PARKER, K. D., CRIM, M., ELLIOTT, H. W., WRIGHT, J. A., NOMOF, N. & HINE, C. H. (1970). Blood and urine concentrations of subjects receiving barbiturates, meprobamate, glutethimide or diphenylhydantoin. *Clin. Toxicol.*, **3,** 131–145.

PRESCOTT, L. F., BUHS, R. P., BEATTIE, J. O., SPETH, O. C., TRENNER, N. R. & LASAGNA, L. (1966). Combined clinical and metabolic study of the effects of α-methyldopa on hypertensive patients. *Circulation*, **34,** 308–321.

PRESCOTT, L. F. & NIMMO, J. (1971). Plasma lidocaine concentrations during and after prolonged infusions in patients with myocardial infarction. In: *Lidocaine in the Treatment of Ventricular Arrhythmias*, ed. by Scott, D. B. & Julian, D. G., pp. 168–177. Edinburgh: Livingstone.

PRESCOTT, L. F., STEEL, R. F. & FERRIER, W. R. (1970). The effects of particle size on the absorption of phenacetin in man. A correlation between plasma concentration of phenacetin and effects on the central nervous system. *Clin. Pharmacol. Therap.*, **11,** 496–504.

PRESCOTT, L. F., WRIGHT, N., ROSCOE, P. & BROWN, S. S. (1971). Plasma-paracetamol half-life and hepatic necrosis in patients with paracetamol overdosage. *Lancet*, **1,** 519–522.

PRICE, L. A. (1971). Liver damage and methotrexate. *Brit. med. J.*, **2,** 464.

REIDENBERG, M. M., ODAR-CEDERLÖF, I., VON BAHR, C., BORGÅ, O. & SJÖQVIST, F. (1971). Protein binding of diphenylhydantoin and desmethylimipramine in plasma from patients with poor renal function. *New Eng. J. Med.*, **285,** 264–267.

ROYDS, R. B. & KNIGHT, A. H. (1970). Tricyclic antidepressant poisoning. *Practitioner*, **204,** 282–286.

SCHANKER, L. S., NAFPLIOTIS, P. A. & JOHNSON, J. M. (1961). Passage of organic bases into human red cells. *J. Pharmacol. exp. Therap.*, **133,** 325–331.

SCHREINER, G. E. (1970). Dialysis of poisons and drugs—annual review. *Trans. Amer. Soc. Artif. Organs.*, **16,** 544–568.

SCOTT, J. L., FINEGOLD, S. M., BELKIN, G. A. & LAWRENCE, J. S. (1965). A controlled double blind study of the haematologic toxicity of chloramphenicol. *New. Eng. J. Med.*, **272,** 1137–1142.

SETTER, J. G., MAHER, J. F. & SCHREINER, G. E. (1966). Barbiturate intoxication, *Arch. Intern. Med.*, **117,** 224–236.

SMITH, T. W. (1971). Measurement of serum digitalis glycoside concentration—clinical implications. *Circulation*, **43,** 179–182.

SMITH, T. W. & HABER, E. (1970). Digoxin intoxication: The relationship of clinical presentation to serum digoxin concentration. *J. Clin. Invest.*, **49,** 2377–2386.

SMITH, T. W. & HABER, E. (1971). The clinical value of serum digitalis glycoside concentrations in the evaluation of drug toxicity. *Ann. N.Y. Acad. Sci.*, **179,** 322–337.

SMITH, T. W. & WILLERSON, J. T. (1971). Suicidal and accidental digoxin ingestion. Report of five cases with serum digoxin level correlations. *Circulation*, **44,** 29–36.

STENSRUD, P. A. & PALMER, H. (1964). Serum phenytoin determinations in epileptics. *Epilepsia*, **5,** 364–370.

STONE, N., KLEIN, M. D. & LOWN, B. (1971). Diphenylhydantoin in the prevention of recurring ventricular tachycardia. *Circulation*, **43,** 420–427.

SUHRLAND, L. G. & WEISBERGER, A. S. (1963). Chloramphenicol toxicity in liver and renal disease. *Archs. intern. Med.*, **112,** 747–754.

SUNSHINE, I., MAES, R. & FARACCI, R. (1968). Determination of glutethimide (Doriden) and its metabolites in biologic specimens. *Clin. Chem.*, **14,** 595–609.

SVEDMYR, N., HARTHON, L. & LUNDHOLM, L. (1969). The relationship between the plasma concentration of free nicotinic acid and some of its pharmacologic effects in man. *Clin. Pharmac. Ther.*, **10,** 559–570.

TOMPSETT, S. L. (1969). Interference from the presence of other substances in detecting and determining barbiturates in biological material. *J. Clin. Path.*, **22,** 291–295.

VON BAHR, C. & BORGÅ, O. (1971). Uptake, metabolism and excretion of desmethylimipramine and its metabolites in the isolated perfused rat liver. *Acta. pharmac. tox.*, **29,** 359–374.

WERT, E. G. (1970). Suicide in relation to toxic agents. In: *Laboratory Diagnosis of Diseases Caused by Toxic Agents*, ed. by Sunderman, T. W. & Sunderman, F. W. pp. 558–571. St. Louis: Warren H Green.

WIKINSKI, J. A., USUBIAGA, J. E. & WIKINSKI, R. W. (1970), Cardiovascular and neurological effects of 4000 mg of procaine. *J. Amer. med. Ass.*, **213,** 621–623.

WINEK, C. L. (1971). The role for the hospital pharmacist in toxicology and drug blood level information. *Amer. J. Hosp. Pharm.*, **28,** 351–356.

WOTMAN, S., BIGGER, J. T., MANDEL, I. D. & BARTELSTONE, H. J. (1971). Salivary electrolytes in the detection of digitalis toxicity. *New. Eng. J. Med.*, **285**, 871–876.

WRIGHT, N. & ROSCOE, P. Acute glutethimide poisoning. Conservative management of 31 patients. *J. Amer. Med. Ass.*, **214**, 1704–1706.

SIX

# Relationship between Pharmacological Effects and Plasma or Tissue Concentration of Drugs in Man

G. LEVY

*Department of Pharmaceutics,*
*School of Pharmacy,*
*State University of New York at Buffalo,*
*Buffalo, N.Y. 14214, USA*

## Introduction

Rationally designed dosage regimens of reversibly acting drugs are supposed to yield drug concentrations at the site of drug action which will elicit a desired intensity and duration of pharmacologic effect. It is ordinarily not possible to determine drug concentrations at the site of action (i.e. at the receptor) in man, and the focus has therefore been on drug concentrations in plasma (or serum), as it has been realized that there is likely to be some relationship between the drug concentrations in this more accessible fluid and the concentration in the fluid which is in direct contact with the receptor. Pharmacokinetic studies of drug absorption, distribution, metabolism and excretion, and investigations of the effects of age, disease, genetic characteristics and environment (including exposure to other drugs) on these processes, have been motivated largely by the realization that changes in the time course of drug concentrations in the body will affect the time course of drug action. However, until recently very little has been done to relate the two quantitatively. Without such knowledge it is difficult to assess the clinical relevance of changes in drug absorption, distribution, metabolism, and excretion and to design dosage regimens which will elicit a particular intensity and duration of effect. Recent advances in drug analysis, pharmacokinetic theory and clinical pharmacology (particularly in the ability to quantitate drug effects in man) have made it possible to develop an integrated rigorous approach toward defining the pharmacokinetics of drug action in man (Levy, 1966; Gibaldi, Levy and Weintraub, 1971; Levy & Gibaldi, 1972).

In relating drug concentration in the plasma to the concentrations elsewhere in the body (including the site of action), the body has been

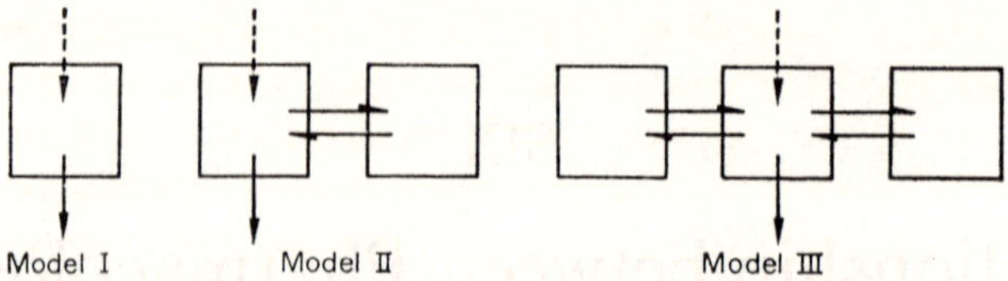


FIG. 1. The most commonly used pharmacokinetic models to describe the time course of drug concentrations in the body. Model I represents the body as a single compartment; Model II consists of a central compartment (which includes the blood plasma and the site(s) of drug elimination) and a peripheral compartment; Model III has two peripheral compartments and a central compartment.

described pharmacokinetically as a system of one or more apparent compartments (Figure 1). In the simplest case, i.e. when a drug is distributed very rapidly, the body may be represented as a single compartment. More often, the body must be described as a system consisting of a central compartment (which includes the blood plasma) and one or two peripheral or 'tissue' compartments. Transfer of drug between compartments and drug elimination (usually, but not always, assumed to occur in the central compartment) may or may not be linear processes. This discussion is limited to linear systems, non-linear processes having been reviewed elsewhere (Levy, 1968).

If the body has the pharmacokinetic characteristics of a multi-compartment system, the site of drug action may be part of one of the compartments of that system. Figure 2 is a schematic representation of the time

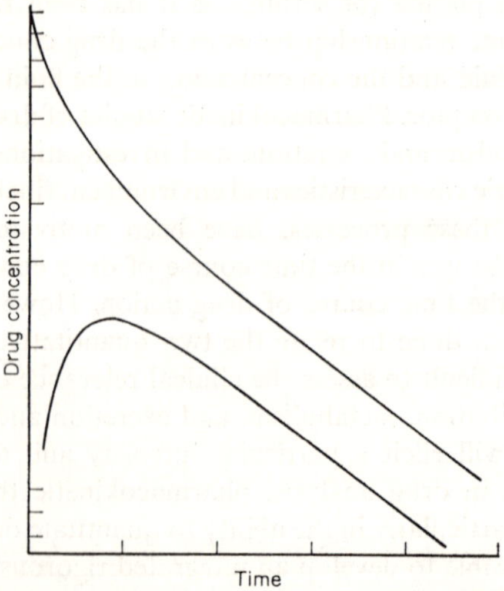


FIG. 2. Schematic representation of the time course of drug concentrations in the central and peripheral compartments of the body when it has the pharmacokinetic characteristics of a two-compartment system. The drug is administered by rapid intravenous injection (i.e. instantaneously into the central compartment). Upper curve, central compartment; lower curve, peripheral compartment.

course of drug concentrations in the central and peripheral compartments of the body when it behaves pharmacokinetically like a two-compartment system. Let it be assumed that a drug acts directly (i.e., without metabolic activation or intermediary reactions which cause a significant delay in the onset of drug action) and reversibly, and that any metabolites which may be formed are pharmacologically inactive. In that case, the maximum intensity of action occurs immediately after rapid intravenous injection if the site of action is part of the central compartment. If, on the other hand, the site of action is part of the peripheral compartment, the intensity of drug action after intravenous injection will first increase and then decrease. The drug concentrations in the central and peripheral compartments decline in parallel after the distribution phase, i.e., when a pseudo distribution equilibrium is reached (Figure 2). It is therefore possible to relate pharmacological effects to the drug concentration in the central compartment (and therefore to the plasma concentration) during the pseudo distribution equilibrium even if the site of action is in a peripheral compartment. Such correlation is not possible in the distributive phase. It is during the pseudo equilibrium phase that the data will reveal the existence of a correlation between effect and drug concentration in the peripheral compartment. The drug concentration in the peripheral compartment first increases and then decreases after drug administration (Figure 2). Consequently, a given drug concentration in that apparent compartment occurs at a certain time both before and after the concentration 'peak'. The intensity of a pharmacological effect should be the same at these two points in time if the site of action is part of the peripheral compartment. For example, the concentration of $\gamma$-hydroxybutyric acid in the brain of rats after intravenous administration of this drug or its precursor $\gamma$-butyrolactone is essentially the same when the animals fall asleep and when they awaken while the concentration in the blood is quite different (Giarman & Roth, 1964).

**Single Compartment Model**

The neuromuscular blocking agent succinylcholine is a drug which confers on the body the pharmacokinetic characteristics of a single-compartment system, albeit for rather unique reasons. Succinylcholine is very rapidly hydrolyzed in the blood and its elimination from the neuromuscular junction is apparently rate-limited by diffusion from that site, with the plasma acting as an infinite sink. The disappearance of the drug from the neuromuscular junction should therefore be described by apparent first-order kinetics

$$\log A = \log A_0 - (k/2{\cdot}3)t \qquad (1)$$

where A is the amount of drug at the junction at time $t$; $A_0$ is the amount of drug at that site very soon after injection (assuming very rapid diffusion to the neuromuscular junction, an assumption which is justified by the rapid onset of action after intravenous injection), and k is an apparent first-order constant. The neuromuscular blocking effect should last until A decreases to a minimum effective level $A_{min}$. Substitution of $A_{min}$ for A and rearrangement of equation (1) yields

$$t = (2{\cdot}3/k) \log A_0 - (2{\cdot}3/k) \log A_{min} \tag{2}$$

where $t$ is now the duration of action. Therefore, a graph of $t$ versus log $A_0$ should be linear. Since $A_0$ should be proportional to the dose, a

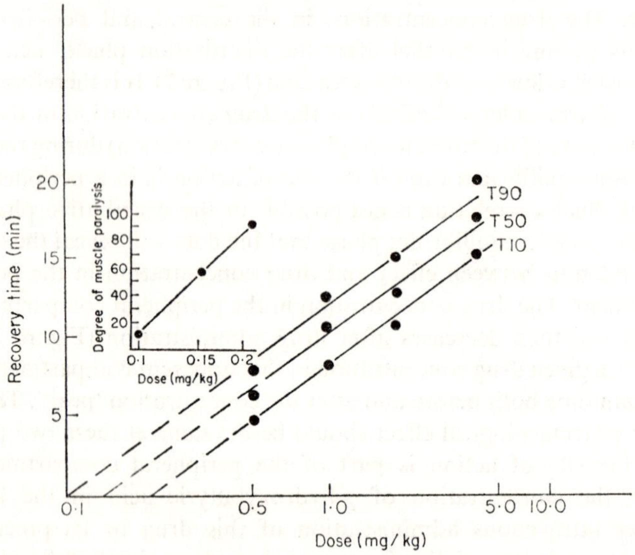


FIG. 3. Relationship between intravenous dose (log scale) of succinylcholine chloride and the duration of various degrees of neuromuscular blocking in human adults (13 to 16 subjects per dose). T10, T50 and T90 are the times required to recover 10, 50 and 90% of normal muscle contraction force. Inset: intensity of effect *v* dose (log scale), based on extrapolation of the duration *v* log dose lines to time = zero. From Levy (1967).

graph of duration of effect versus log of the dose should also be linear, with a slope equal to 2·3/k. Figure 3 shows that such a linear relationship does exist. The slope of the line is independent of the intensity of effect used as the end-point; different end-points result only in different intercept values due to the change in $A_{min}$. This pharmacokinetic model has been verified by determination of the value of k from the slope of the graph of duration of effect versus the log of the dose as well as from the slope of the intensity of effect versus time relationship, with excellent agreement between the two determinations (Levy, 1967). Clinical applications of this pharmacokinetic approach have been described elsewhere (Levy, 1970a & b).

## Multi-compartment Models

The linear relationship between duration of effect and the log of the dose does not obtain if the body has the pharmacokinetic characteristics of a multi-compartment system.

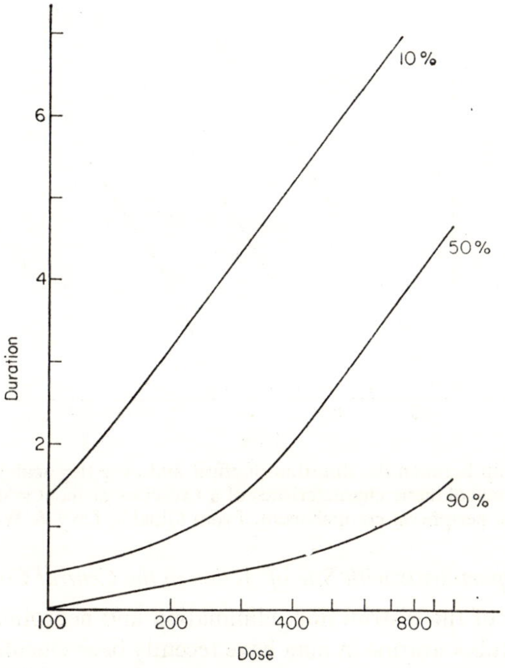


FIG. 4. Relationship between duration of effect and dose (log scale) when the body assumes the pharmacokinetic characteristics of a two-compartment system and the site of action is in the central compartment. The percentage next to each curve indicates the intensity of the pharmacologic effect, assuming that 100% is the maximum attainable effect. From Gibaldi, Levy & Weintraub (1971).

### (*a*) *Two Compartments with Site of Action in the Central Compartment*

Figure 4 shows the nature of the relationship between duration of effect (of various intensities) and log dose for a two-compartment system with the site of action in the central compartment. Examples of such curves based on data reported in the literature have been presented (Gibaldi, Levy & Weintraub, 1971). Figure 5 shows the relationship between duration of effect and log of dose if the site of drug action is in the peripheral compartment of a two-compartment system.

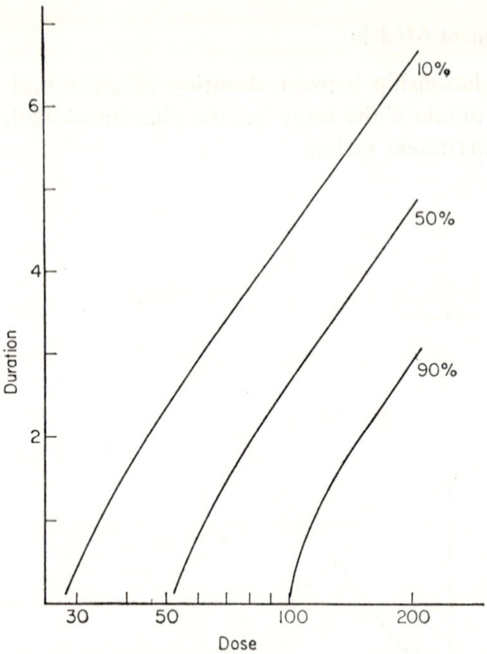


FIG. 5. Relationship between the duration of effect and dose (log scale) when the body assumes the pharmacokinetic characteristics of a two-compartment system and the site of action is in the peripheral compartment. From Gibaldi, Levy & Weintraub (1971).

### (*b*) *Three Compartments with Site of Action in the Central Compartment*

The kinetics of the distribution, elimination and neuromuscular blocking effect of *d*-tubocurarine in man have recently been elucidated (Gibaldi, Levy & Hayton, 1972a). A pharmacokinetic description of the distribution and elimination of this drug requires the use of a three-compartment model as shown in Figure 6. The time courses of the amounts of *d*-tubo-

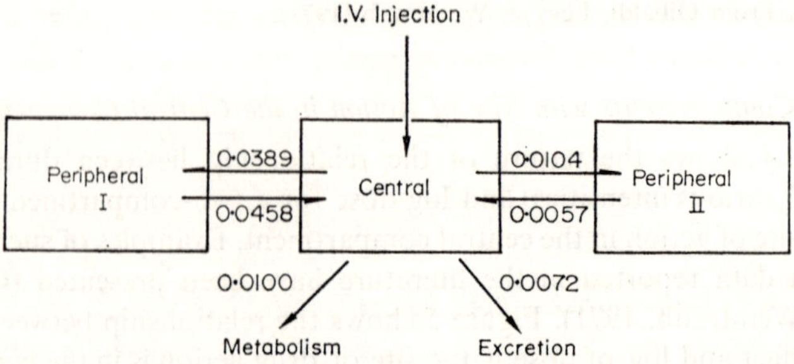


FIG. 6. Pharmacokinetic model for the distribution and elimination of *d*-tubocurarine in man. Rate constants, in reciprocal minutes, are shown next to the arrows, which represent apparent first-order processes for transfer of the drug between compartments and elimination from the central compartment. From Gibaldi, Levy & Hayton (1972b).

curarine in the central compartment of the body after rapid intravenous injection of different doses, computed on the basis of the model, are shown in Figure 7. Also shown are the durations of effect of these different

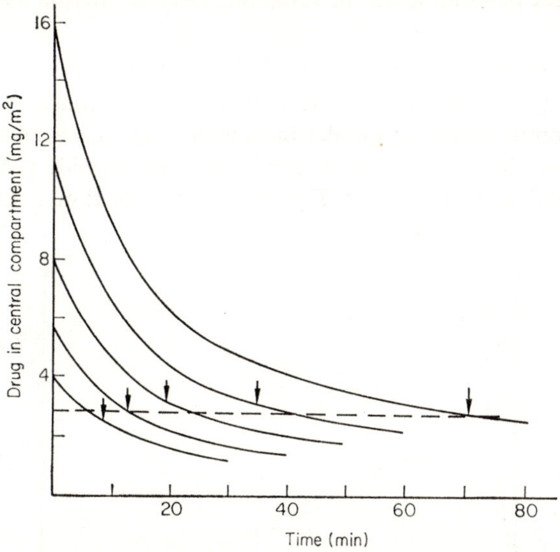


FIG. 7. Computer-simulated time course of the amount of *d*-tubocurarine in the central compartment of the body after rapid intravenous injection of 4·0, 5·6, 8·0, 11·2 or 16·0 mg/m². The arrows show the duration of the neuromuscular blocking effect (to 10% recovery) of these doses, as reported by Walts & Dillon (1968). From Gibaldi, Levy & Hayton (1972a).

doses. The amount of drug in the central compartment (but not in the two peripheral compartments) is essentially the same at the time of recovery, independent of dose. This indicates that the site of action is part of the central compartment. The pharmacokinetic model has been verified by calculating the duration of action obtained by administering various second doses upon recovery from the effect of an initial dose. Excellent agreement between these theoretical predictions and experimental results

TABLE 1. *Predicted and observed duration of effect of a second dose of d-tubocurarine administered after recovery from the effect of an initial dose of* 8 *mg/m²*

| | Duration of effect (min) | | | |
|---|---|---|---|---|
| Second dose | Recovery to 10% of control | | Recovery to 50% of control | |
| mg/m² | predicted* | observed† | predicted* | observed† |
| 2 | 18 | 18 | — | — |
| 4 | 32 | 36 | 51 | 41 |
| 8 | 61 | 69 | 90 | 90 |

* From Gibaldi, Levy & Hayton (1972a).
† From Walts & Dillon (1968).

has been achieved (Table 1). It is therefore feasible to predict the duration of effect obtained by different dosage regimens of clinical interest and to assess the likely effect of renal failure on the duration of the neuromuscular blocking effect of *d*-tubocurarine (Gibaldi, Levy & Hayton 1972a & b).

## (*c*) *Models with Site of Action in Peripheral Compartment*

A correlation between the time course of drug concentrations in a peripheral compartment and a pharmacologic effect has been noted in the case of a behavioural effect of lysergic acid diethylamide (LSD) in man (Levy, Gibaldi & Jusko, 1969). Figure 8 shows the time course of LSD

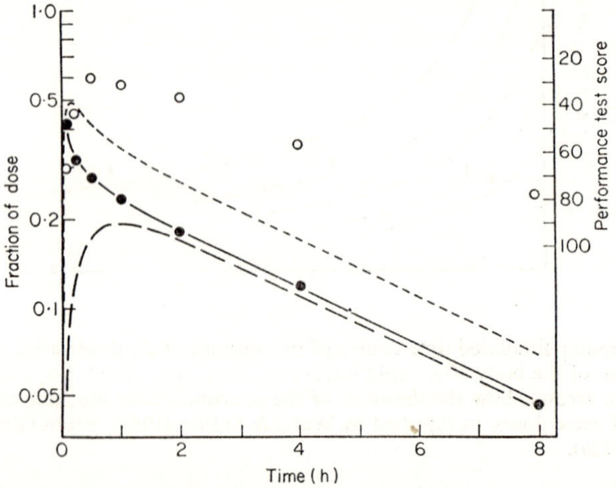


FIG. 8. The time course of the amounts of lysergic acid diethylamide (LSD) in the central compartment (——); rapidly accessible peripheral compartment (- - - - -); and slowly accessible peripheral compartment (– – –) of the body after rapid intravenous injection of 2 $\mu$g LSD per kg body weight, assuming the body to be a three-compartment system. ●, relative concentration of LSD in the plasma; ○, mathematical performance of test scores. Experimental data on five normal human subjects from Aghajanian & Bing (1964). From Levy, Gibaldi & Jusko (1969).

levels in the central and peripheral compartments of the body as calculated from plasma concentrations of LSD after rapid intravenous injection. Also shown in the figure is the time course of performance test scores (as a percent of normal) in solving mathematical problems. A very good correlation between impairment of performance and the amount of drug in one of the peripheral compartments was found (Figure 9), but the pharmacokinetic model has not been verified by additional coordinated mathematical and experimental studies.

Reasonably accurate predictions of the time course of drug levels in peripheral compartments require accurate determinations of drug distribution rate constants. These are quite difficult to obtain because of the rapid changes in drug concentration during the distributive phase. Good quantitative correlations of pharmacological effects with drug levels in an apparent peripheral compartment are, therefore, not easily achieved. Fortunately, a correlation between drug concentrations in the plasma (representing the central compartment) and pharmacological effects can be obtained in the post-distributive phase even if the site of drug action is in a peripheral compartment. However, such correlation will not permit predictions concerning the rate of onset and decline of the drug effect at the beginning and end, respectively, of a course of therapy.

*Kinetics of Indirect Pharmacological Effects*

There are instances when, despite very precise and extensive data on plasma concentration and intensity of effect, a correlation between effect

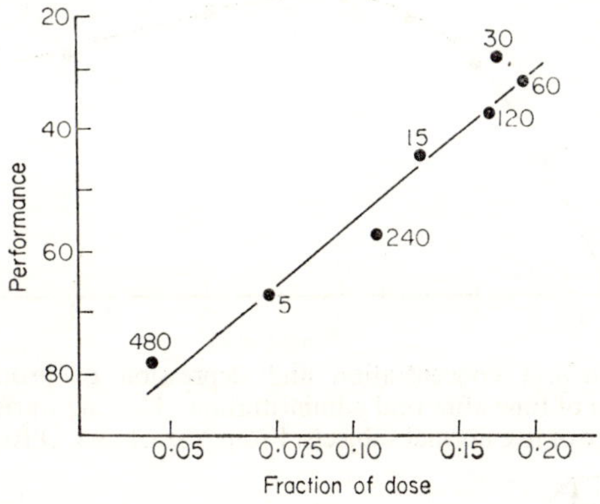


FIG. 9. Relationship between the amount of LSD (expressed as the fraction of a 2 μg/kg dose) in the slowly accessible peripheral compartment of the body and the intensity of the pharmacologic effect. The number next to each data point represents the time (minutes) after injection when the measurements were made. From Levy, Gibaldi, & Jusko (1969).

and drug concentration in one of the pharmacokinetically recognizable apparent body compartments is not (or does not appear to be) feasible. There are many possible reasons for this lack of correlation. One likely reason is that the site of action may represent a distinct compartment of its own, but one so small that it does not affect the time course of drug concentrations in the plasma and, therefore, is not recognizable pharmacokinetically. Another possible reason is that the observed pharmacological effect is not the 'real' effect of the drug but rather a consequence of the drug's direct effect. A case in point is the anticoagulant effect of warfarin and other coumarin anticoagulants.

Warfarin inhibits the synthesis of vitamin K-dependent clotting factors

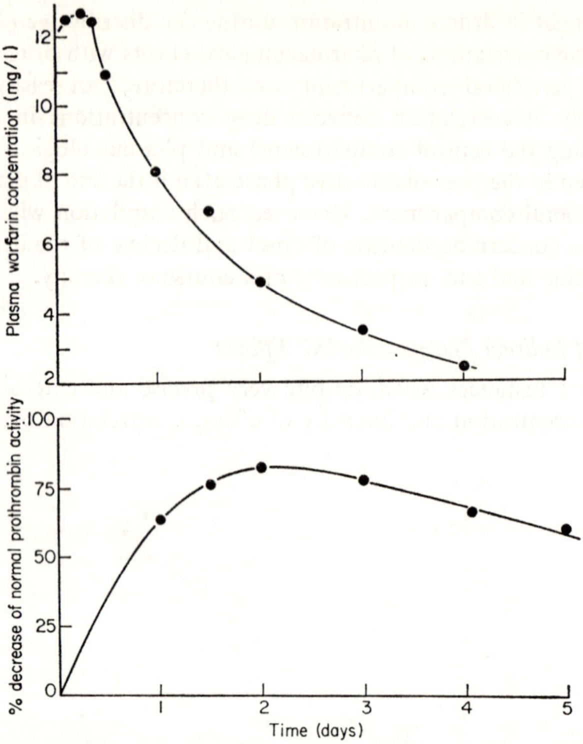


FIG. 10. Plasma-warfarin concentration and depression of prothrombin complex activity as a function of time after oral administration of 1·5 mg warfarin sodium per kg body weight. Average of five normal subjects. From Nagashima, O'Reilly & Levy (1969).

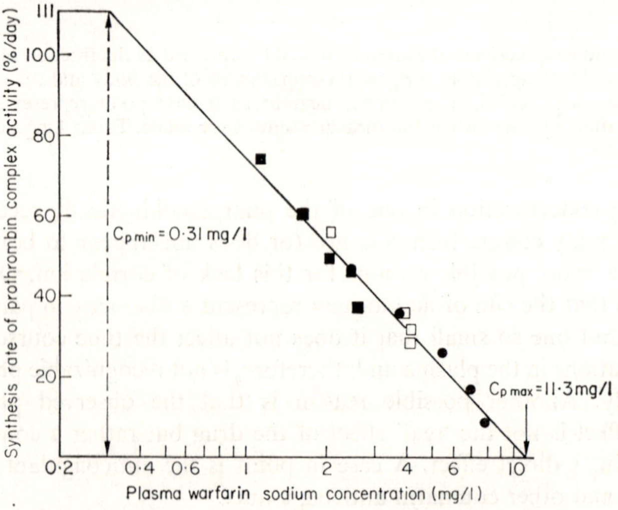


FIG. 11. Relationship between synthesis rate of prothrombin complex activity and plasma warfarin concentration in six normal subjects after a single oral dose of 1·5 mg/kg (●); 10 mg daily for 5 days (■); and 15 mg daily for 4 days (□). From Nagashima, O'Reilly & Levy (1969).

(factors II, VII, IX and X). The observed effect is the decrease of prothrombin complex activity (reflected by increased blood-clotting time) which is a function not only of the synthesis rate of clotting factors but also of their rates of degradation. Consequently there is no direct correlation between the time course of warfarin concentrations in the plasma and prothrombin complex activity (Figure 10). If, however, the change in prothrombin complex activity is converted, by appropriate calculations, to synthesis rate of prothrombin complex activity, an excellent correlation between the logarithm of warfarin concentrations in the plasma and the inhibition of synthesis rate can be demonstrated (Figure 11). The model has been tested by increasing the rate of warfarin elimination by pretreatment with heptabarbital which induces the warfarin-metabolizing enzyme system. The relationship between drug concentration and effect is not affected despite the more rapid elimination of warfarin after hexobarbital pretreatment (Figure 12; Levy, O'Reilly, Aggeler & Keech, 1970). On the other hand, a change in the distribution of warfarin in the body due to displacement of the drug from plasma proteins by phenylbutazone changes profoundly the relationship between plasma–warfarin concentration and the pharmacological effect (O'Reilly & Levy, 1970).

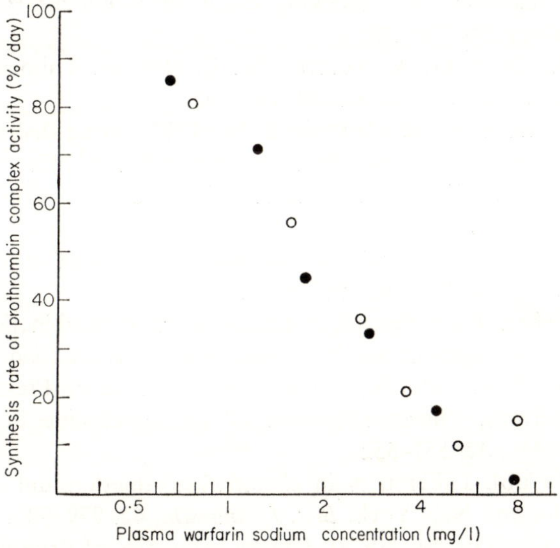


FIG. 12. Effect of heptabarbital (400 mg daily for 15 days, starting 10 days before warfarin) on the relationship between synthesis rate of prothrombin complex activity and plasma-warfarin concentration in a 21-year-old normal male subject; control experiment on 10-2-1967 (○); with heptabarbital on 11-21-1968 (●). From Levy, O'Reilly, Aggeler & Keech (1970).

## Conclusions

The elucidation of the kinetics of drug action in man is the ultimate objective in the pharmacokinetic characterization of a drug. It requires accurate, precise and extensive data on drug concentration and pharmacological effect. With the knowledge of the kinetics of drug elimination and drug action, it is possible to develop the best dosage regimens for safe and effective drug therapy and to make proper adjustments of dosage to account for individual variations in drug metabolism and response.

## REFERENCES

Aghajanian, G. K. & Bing, O. H. L. (1964). Persistence of lysergic acid diethylamide in the plasma of human subjects. *Clin. Pharmac. Ther.*, **5,** 611–614.

Giarman, N. J. & Roth, R. H. (1964). Differential estimation of $\gamma$-butyrolactone and $\gamma$-hydroxybutyric acid in rat blood and brain. *Science*, **145**, 583–584.

Gibaldi, M., Levy, G. & Hayton, W. L. (1972a). Kinetics of the elimination and neuromuscular blocking effect of *d*-tubocurarine in man. *Anesthesiology*, **36,** 213–218.

Gibaldi, M., Levy, G. & Hayton, W. L. (1972b). Tubocurarine and renal failure. *Brit. J. Anaesth.*, **44,** 163–165.

Gibaldi, M., Levy, G. & Weintraub, H. (1971). Drug distribution and pharmacologic effects. *Clin. Pharmac. Ther.*, **12**, 734–742.

Levy, G. (1966). Kinetics of pharmacologic effects. *Clin. Pharmac. Ther.*, **7**, 362–372.

Levy, G. (1967). Kinetics of pharmacologic activity of succinylcholine in man. *J. Pharm. Sci.*, **56**, 1687–1688.

Levy, G. (1968). Dose-dependent effects in pharmacokinetics. In: *The Importance of Fundamental Principles in Drug Evaluation*, ed. D. H. Tedeschi & R. E. Tedeschi, p. 141. New York: Raven Press.

Levy, G. (1970a). Pharmacokinetics of succinylcholine in newborns. *Anesthesiology*, **32**, 551–552.

Levy, G. (1970b). Differences in effect of suxamethonium in London, Los Angeles and New York. *Brit. J. Anaesth.*, **42**, 979–980.

Levy, G. & Gibaldi, M. (1972). Pharmacokinetics of drug action. *Ann. Rev. Pharmacol.*, **12,** 85–98.

Levy, G., Gibaldi, M. & Jusko, W. J. (1969). Multicompartment pharmacokinetic models and pharmacologic effects. *J. Pharm. Sci.*, **58,** 422–424.

Levy, G., O'Reilly, R. A., Aggeler, P. M. & Keech, G. M. (1970).

Pharmacokinetic analysis of the effect of barbiturate on the anticoagulant action of warfarin in man. *Clin. Pharmac. Ther.*, **11**, 372–377.

NAGASHIMA, R., O'REILLY, R. A., LEVY, G. (1969). Kinetics of pharmacologic effects in man: The anticoagulant action of warfarin. *Clin. Pharmac. Ther.*, **10**, 22–35.

O'REILLY, R. A. & LEVY, G. (1970). Pharmacokinetic analysis of potentiating effect of phenylbutazone on anticoagulant action of warfarin in man. *J. Pharm. Sci.*, **59**, 1258–1260.

WALTS, L. F. & DILLON, J. B. (1968). Durations of action of *d*-tubocurarine and gallamine. *Anesthesiology*, **29**, 499–504.

SEVEN

# Are we Measuring the Right Things? The Role of Active Metabolites

J. A. OATES AND D. G. SHAND

*Departments of Medicine and Pharmacology, Vanderbilt University, Nashville, Tennessee, USA*

## Introduction

As teachers of pharmacology we emphasize the relationship of the concentration of free drug in plasma to the effect of certain drugs. As investigators, however, we are interested when a lack of correlation is found between plasma level and effect; this raises the possibility that the fate of the drug in the body and its effect(s) are interrelated in a unique way.

There are a number of mechanisms whereby plasma levels do not correlate appropriately with effect in a given individual even when other variables are constant:

(1) The plasma assay may be too insensitive to reflect an important pool of the drug, such as that for guanethidine stored in adrenergic neurones (Oates, Mitchell, Feagin, Kaufmann & Shand, 1971). In such instances it may be necessary to forsake kinetic analysis based on the concentration of drug in plasma and examine urinary excretion as it reflects the kinetics of the drug in plasma.

(2) Levels of drug in plasma are unlikely to reflect non-reversible binding to tissue or frank cellular alteration that persists after the drug is removed.

(3) When the effect of a drug is mediated by an active metabolite, the plasma level-effect relationship may also go awry. Whereas such a dissociation is not always the case with active metabolites, its occurrence should call attention to this possibility.

Thus, for the pharmacologist, consideration of the possibility of an active metabolite often begins with a finding that levels of drug in plasma do not correlate with pharmacological response.

## I. Active Metabolites with Kinetics of Formation and Disposition that are not a Function of the Levels of Parent Drug in Plasma

Drug concentration usually relates to receptor response according to the law of mass action. Variation from this relationship as a function of time may reflect a pharmacologically active metabolite which has kinetics different from the parent drug. This difference may result from distribution of the active metabolite to a pool from which it is released more slowly than the disposition of the parent drug, or the active metabolite may be formed primarily during passage of the drug from the gut into the systemic circulation rather than as a continuing function of the plasma level of parent drug.

### A. *Active Metabolite Storage in a Pool from which it is Released more slowly than the Rate of Disposition of the Parent Drug*

Methyldopa was introduced into clinical studies because of its known inhibition of aromatic amino acid decarboxylase. This is a competitive inhibition, and as such should be a function of the concentration of available drug. The hypotension produced by methyldopa in man however had a quite different time course from the concentration of methyldopa in plasma. With a half-life of 1·4 to 1·8 h, exceedingly small concentrations of methyldopa are present in plasma after 8 h (Sjoerdsma, Vendsalu &

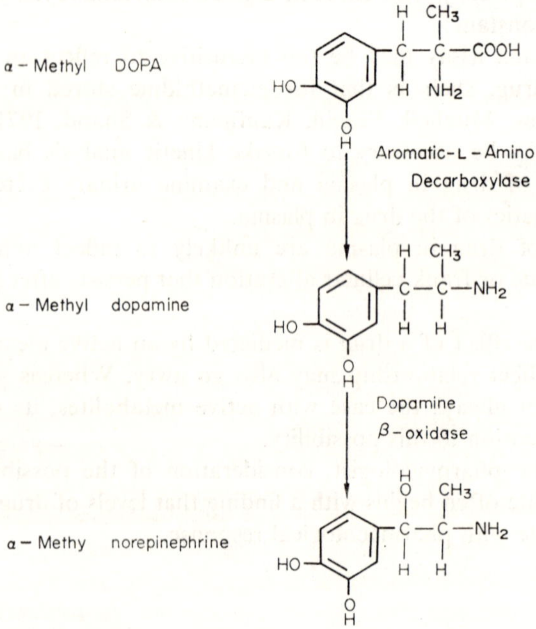


FIG. 1. Biotransformation of methyldopa to its active metabolite.

Engelman, 1963). However, substantial hypotension persists beyond 24 h. This, together with other evidence, raised the question of a unique fate for this drug. Possibilities included storage of the drug at its cellular site of action or formation of an active metabolite which had a longer half-life than the parent drug. It was found that levels of methyldopa in the guinea pig brain were reduced to less than one-half per cent of maximum at 15 h whereas noradrenaline depletion from brain was still near maximum at this time (Hess, Connamacher, Osaki & Udenfriend, 1961). Thus a tissue storage pool of methyldopa did not exist and the effects of the drug on noradrenaline levels could not be explained simply on the basis of competitive inhibition of noradrenaline synthesis. Further studies demon-

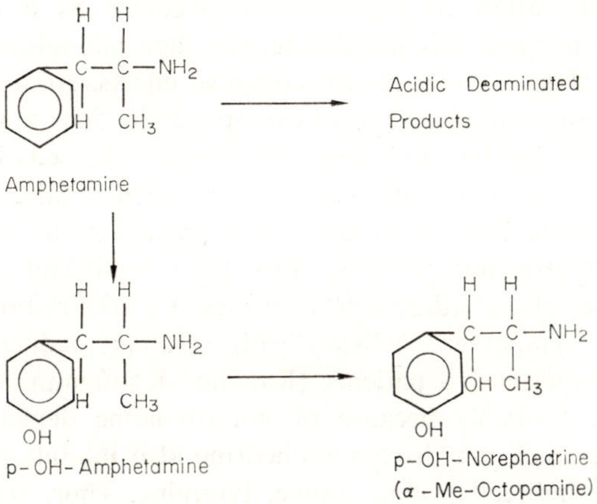


FIG. 2. Biotransformation of *d*-amphetamine to an active metabolite, *p*-hydroxynorephedrine.

strated that methyldopa and its congener, methyl-meta-tyrosine, are themselves decarboxylated by aromatic amino acid decarboxylase to amine metabolites which deplete catecholamines (Lovenberg, Weissbach & Udenfriend, 1962; Porter, Totaro & Leiby, 1961). Further metabolism of the amine metabolites by $\beta$-hydroxylation (Figure 1) yields amines ($\alpha$-methylnoradrenaline and metaraminol) which can replace noradrenaline in the neurosecretory vesicles and are released in its place (Carlsson & Lindqvist, 1962; Muscholl & Maitre, 1963). After administration of methyldopa, $\alpha$-methylnoradrenaline persists in the adrenergic neurone long after the parent drug has disappeared. For this reason, plasma levels of methyldopa do not relate appropriately to effect because the active metabolite is stored in a neuronal pool from which it is released more slowly than the rate of disposition of methyldopa itself.

Similarly, an active metabolite of amphetamine also is stored within the adrenergic neurone from which it is released more slowly than the rate of disposition of its parent drug. As shown in Figure 2, amphetamine is converted in man to *p*-hydroxynorephedrine (Cavanaugh, Griffith & Oates, 1970); *p*-hydroxylation of amphetamine occurs in the liver (Dring, Smith & Williams, 1965), and the *p*-hydroxyamphetamine formed is transported into the adrenergic neurone by the noradrenaline pump where it is β-hydroxylated to *p*-hydroxynorephedrine (Goldstein & Anagnoste, 1965). *p*-Hydroxynorephedrine is then stored within the neurosecretory vesicle where it replaces noradrenaline and is released in its stead as a false neurotransmitter. Thus, the specialized transport of its precursor into the neurone, synthesis within the neurone, and the capacity of neurosecretory vesicles to store amines all contribute to a remarkable localization of this minor active metabolite at its site of action.

Upon identification of *p*-hydroxynorephedrine as a metabolite of amphetamine in man, this metabolite was then administered to human volunteers to determine its pharmacological effects. As it is much more polar than amphetamine, *p*-hydroxynorephedrine does not readily cross the blood brain barrier, and does not produce the sedation-depression effect on the central nervous system seen when a false transmitter is introduced into the body as an amino acid precursor such as methyldopa. However, *p*-hydroxynorephedrine does have significant effects on the function of peripheral adrenergic neurones. Its administration produces inhibition of sympathetic reflexes with resultant reduction of blood pressure in hypertensive patients (Rangno, Kaufmann, Cavanaugh & Oates, 1970). Probably because of noradrenaline depletion from the adrenergic neurone, *p*-hydroxynorephedrine also inhibits the pressor response to the indirectly acting amine, tyramine. Thus, accumulation of neuronal *p*-hydroxynorephedrine following repeated administration of amphetamine by abusers of this drug could account for the tachyphylaxis which they develop to the cardiovascular effects of amphetamine.

Studies on the disposition of *p*-hydroxynorephedrine indicate that this metabolite should accumulate following continuing administration of amphetamine. Following the discontinuation of *p*-hydroxynorephedrine administration, it is excreted in the urine in two phases. The late phase pool of the drug has a half-life of approximately 55 h. That this late phase pool represents storage of *p*-hydroxynorephedrine in the adrenergic neurone is suggested by the duration of the hypotensive effect, its known site of synthesis within the neurone and the analogy to the kinetics of guanethidine which is also stored in the adrenergic neurone. The long half-life of this pool permits accumulation of *p*-hydroxynorephedrine for longer than amphetamine itself. Thus maximal catecholamine depletion from the neurone would not be expected to occur for an additional 11 days after when the parent drug had accumulated to plateau levels. In studies on the chronic ingestion of amphetamine (Cavanaugh, Griffin & Oates, 1970), maximal depression of tyramine's pressor effect had not been reached after 5 days of amphetamine administration. It is predicted that the accumulation of *p*-hydroxynorephedrine in adrenergic neurones on more chronic use of the drug will lead to a profound inhibition of pressor responses to indirectly acting amines and perhaps inhibition of sympathetic reflexes as well. The blockade of the pressor effect of tyramine could have diagnostic value in the paranoid patient suspected of amphetamine abuse.

B. *Active Metabolite Formation Primarily During the Passage of Drug from the Gut into the Systemic Circulation*

Most of the metabolites formed in the liver are removed from the body more rapidly than their parent compounds. If formation of the metabolite is a continuing function of the levels of parent drug, then the effect of the more rapidly eliminated metabolite should mirror the level of parent drug. In such a situation, plasma level will be related to effect. When the metabolite is formed only (or largely) during the first passage of the drug into the circulation after oral administration, however, the effect of the metabolite will diminish more rapidly than the levels of parent drug.

Propranolol is an example of a drug from which an active metabolite is formed chiefly during the absorption process. When administered intravenously the effect of propranolol on exercise tachycardia is a linear function of the log of its plasma level, and the ratio of log-plasma level to effect remains constant with time after administration (Coltart & Shand, 1970). However, at 2 h after *oral* administration of propranolol there was a much greater effect for a given plasma level than seen with the intravenous dose. This finding is in line with observation of Paterson, Conolly, Dollery, Hayes & Cooper (1970) that propranolol is converted to at least one metabolite with beta blocking activity, 4-hydroxypropranolol, but only after oral administration. Further, this metabolite disappears more rapidly than parent drug, suggesting formation primarily during the first pass into the systemic circulation. This rapid disappearance of 4-hydroxypropranolol is reflected in the time course of the observed beta blockade (Cleaveland & Shand, 1972). Propranolol's inhibition of isoproterenol-induced tachycardia was quantified by determining the dose of isoproterenol required to raise the cardiac rate 25 per min (chronotropic $dose_{25}$) as measured from a partial dose response curve before and after propranolol. The 'predicted effect' for propranolol alone was taken as the chronotropic $dose_{25}$ associated with a given plasma level after intravenous administration (a situation in which 4-OH propranolol is not detectable). Again, at 2 h after the oral dose the observed effect was about twice the predicted effect for propranolol administered intravenously. By the end of the six-hour period, however, beta blockade is appropriate for the plasma level, indicating that the active metabolite is no longer present in significant amounts (Figure 3). After a given single dose, the higher was an individual's level of propranolol in plasma, the more the observed effect of propranolol exceeded that predicted from the plasma level after intravenous administration. This suggests that after a single oral dose, metabolite formation is greater in those individuals in whom an alternate pathway of metabolism is more readily saturated, leading to more parent drug reaching the systemic circulation as well as more available as substrate for 4-hydroxylation to the active metabolite.

There is also some evidence that the duration of drug administration

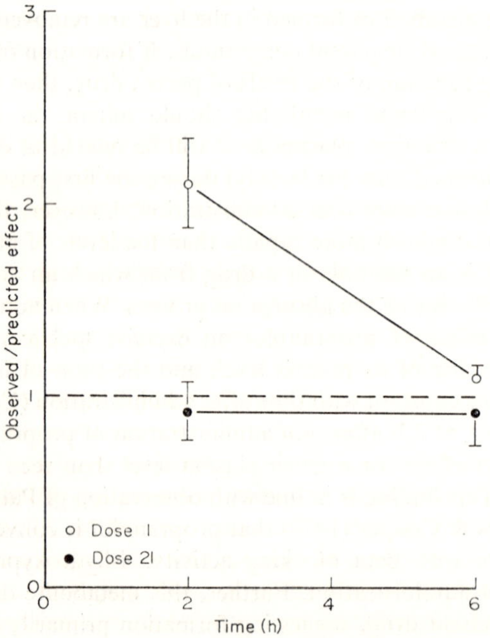


FIG. 3. The observed/predicted effect of propranolol 2 and 6 h after oral administration of one (○–○) and 21 (●–●) doses.

can alter the contribution of this active metabolite to the overall pharmacological effect. Thus during chronic administration (Figure 3), the observed and predicted effects were the same and, in this case, no change was observed with time. In addition, plasma levels of the parent drug increased during chronic administration to a greater extent than would have been predicted from its rate of elimination. These data suggest that, as a result of prolonged administration, the relative amounts of parent drug and active metabolite are altered in such a way that the effect of any circulating active metabolite is biologically of much less significance than following a single dose.

Thus, propranolol is an example of a drug having only part of its action mediated by way of an active metabolite. This active metabolite is formed during the first pass of the drug into the systemic circulation after oral administration and therefore exists for only a portion of the time during which the parent drug exerts an effect.

Present evidence suggests that 4-hydroxypropranolol is formed primarily in the liver after oral administration (Hayes & Cooper, 1971). The predominant formation of an active metabolite during the absorptive process might also result from metabolism of the parent drug within the intestinal wall or by intestinal flora.

## II. Importance of Species Differences in Formation of Active Metabolites to Drug Evaluation in Man

The variation between species in the pathways to active metabolites must be considered in attempts to predict whether pharmacological or toxicological data obtained in experimental animals can be extrapolated to man. Thus when an active metabolite mediates pharmacological or toxic effects in an experimental animal, no conclusions may be made on the clinical relevance of the findings until the metabolic pathways or the pharmacological effects of the drug are determined in the human.

A number of monoamine oxidase inhibitors such as iproniazid are known to act via metabolism to hydrazines which are potent non-reversible inactivators of the enzyme. Furazolidone, an intestinal anti-bacterial agent said not to produce significant plasma levels after oral administration, was found incidentally to inhibit monoamine oxidase *in vivo* in the rat but not to inhibit this enzyme *in vitro* (Stern, Hollifield, Wilk & Buzard, 1967). This suggested that an active metabolite of furazolidone inhibited monoamine oxidase in the rat and indeed among the potential metabolites 2-hydroxyethyl hydrazine was found to be a potential monoamine oxidase inhibitor. In order to determine the clinical relevance of these findings, however, it was necessary to ascertain whether furazolidone was converted to a metabolite capable of inhibiting significantly monoamine oxidase in man. Monoamine oxidase in human intestinal biopsy samples was not inhibited by furazolidone *in vitro,* but was inhibited by administration of furazolidone (Pettinger, Soyangco & Oates, 1968). This finding in intestinal mucosa, together with a markedly increased sensitivity to the pressor effect of tyramine, indicated that man, like the rat, converted furazolidone to an active monoamine oxidase inhibitor. Thus the metabolism of this antibacterial confers on it a clinically significant potential for pressor reactions to indirectly acting amines such as amphetamine and tyramine (in cheese).

In contrast, the metabolism of amphetamine to *p*-hydroxynorephedrine is highly dependent upon the species (Axelrod, 1954; Dring, Smith & Williams, 1966) and illustrates how studies limited to an experimental animal might predict the human pharmacology erroneously. The variable step in *p*-hydroxynorephedrine formation is *p*-hydroxylation of amphetamine which is a major pathway in the rat, negligible in the guinea pig and intermediate in man. Studies on the protracted depletion of catecholamines by amphetamine and tachyphylaxis to this drug in the guinea pig certainly could not be relevant to man. In contrast, use of the rat as the experimental model would exaggerate the importance of *p*-hydroxynorephedrine in the pharmacology of a single dose of amphetamine in man.

## III. Paradoxical Relation of Plasma Level to Effect

In addition to having a different time course of action from the parent drug, active metabolites may actually vary in the opposite direction from plasma levels of parent drug during treatment with agents that induce or inhibit formation of the active metabolite. This creates a plasma level-effect paradox which has more than theoretical significance.

Cyclophosphamide produces very little cytotoxicity itself. Its pharmacological effect is mediated primarily by one or more active metabolites formed by hepatic microsomal enzymes. One such metabolite, 4-ketocyclophosphamide, has been isolated from microsomal incubations of the parent drug, and has more than fifty times the potency as cyclophosphamide itself (Hohorst, Ziemann & Brock, 1971). Phenobarbital, by inducing the formation of the active metabolite(s), more than doubles the toxicity of cyclophosphamide in the rat (Cohen & Jao, 1969).

Phenobarbital has been shown to lower plasma levels of cyclophosphamide in man, and were this the limit of our information on the drug, it might be erroneously predicted that cyclophosphamide would be less toxic after phenobarbital. Although definitive studies have not yet been done to show that the phenobarbital induced decrease in cyclophosphamide levels in man is accompanied by an increase in formation of the active metabolite, there are clinical reports of cyclophosphamide toxicity when the drug has been given in usual doses to patients who are also on phenobarbital and other anticonvulsants (Drummond, Hillman, Marchessault & Feldman, 1968).

This paradoxical relation between plasma levels and toxicity is also likely to be seen with other drugs whose toxicity is mediated by an active metabolite formed by the mixed function oxygenase system. The arene oxides discussed by Drs. Mitchell and Brodie (see page 8) provide an excellent example of how this can occur if the inducer has its primary effect on epoxide formation (as opposed to its disposition by epoxide hydrase). The anaesthetic drug, methoxyflurane, produces nephrotoxicity that appears to result from its one or more metabolites (Mazze, Trudell & Cousins, 1971). Thus environmental or genetic factors that enhance biotransformation to toxic metabolites would lead to greater toxicity in association with lower plasma levels of parent drug.

## IV. Conclusions

Plasma levels may not maintain the expected relationship to pharmacological effect throughout the time course of drug action. In certain cases this may result from formation of an active metabolite which has a slower rate of disposition than the parent drug, or, in the case of orally administered drug, formation of active metabolite that is not a continuing function of plasma levels.

Paradoxical relationships between plasma level of parent drug and toxicity may result from induction or inhibition of the formation of active metabolites.

Because of the known potential for species difference in the formation of active metabolites, inferences from animal species are no substitute for data from man. This has important implications in the development of new drugs and in the assessment of their toxicity.

## REFERENCES

CARLSSON, A. & LINDQVIST, M. (1962). *In vivo* decarboxylation of α-methyldopa and α-methyl meta-tyrosine. *Acta. Physiol. Scand.*, **54,** 87–94.

CAVANAUGH, J. H., GRIFFITH, J. D. & OATES, J. A. (1970). Effect of amphetamine on the pressor response to tyramine: Formation of *p*-hydroxynorephedrine from amphetamine in man. *Clin. Pharmacol. & Ther.*, **11,** 656–664.

CLEAVELAND, C. R. & SHAND, D. G. (1972). The effect of duration of drug administration on the relationship between β-adrenergic blockade and plasma propranolol concentration. *Clin. Pharmacol. & Ther.*, **13,** 181–189.

COHEN, J. L. & JAO, J. Y. (1969). Enzymatic basis of cyclophosphamide activation by rat liver. *Proc. Am. Assoc. Cancer Res.*, **10,** 14.

COLTART, D. J. & SHAND, D. G. (1970). Plasma propanolol levels in the quantitative assessment of β-adrenergic blockade in man. *Brit. Med. J.*, **3,** 731–734.

DRING, L. G., SMITH, R. L. & WILLIAMS, R. T. (1965). The fate of amphetamine in man and other mammals. *J. Pharm. Pharmacol.*, **18,** 402–404.

DRUMMOND, K. N., HILLMAN, D. A., MARCHESSAULT, J. H. V. & FELDMAN, W. (1968). Cyclophosphamide in the nephrotic syndrome of childhood. *Can. Med. Assn. J.*, **98,** 524–531.

GOLDSTEIN, M. & ANAGNOSTE, B. (1965). The conversion *in vivo* of *d*-amphetamine to (+)-*p*-hydroxynorephedrine. *Biochim. Biophys. Acta*, **107,** 166–168.

HAYES, A. & COOPER, R. G. (1971). Studies on the absorption, distribution and excretion of propranolol in rat, dog and monkey. *J. Pharmacol. Exp. Therap.*, **176,** 302–311.

HESS, S. M., CONNAMACHER, R. H., OSAKI, M. & UDENFRIEND, S. (1961). The effects of α-methyldopa and α-methyl-meta-tyrosine on the metabolism of norepinephrine and serotonin *in vitro*. *J. Pharmacol. Exp. Therap.*, **134,** 129–138.

HOHORST, H. J., ZIEMANN, A. & BROCK, M. (1971). 4-Ketocyclophosphamide, a metabolite of cyclophosphamide. *Arzniem. Forsch.*, **21,** 1254–1257.

LOVENBERG, W., WEISSBACH, H. & UDENFRIEND, S. (1962). Aromatic L-amino acid decarboxylase. *J. Biol. Chem.*, **237,** 89–93.

MAZZE, R. I., TRUDELL, J. R. & COUSINS, M. J. (1971). Methoxyflurane metabolism and renal dysfunction. *Anesthesiology*, **35,** 247–252.

MUSCHOLL, E. & MAITRE, L. (1963). Release by sympathetic stimulation of α-methyl noradrenaline stored in the heart after administration of α-methyldopa. *Experientia*, **19,** 658–659.

OATES, J. A., MITCHELL, J. R., FEAGIN, O. T., KAUFMANN, J. S. & SHAND, D. G. (1971). Distribution of guanidinium antihypertensives: Mechanism of their selective action. *Ann. N.Y. Acad. Sci.*, **179,** 302–309.

PATERSON, J. W., CONOLLY, M. E., DOLLERY, C. T., HAYES, A. & COOPER, R. G. (1970). The pharmacodynamics and metabolism of propranolol in man. *Pharmacologia Clinica*, **2,** 127–133.

PETTINGER, W. A., SOYANGCO, F. G. & OATES, J. A. (1968). Inhibition of monoamine oxidase in man by furazolidone. *Clin. Pharmacol. & Therap.*, **9,** 442–447.

PORTER, C. C., TOTARO, J. A. & LEIBY, C. M. (1961). Some biochemical effects of α-methyl-dihydroxyphenylalamine and related compounds in mice. *J. Pharmacol. Exp. Therap.*, **134,** 139–145.

RANGNO, R. E., KAUFMANN, J. S., CAVANAUGH, J. S. & OATES, J. A. (1970). Reduction of arterial pressure by the amphetamine metabolite, *p*-hydroxynorephedrine. *Clin. Res.*, **18,** 342.

STERN, I. J., HOLLIFIELD, R. D., WILK, S. & BUZARD, J. A. (1967). The anti-monoamine oxidase effects of furazolidone. *J. Pharmacol. Exp. Therap.*, **156,** 492–499.

SJOERDSMA, A., VENDSALU, A. & ENGELMAN, K. (1963). Studies on the metabolism and mechanism of action of methyldopa. *Circulation*, **28,** 492–502.

**Session 2**

Chairman: Professor L. I. Goldberg, Atlanta, U.S.A.

Therapeutic Use of Cardiovascular Drugs

EIGHT

# Clinical Implications of the Disposition of Lidocaine in Man: a Multidisciplinary Study

K. L. MELMON, M. ROWLAND, L. SHEINER AND W. TRAGER

*Schools of Medicine and Pharmacy, Division of Clinical Pharmacology, University of California, San Francisco, California 94122*

## Introduction

Lidocaine is a commonly used and efficacious antiarrhythmic agent. It is generally considered safe despite wide swings in its plasma concentration after intravenous administration. However, cautious administration is necessary because: (a) the rates and overall consequences of toxicity of most drugs are difficult to assess, are usually underestimated, and are avoidable (Melmon, Sheiner & Morrelli, 1971); (b) the pharmacological effects of lidocaine are similar to those that may cause threatening re-entrant arrhythmias; (c) such arrhythmias may be difficult to distinguish from spontaneous ones which would respond to lidocaine therapy; and (d) the chemical characteristics of the drug make it likely that its disposition kinetics may be altered in at least some of the cardiovascular disease states in which it is used.

## Pharmacokinetics of Lidocaine

As a prelude to the investigation of the pharmacokinetics of lidocaine in patients with disease, population data were derived in normals (Rowland, Thomson, Guichard & Melmon, 1971). Figure 1 and Table 1 summarize the results obtained following a 50 mg intravenous bolus.

Concentration of lidocaine in plasma, analysed by a gas–liquid chromatographic method, declined with a bi-exponential character. An early rapid decay in lidocaine plasma levels (mean half-life 8·3 min, Table 1) correlates with the rapid decline in pharmacological activity after an i.v. bolus of the drug. However, there is also a much shallower phase (mean half-life 107 min), which relates to the elimination of this drug from the body. The average value of 107 min (Table 1) agrees closely with the elimination half-life found by Boyes, Scott, Jebsson, Godman & Julian (1971), Hayes (1971) and Tucker & Boas (1971) from blood data, and earlier values from urinary data by Beckett, Boyes & Appleton (1966).

We found no differences in the disposition kinetics of lidocaine between young (24–34 years) and older (52–57 years) normal subjects. The latter were age-matched with patients commonly having ventricular arrhythmias.

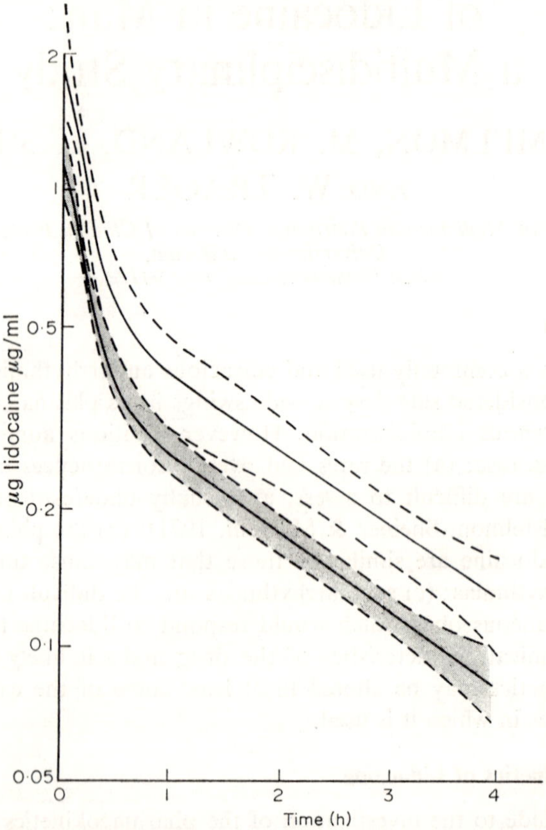


FIG. 1. Population estimates for the plasma levels of lidocaine with 95% confidence intervals in normal volunteers (shaded) and in patients with heart failure receiving a single intravenous bolus of 50 mg lidocaine hydrochloride. Reproduced by permission of the *Annals of Internal Medicine*.

TABLE 1. *Population data for lidocaine disposition in various groups of patients**

| | Half-life shorter phase (min) | Half-life longer phase (min) | Initial dilution volume (Vp; l) | Volume of distribution (Vdss; l) | Plasma clearance (Cl; l/min) | Vp/kg (l/kg) | (Vdss/kg) (l/kg) | Cl/kg (ml/min/kg) |
|---|---|---|---|---|---|---|---|---|
| Total (N = 32) | 8·2 | 97·6 | 35·8 | 90·6 | 0·78 | 0·51 | 1·29 | 11·1 |
| Normal (N = 10) | 8·3 | 107·8 | 37·0 | 92·8 | 0·703 | 0·53 | 1·32 | 10·0 |
| Heart (N = 8) | 7·3 | 115 | 21·3 | 62·0 | 0·443 | 0·30 | 0·88 | 6·3 |
| Renal (N = 6) | 9·3 | 77·4 | 38·3 | 84·0 | 0·959 | 0·55 | 1·20 | 13·7 |
| Liver (N = 8) | 8·8 | 296 | 43 | 162 | 0·419 | 0·61 | 2·31 | 6·0 |

* Reproduced by permission of the *Annals of Internal Medicine*.

Also, ours and other data do not suggest dose-dependent kinetics of lidocaine used in 100–200 mg doses. The bi-exponential character of the decay curve may be interpreted as lidocaine distributing initially into a pool (volume *Vp*) composed of blood and well-perfused tissue, from which further distribution and elimination later occur.

In man lidocaine is primarily eliminated via the liver, though renal clearance plays a minor role. Metabolism by other tissues is minimal. Less than 5% of the dose is normally excreted unchanged in the urine. Although lidocaine, a weak base, is reabsorbed from the kidney tubules by non-ionic diffusion (Eriksson & Granberg, 1965), even when the urine is maximally acidic, renal clearance of the drug accounts for less than 20% of total body clearance. The high initial dilution space (0·53 l/kg) and the volume of distribution at steady state[1] (1·32 l/kg), also noted by others in man (Boyes *et al.*, 1971) and dog (Boyes, Adams & Duce, 1970), indicate the marked extravascular concentration of this drug. Because lidocaine is lipid soluble, its equilibration between plasma and brain and heart probably is very rapid. It is probable that the high partition of lidocaine into most major organs, including kidney, liver and brain in rats and mice (Sun & Truant, 1954) also occurs in man.

Patients in heart failure exhibited higher plasma concentrations of lidocaine than normal subjects receiving the same intravenous dose (Figure 1) (Thomson, Rowland & Melmon, 1971). In these bolus studies both the initial volume and volume of distribution were lower than in normal subjects and the clearance was markedly reduced (Table 1). Interestingly enough, in many instances the half-life of the slower phase differed little from that seen in normals, the fall in clearance being matched by the reduction in volume of distribution (as a reasonable approximation the half-life ($T\frac{1}{2}$) of the slower phase is given by $0{\cdot}693 \times \text{Vdss}/\text{Clearance}$). We found similar findings in patients with heart failure receiving an initial bolus immediately followed by a short term (2 h) infusion (Thomson *et al.*, 1971).

We calculated that the hepatic extraction ratio for lidocaine is 0·6 (Rowland *et al.*, 1971); it was found to be 0·72 when measured by Stenson, Constantino & Harrison (1971) who found a good correlation between hepatic blood flow and lidocaine clearance—the lower the flow the lower the clearance. They also noted good correlation between lidocaine clearance and cardiac index, an indirect, but a clinically related and more easily measured function than hepatic blood flow. Hence, lidocaine

[1] Volume parameters were calculated assuming a two-compartment open body model. The volume of distribution at steady state is calculated assuming this model and should not be confused with the estimates derived by extrapolating the slow phase on semi-logarithmic paper to zero time and dividing this intercept into the dose administered (Riegelman, Loo & Rowland, 1968).

clearance should be significantly influenced by hepatic blood flow. The decrease in the volume of distribution in patients with heart disease studied for short terms may be rationalized by decreased perfusion to various tissues and perhaps by alterations in the partition of lidocaine between blood and tissue components. A decreased volume of distribution of procainamide was also noted by Koch-Weser & Klein (1971) using the drug in patients with heart failure. Higher than usual blood levels of quinidine have been produced in patients with congestive heart failure who were given standard doses of the drug (Ditlefsen, 1957). It is also accepted that lower than ordinary doses of barbiturates should be given to patients in shock when, because of diminished perfusion to many organs, a greater fraction of the dose initially exists in the vascular system. Under these circumstances the brain, which is still being well perfused, may receive excessively high total amounts of drug resulting in CNS-related toxicity following standard doses of a drug.

Whether abnormalities in drug distribution in heart disease patients disappear when lidocaine is used for long terms is not known. The data of Prescott & Nimmo (1971) suggest that distribution takes many hours. After infusion for a day or longer, they observed that patients with heart disease had a low lidocaine clearance, but the volume of distribution was somewhat larger and was accompanied by a longer half-life (T $\frac{1}{2}$) than we had observed. Hayes (1971) also indicated that the half-life may be as long as 10 h following long-term infusion. Certainly these last observations should be repeated and confirmed because toxicity is related to plasma lidocaine levels, and cessation of a protracted infusion after the first signs of toxicity may not lead to as rapid a decline in plasma levels as are needed and would be suggested from the short-term studies. Thus the need to determine concentrations of lidocaine in blood during ongoing therapy if toxicity is to be avoided is stressed. Furthermore, if clinical improvement during therapy changes clearance and distribution of the drug towards normal, dosages may need to be readjusted in order to insure continued efficacy of the drug.

Patients with liver disease, particularly severe cirrhosis, have a lower lidocaine clearance and higher volume of distribution than normals (Thomson *et al.*, 1971) (Table 1). In short-term (4 h) experiments, although confidence in the estimate of the half-life (T $\frac{1}{2}$) of the slower phase was poor, it appeared to be longer than in normal subjects. Severe destruction of hepatic tissue and alterations in the pattern of blood perfusion within the liver may be responsible for the lower clearance. The apparent increase in the volume of distribution requires further investigation. Alterations in plasma or tissue binding of lidocaine may be the reason for this observation. Also, like many of our initial studies, base-line measurements in this group were made following a single intravenous bolus of drug. Different values may be observed after long-term infusions in actual clinical settings.

As expected, because renal clearance accounts for a small fraction of total body clearance of lidocaine, the disposition kinetics of the drug in anephric and oliguric patients did not differ from those in normal subjects (Table 1). However, polar metabolites predominantly cleared by the kidneys will accumulate and may produce toxicity during prolonged infusion. This possibility deserves careful study.

The volume of distribution is defined with respect to plasma (or blood). Lidocaine is significantly protein bound, and if diseases change the nature and extent of the protein(s) responsible for binding, alterations in the volume of distribution would be expected. This point is being actively considered. Lidocaine has a large volume of distribution (60–120 l) and only 6% of that in the body is present in the blood. Accordingly, any changes in plasma protein binding, while affecting the calculated volume of distribution, may have little effect on the concentration of unbound lidocaine and therefore on its biological action. Presumably it is this 'free drug' which penetrates tissues and which should be more closely correlated with its pharmacological effect and toxicity. Conversely, because most of the drug is in the tissues, diseases which alter tissue binding could profoundly influence the total unbound circulating drug levels and therefore the pharmacological effects. There has not been a systematic study of the disease states in which altered tissue binding may be an important factor contributing to changes in the pharmacokinetics and pharmacological effects of lidocaine.

## Dosage Regimens

Lidocaine is the most widely used parenterally administered agent for the control of ventricular arrhythmias. Usually the drug is administered in from one to three intravenous boluses, given 5 to 10 min apart until the arrhythmia stops or toxicity ensues. Each bolus generally contains about 1 mg lidocaine per kg of body weight. Therapeutic blood levels of lidocaine are considered to be between 1·2 and 5·5 μg/ml (Gianelly, Von Der Groeben, Spivack & Harrison, 1967; Jewitt, Kishon & Thomas, 1968). Levels in excess of 9 μg/ml are associated with a high incidence of convulsions, central nervous system depression or hypotension. Similar toxicity occasionally occurs at plasma levels below 9 μg/ml (Binnion, Murtagh, Pollock & Fletcher, 1969; Flensted-Jensen & Sandoe, 1969). To sustain plasma concentrations within the therapeutic dose range, the boluses commonly are followed by constant infusion controlled either by gravity, an infusion drip, or for accurate control, by using a constant rate infusion pump. The recommended infusion rates for lidocaine suggested by Gianelly *et al.* (1967) and now recommended in the package inserts of the drug range from 20 to 50 $\mu$g/kg/min or 1·4 to 3·5 mg/min in a 70 kg patient.

The antiarrhythmic effects of a 50 mg bolus of lidocaine usually last 10–20 min. It is common practice to give a second 50 mg bolus of this drug if the first dose is ineffective or if the arrhythmias reappear. In the earliest periods of drug administration, the decline in the plasma levels of drug is due predominantly to distribution from plasma into other tissues, although some elimination takes place (Rowland *et al.*, 1971). Administration of the second dose adds to the existing amount of drug in blood, and if this procedure is repeated too frequently toxicity may occur as drug accumulates. Accordingly, it may be prudent to reduce the size of repetitive injections (given at intervals of less than a half-life) to avoid the problem of gradual drug accumulation. It should be noted that despite marked differences in the elimination half-lives of some commonly used anti-arrhythmic agents, e.g. procainamide—2 h (Koch-Weser & Klein, 1971) and dilantin—10–25 h (Bigger, Schmidt & Kutt, 1968), the duration of effect of a single intravenous therapeutic dose of each is essentially the same. With these, as with lidocaine, the acute pharmacological effect is seen during the distributive phase of the drug. Repeated doses of any of the agents at intervals shorter than their average chemical half-lives will increase mean concentration of drug and can result in toxicity; under normal circumstances the tendency toward protracted toxicity is greater with dilantin and less with procainamide and lidocaine. Thus, the correct assessment of doses or infusion rate needed to maintain therapeutic blood levels without danger of toxicity is made with knowledge of the elimination half-life and clearance of the drug and independent of the 'half-life' of its therapeutic effect. Similar considerations may be important with a variety of other drugs; such examples serve to emphasize the value of knowing the concentration of drug in the blood in order to use the drug properly in clinical settings. The examples also emphasize the fallacy of assuming that the duration of a drug's pharmacological effect following an intravenous bolus can be used as an index of its chemical half-life.

Lidocaine is occasionally given by infusion only. It takes approximately 3 to 4 half-lives to approach plateau levels in the body (Goldstein, Aronow & Kalman, 1968), which for lidocaine in normal subjects and in patients with renal disease is between 5–7 h. However, during liver disease and severe cardiac failure, the half-life is prolonged and it will take many more hours to reach the plateau concentration. Indeed, Prescott & Nimmo (1971) have observed continually rising lidocaine concentrations in blood over 24 h during continual infusion in a patient with severe cardiac failure. They obtained no evidence that a plateau concentration had been reached during this unusually long period. Although the time needed to reach the plateau is dependent solely on the elimination half-life of the drug, the plateau concentration is a function of the infusion rate and clearance of the drug. The clearance of lidocaine is exceedingly high in normal subjects and in those with renal impairment. We have found it to be 720 ml/min/70 kg body weight, and even higher values have been reported (Boyes *et al.*, 1971). Most of this is due to hepatic metabolism. If a plasma concentration of 1 μg/ml is desired, an infusion rate of 0·85 mg/min/70 kg man, or 12 μg/min/kg, is required. The predicted plateau concentration for the group of normal subjects and those in renal failure at commonly accepted

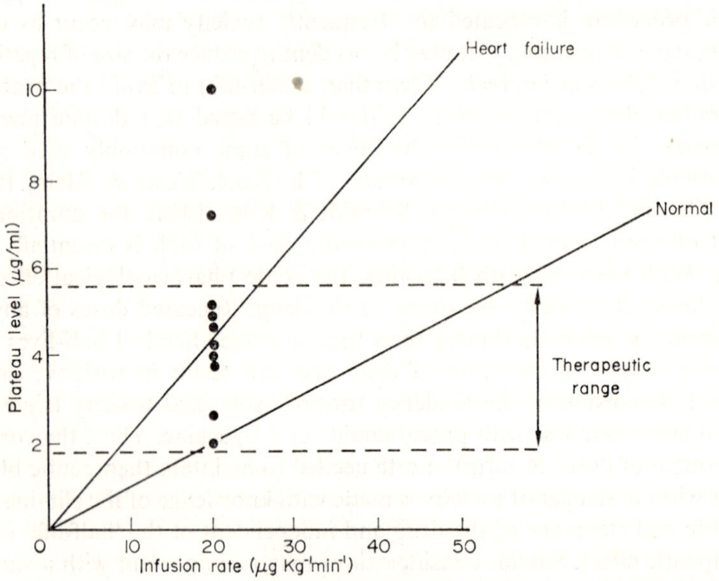


FIG. 2. Relationship between infusion rate and mean plateau lidocaine plasma concentration in normal volunteers and patients in heart failure.* Solid lines represent mean data; solid dots are the predicted plateau concentrations for heart failure subjects calculated from individual lidocaine clearance values.

infusion rates 20, 35 and 50 μg/min/kg, which correspond to 1·4, 2·5 and 3·5 mg/min/70 kg man, are given in Figure 2. The predicted plateau concentrations of lidocaine in plasma were satisfactory at all three infusion rates and agree with those found by Gianelly *et al.* (1967). To overcome the delay in reaching desirable levels, a bolus immediately precedes the infusion. The dosage regimen ascertained from the kinetic data in normal subjects and those in renal failure is in accord with that recommended in the literature (Gianelly *et al.*, 1967; Binnion, 1969; Spracklen, Kimmerling, Besteman & Litchfield, 1968). For example, to achieve and maintain a

* Reproduced by permission of the *Annals of Internal Medicine.*

level of 2 μg/ml, the bolus should be about 2 mg/kg (product of volume of distribution and desired concentration) followed by an infusion rate of 20 μg/min/kg. In practice, the desired concentration is achieved with a smaller bolus (1 mg/kg produces an initial concentration of 2 μg/ml) or, as mentioned earlier, it is given as divided doses, 0·8–1·5 mg/kg to start and then another 1 mg/kg dose within 30 min. This procedure will achieve the desired lidocaine concentration without the initial extremely high and potentially undesirable levels.

The low lidocaine clearance in patients with heart failure necessitates lower infusion rates of lidocaine than those needed in normal subjects. The mean data would suggest that infusion rates of 30 μg/min/kg should not be exceeded (Figure 2). The patient should always be closely observed for signs of toxicity. Periodic analysis of plasma lidocaine could greatly decrease the chance of toxicity by allowing proper readjustment of the therapeutic regimen. A decreased clearance has also been noted in patients with myocardial infarction (Prescott & Nimmo, 1971) with no obvious (but perhaps occult) or only mild cardiac failure. The latter observations emphasize the need to make measurements of objective signs of congestive heart failure and to integrate these data with pharmacokinetic information to choose a proper dosage regimen of the drug. The present data also suggest that patients with severe liver disease may require lower than ordinary infusion rates if toxicity is to be avoided. Since the severity of an illness varies between patients and the process may change in an individual, adjustments of dosage regimens are necessary at varying time intervals dependent on the stage of the disease and the rapidity of its progress or cure, if satisfactory lidocaine levels are to be maintained.

Sometimes arrhythmias reappear in a patient previously stabilized on a plateau concentration of lidocaine. To control the arrhythmias promptly, a lidocaine bolus may be considered necessary, but if the infusion rate is simultaneously increased and continued, it should be remembered that many hours must pass before a new plateau concentration is reached. Failure to appreciate and use this last point could lead to excessively high concentrations of drug in plasma. Also, when 'tapering' a patient off lidocaine, 5 to 7 h, or longer, are required to move from one plateau level to the new steady state produced by alteration of the infusion rate.

Because many patients die from serious arrhythmias before admission to hospital, some investigators have been prompted to examine routes of administration of lidocaine which avoid the need for careful supervision when the intravenous mode is used and yet produce efficacious concentrations of drug in blood. Both the intramuscular and oral route have been examined. Lidocaine is generally rapidly absorbed from the intramuscular site with peak plasma concentrations of 2–3 μg/ml being achieved within 30 min following 200–300-mg doses, respectively (Scott, Jebson, Vellani &

Julian, 1970; Bellet, Roman, Kostis & Fleischmann, 1971). The site of administration can influence the blood level time curve (Meyer & Zelechowski, 1971). Assuming complete absorption and small loss at the time of maximum levels, these last data suggest a volume of distribution of approximately 100 l which agrees with that observed in the normal subjects in our studies (Rowland *et al.*, 1971). Bellet *et al.* (1971) have found that 300 mg was effective in suppressing ventricular arrhythmias for at least 45 min without noticeable side effects. The data would suggest that to maintain a plasma level of approximately 3 μg/ml, 75 mg of lidocaine should be injected every 45 min.

The rapid absorption of lidocaine from the I.M. sites suggests oral administration might be reasonable for a patient outside the hospital. The relatively short half-life would necessitate frequent dosing. A serious argument against this route is the high total body clearance of the drug. With a hepatic extraction ratio of around 0·6, 60% or more of the lidocaine could be cleared in its first passage through the liver. This is verified by the lower availability of oral lidocaine (0·24–0·48) noted by Boyes *et al.* (1971) and Scott (1971). They found that doses as large as 500 mg barely produced peak plasma levels in excess of 1 μg/ml. The variable availability of oral lidocaine between the subjects studied makes prediction of the desirable oral regimen extremely difficult. Moreover, as suggested by Boyes *et al.* (1971), the dizziness noted in some subjects taking 500 mg orally cannot be explained by the lower lidocaine concentration and probably arises from a high circulating concentration of metabolites after this rather large dose.

## General Considerations of the Practical Management of a Dosage Regimen

A convincing relationship between the concentration of a drug in blood and its pharmacological effect, and knowledge of normal and disease-induced changes in the pharmacokinetics of the drug, are often not enough to help a doctor decide how much of an agent, and by what temporal pattern it should be given.

We have begun the construction of algorithmic techniques for the drug dosage problem and have reported some success with digoxin (Sheiner, Rosenberg & Melmon, 1972). To provide a notion of how such a scheme might operate, we will discuss our approach and results with reference to digoxin; application to lidocaine is expected to yield similar results.

Our conceptual scheme relates routinely available clinical observations successively to measures of underlying physiological and pharmacokinetic factors and, ultimately, to pharmacokinetic parameters. These can be used in a pharmacokinetic model to produce optimal initial dosage suggestions tailored to individual needs. Statistical methodology will enable us to adjust and improve our individual estimates in the light of subsequent response data.

Our scheme is highly general; most of the definable influences on drug absorption, distribution, metabolism and elimination can be represented, quantified, merged with others and tested in relation to blood level data. As a consequence of the statistical techniques and the degree to which extensive exploitation of prior information is possible, determination of even a single blood level for an individual should markedly enhance the system's predictive accuracy for him. Drug levels determined in order to improve performance for an individual also contribute to the underlying data base which is used to update the various estimated population coefficients. Thus, the system can learn. A broad definition of what constitutes an observation will allow us to use the pharmacokinetic variables determined for one drug, for one patient, in the estimation of the pharmacokinetic parameters for another drug for him, if a meaningful general relationship holds between them. Hence, the system is also a research tool.

With the scheme set for digoxin and necessary parameter values obtained from regression using the data available to us, we examined the ability of the scheme to predict blood levels of patients without feedback utilization of measured blood levels. The prediction error for a group of 161 patients (305 blood levels) was 0·6 ng/ml. The contribution of feedback adjustment was studied for a subgroup of patients. It was found that knowledge of the preceding four blood levels of digoxin allowed prediction of a fifth level (a few days after the last previous level) with a prediction error of less than 0·3 ng/ml, only 30% higher than the theoretical minimum prediction error, and one half of the non-feedback error.

If future clinical trials confirm the usefulness of the improved predictions, our system can be used by physicians in the following manner: an interactive programme, to run in a time-shared mode (for use via a remote access terminal), would accept clinical observations on a patient as well as the (physician determined) target blood level (TBL) and deliver a dosage scheme adjusted for the individual, and designed to produce the TBL. In addition, as clinical characteristics change or blood levels are measured, the suggested dosage scheme can be improved automatically to reflect this information.

**Metabolism of Lidocaine**

The accuracy of any predictive system relating plasma concentration of a drug with its effect depends on the proper drug being analysed. Even when there are apparent effects of drug concentration, systematic search for active metabolites of the drug must be made. In the case of lidocaine, in addition to previously reported metabolites, we discovered two new ones. These are N′-ethyl-2-methyl-N$^3$-(2,6-dimethylphenyl)-4-imidazolidinone (Breck & Trager, 1971) and N′-ethyl-N$^3$-(2,6-dimethylphenyl)-4-imidazolidinone (Breck & Trager, unpublished results), 1 and 2, respectively. Preliminary pharmacological testing indicates that these

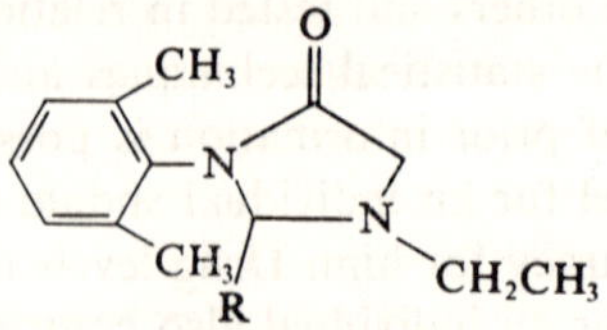

1. R, $CH_3$
2. R, H

materials are equipotent to lidocaine in the rat sciatic nerve test. Their activities as antiarrhythmic agents are as yet unknown. They can be obtained synthetically by the reaction of an appropriate secondary amine, in this case ω-ethylamino-2,6-dimethylacetanilide, 3, and either acetaldehyde to yield 1, or formaldehyde to yield 2. The synthetic material arises presumably via a Mannich type of intermediate as shown below.

There is considerable evidence that enzymatic N-dealkylations occur via a carbinolamine intermediate such as that shown below, which then either spontaneously or enzymatically rearranges to an amine and an aldehyde.

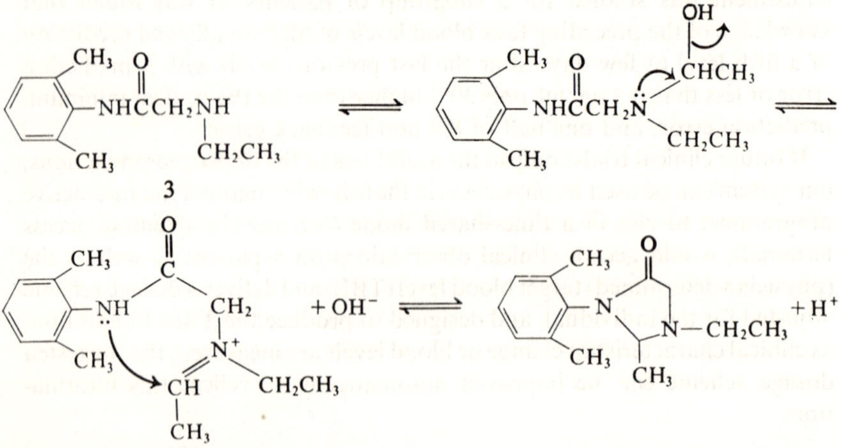

Since both of these reactions involve a common intermediate, it would seem probable that the *in vivo* production of 1 follows a similar pathway. In the case of lidocaine, a nucleophilic centre, the amide nitrogen, is built into the molecule 5 atoms away from the reactive centre and is thus ideally situated to 'scavenge' the reactive intermediate and lead to a neutral, stable molecule. Normally an amide nitrogen is a very weak nucleophile, and in the case of lidocaine this problem is compounded by the steric hindrance provided by the ortho methyl groups of the aromatic ring. This implies that good nucleophiles such as the sulphydryl group of cysteine, or the ring nitrogen of histidine, could effectively compete for reaction with this reactive intermediate provided such groups are at the enzymatic site. If the formation of such a reactive electrophilic intermediate is a general phenomenon in N-dealkylation processes, perhaps the biological responses, either efficacious or toxicological, of various amine drugs may, at least partially, be explained in terms of reaction of such an intermediate with nucleophiles at a critical enzymatic site.

The *in vivo* formation of 2 from either lidocaine or 1 cannot be rationalized chemically in any simple fashion. One possible way this metabolite might arise is by lidocaine first being metabolized to 3 and 3 then reacting

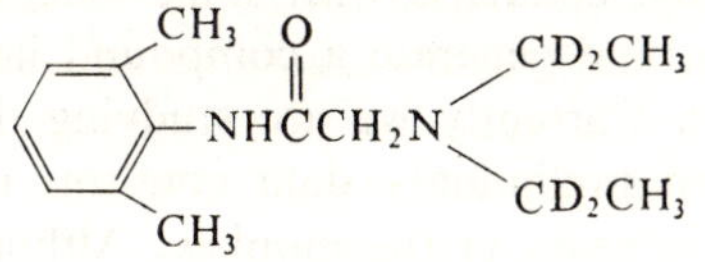


4

with an endogenous source of formaldehyde or at least some activated C 1 unit at the oxidation level of formaldehyde to generate 2 via a mechanism analogous to that presented above. In an attempt to answer the question of whether the carbon atom between the two nitrogen atoms in 2 comes from the originally administered lidocaine or from some *in vivo* source, we prepared the tetradeuteriolidocaine derivative 4 (Boyes *et al.*, 1971). This material was administered i.v. to a *Rhesus* monkey, since in previous studies we had established that the monkey produced both 1 and 2. In the present study both metabolites were collected from the urine and analysed by mass spectrometry. If the carbon atom between the

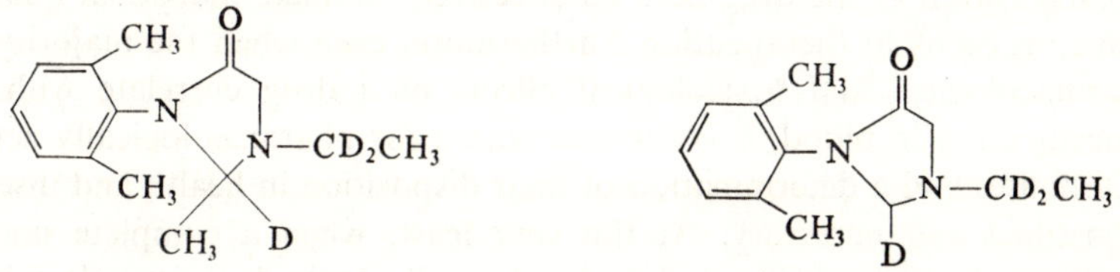


two nitrogen atoms came from the originally administered lidocaine, then both compounds should contain three atoms of deuterium as shown above provided some sort of exchange process was not occurring. On the other hand, if this carbon atom was coming from an endogenous source, 'acetaldehyde' in the case of 1 and 'formaldehyde' in the case of 2, then the isolated metabolites should contain only two atoms of deuterium. The mass spectra of these compounds were determined and in both cases were found to contain only two atoms of deuterium. These results strongly imply that both metabolites, at least to a significant extent, are formed by the reaction of 3 with an endogenous source of a reactive C 1 and C 2 unit (Breck & Trager, unpublished results). To be absolutely sure this result is not an artifact, we are currently synthesizing lidocaine containing $^{14}C$ specifically in the critical carbon position.

These results suggest that secondary amines can react with *in vivo* materials at the oxidation state of aldehydes. This further means metabolism must be considered from the viewpoint of synthesis. A tertiary amine drug, e.g. lidocaine, may undergo N-dealkylation in the liver to form the secondary amine; the secondary amine may then recondense with 'acetaldehyde' to generate the cyclic metabolite or circulate to some other site in the body, condense with some aldehyde product of intermediary metabolism, and generate a compound having totally different biological properties. Currently we are studying the disposition of the cyclic metabolite and preliminary data confirms its presence in blood following lidocaine infusion in the monkey. Although its concentration in blood is much lower than that of lidocaine, its concentration in tissues, e.g., brain, kidney, liver, is comparable to that of lidocaine (Benowitz, Rowland & Melmon, unpublished data). Evidently the metabolite partitions more extensively into tissue than lidocaine. Hence care should be exercised before conclusions are drawn as to the pharmacological or toxicological consequences of the metabolite based solely on its blood levels.

In summary, we have tried to illustrate how therapeutic implications of a concentration of a drug in blood are only partially elucidated by study of the pharmacokinetics of the drug. Only when blood levels are related to a full understanding of the pharmacokinetics and to easily and routinely recorded patient data can the normal and disease-induced alterations in the disposition of the drug be used effectively to make individual quantitative decisions in therapeutics. Furthermore, even when the majority of pharmacological and toxicological effects of a drug correlate with its concentration in blood, a systematic search for pharmacologically active metabolites and a determination of their disposition in health and disease is justified and necessary. At the very least, when a complete understanding of a commonly used and potentially toxic drug is undertaken, its proper use will be defined. The pragmatic implications of such definition will be more frequently efficacious and less frequently toxic experiences with the drug. As in the case of digoxin, just how much clinical benefit comes from such an approach remains to be shown. At the most, general concepts of drug metabolism, of *in vivo* drug synthetic processes and of structure action relationships of a class of drugs will be revealed. We have tried to summarize evidence proving that the integrated efforts of the scientific community to understand the disposition of lidocaine have been amply rewarded by approaching the extremes of such goals.

The work reported has been supported by grants from the US Public Health Service—GM-16496 and 01791.

## REFERENCES

BECKETT, A. N., BOYES, R. N. & APPLETON, P. J. (1966). The metabolism and excretion of lidocaine in man. *J. Pharm. Pharmacol.*, **18** (Supp.), 76–81.

BELLET, S., ROMAN, L., KOSTIS, T. B. & FLEISCHMANN, D. (1971) Intramuscular lidocaine in the therapy of ventricular arrhythmias. *Amer. J. Cardiology*, **27**, 291–293.

BIGGER, J. T., SCHMIDT, D. M. & KUTT, H. (1968). Relationship between the plasma level of diphenylhydantoin sodium and its cardiac antiarrhythmic effects. *Circulation*, **38**, 363–374.

BINNION, P. F., MURTAGH, G., POLLOCK, A. M. & FLETCHER, E. (1969). Relation between plasma lignocaine levels and induced haemodynamic changes. *Brit. Med. J.*, **3**, 390–392.

BOYES, R. N., ADAMS, H. J. & DUCE, B. R. (1970). Oral absorption and disposition kinetics of lidocaine hydrochloride in dogs. *J. Pharmacol. Exptl. Ther.*, **174**, 1–8.

BOYES, R. N., SCOTT, D. B., JEBSSON, P. J., GODMAN, M. J. & JULIAN, D. G. (1971). Pharmacokinetics of lidocaine in man. *Clin. Pharmacol. Ther.*, **12**, 105–116.

BRECK, G. D. & TRAGER, W. F. (1971). Oxidative N-dealkylation. A Mannich intermediate in the formation of a new metabolite of lidocaine in man. *Science*, **173**, 544–545.

DITLEFSEN, E. L. (1957). Quinidine concentration in blood and excretion in urine following parenteral administration as related to congestive heart failure. *Acta Med. Scand.*, **159**, 105–109.

ERIKSSON, E. & GRANBERG, P. (1965). Studies on the renal excretion of Citanest® and Xylocaine®. *Acta Anaesth.* (Supp.), **16**, 79–85.

FLENSTED-JENSEN, E. & SANDOE, E. (1969). Lidocaine as an antiarrhythmic agent. *Acta Med. Scand.*, **185**, 297–302.

GIANELLY, R., VON DER GROEBEN, J., SPIVACK, A. P. & HARRISON, D. C. (1967). Effect of lidocaine on ventricular arrhythmias in patients with coronary heart disease. *New Eng. J. Med.*, **277**, 1215–1221.

GOLDSTEIN, A., ARONOW, L. & KALMAN, S. M. (1968). Principles of Drug Action; The Basis of Pharmacology, pp. 292–309, New York: Hoeber, Harper & Row.

HAYES, A. H. (1971). Intravenous infusion of lidocaine in the control of ventricular arrhythmias. In: *Lidocaine in the Treatment of Ventricular Arrhythmias*, ed. by Scott & Julian, p. 189. Edinburgh: Livingstone.

JEWITT, D. E., KISHON, Y. & THOMAS, M. (1968). Lidocaine in the management of arrhythmias after acute myocardial infarction. *Lancet*, **2,** 266–268.

KOCH-WESER, J. & KLEIN, S. W. (1971). Procainamide dosage schedules, plasma concentrations and clinical effects. *JAMA*, **215,** 1454–1460.

MELMON, K. L., SHEINER, L. & MORRELLI, H. F. (1971). Preventable drug reactions: causes and cures. *New Eng. J. Med.*, **284,** 1361–1368.

MEYER, M. B. & ZELECHOWSKI, K. (1971). Intramuscular lidocaine in normal subjects. In: *Lidocaine in the Treatment of Ventricular Arrhythmias*, ed. by Scott & Julian, p. 161. Edinburgh: Livingstone.

PRESCOTT, L. F. & NIMMO, J. (1971). Plasma lidocaine concentrations during and after prolonged infusion in patients with myocardial infarction. In: *Lidocaine in the Treatment of Ventricular Arrhythmias*, ed. by Scott & Julian, p. 168. Edinburgh: Livingstone.

RIEGELMAN, S., LOO, J. & ROWLAND, M. (1968). Concept of a volume of distribution and possible errors in evaluation of this parameter. *J. Pharm. Sci.*, **57,** 128–133.

ROWLAND, M., THOMSON, P. D., GUICHARD, A. & MELMON, K. L. (1971). Disposition kinetics of lidocaine in normal subjects. *Ann. N.Y. Acad. Sci.*, **179,** 383–398.

SCOTT, D. B. (1971). Blood levels of lidocaine following various routes of administration. In: *Lidocaine in the Treatment of Ventricular Arrhythmias*, ed. by Scott & Julian, p. 153. Edinburgh: Livingstone.

SCOTT, D. B., JEBSSON, P. J., VELLANI, C. W. & JULIAN, D. G. (1970). Plasma-lidocaine levels after intravenous and intramuscular injection. *Lancet*, **1,** 41.

SHEINER, L. B., ROSENBERG, B. & MELMON, K. L. (1972). Pharmacokinetic modelling for individual patients: a practical basis for computer-aided therapeusis. *Comp. Biomed. Research* (in press).

SPRACKLEN, F. H. N., KIMMERLING, J. J., BESTEMAN, E. M. M. & LITCHFIELD, J. W. (1968). Use of lignocaine in treatment of cardiac arrythmias. *Brit. Med. J.*, **1,** 89–91.

STENSON, R. E., CONSTANTINO, R. T. & HARRISON, D. C. (1971). Interrelationships of hepatic blood flow, cardiac output and blood levels of lidocaine in man. *Circulation*, **43,** 205–211.

SUNG, C. Y. & TRUANT, A. P. (1954). Physiological disposition of lidocaine and its comparison in some respects with procaine. *J. Pharmacol. Exptl. ther.*, **112,** 432–443.

THOMSON, P. D., ROWLAND, M. & MELMON, K. L. (1971). The influence of heart failure, liver disease, and renal failure on the disposition of lidocaine in man. *Amer. Heart J.*, **82,** 417–421.

TUCKER, G. T. & BOAS, R. A. (1971). Pharmacokinetic aspects of intravenous regional anesthesia. *Anesthesiology*, **34,** 538–549.

# NINE

# Pharmacological Effects of Propranolol in Relation to Plasma Levels

C. F. GEORGE, T. FENYVESI[1] AND
C. T. DOLLERY

*MRC Clinical Pharmacology Research Group,
Royal Postgraduate Medical School, Ducane Road, London, W12*

## Introduction

Since the introduction of propranolol in 1964, β-adrenoceptor antagonists have become widely used in the treatment of angina pectoris, arterial hypertension and cardiac arrhythmias. Clinical experience indicates that the dose of propranolol must be adjusted in each patient in order to produce a therapeutic response (Gillam & Prichard, 1966) and may range from 60 mg to more than 1g daily (Wolfson & Gorlin, 1967). A possible explanation for these individual differences was provided by Grant *et al.* (1966) who measured blood levels in 22 patients taking propranolol for angina pectoris. These workers found a wide range of blood levels at one and four hours after oral dosing, which they attributed to differences in absorption. This variability has since been confirmed by Shand, Nuckolls & Oates (1970) who reported a seven-fold range in the peak plasma levels attained in different individuals given the same oral dose of propranolol. Although the original explanation for these findings is no longer valid as the absorption of propranolol is virtually complete after oral administration (Paterson *et al.*, 1970), these differences would be of practical importance if the pharmacological and therapeutic effects of propranolol were related to the concentration in blood.

*In vitro* studies on isolated tissues have shown that β-adrenoceptor antagonism produced by propranolol is competitive, and varies according to the concentration in the surrounding medium (Black, Duncan & Shanks, 1965). The same authors also showed that in anaesthetized cats the antagonism of the chrontropic response to intravenous isoprenaline was related to the concentration in blood. Similar correlations have been found in anaesthetized dogs (George & Fenyvesi—unpublished findings).

There is surprisingly little information on the relationship between

[1] 2nd Medical Department, Semmelweis University, Budapest, Hungary.

pharmacological effects and blood levels of propranolol in man. Paterson *et al.* (1970) showed that the degree of antagonism of an isoprenaline-induced tachycardia was related to the level of propranolol in blood, and these findings have since been confirmed by Coltart & Shand (1970). However, isoprenaline is not a physiological stimulus whereas techniques such as inhibition of the tachycardia produced by exercise and tilting to 80° head up are more akin to everyday experience and might be expected to provide information which is relevant to treatment. Unfortunately, most previous studies have been concerned with determining the relative importance of para-sympathetic and sympathetic nervous control in the tachycardia produced by these manœuvres (*cf.* Epstein, Robinson, Kahler & Braunwald, 1965; Robinson, Epstein Beiser & Bruanwald, 1966; Leon, Shaver & Leonard, 1970). Since blood levels were not measured and in many instances only one dose level of propranolol was used few conclusions can be drawn. The aim of the present study was, therefore, to re-evaluate four tests of B-adrenoceptor blockade by relating pharmacological response to the concentration of propranolol in plasma, and hence to derive further information on the value of measurements of plasma propranolol.

## Methods

Five volunteers (four male and one female) were studied after oral dosing with propranolol (Inderal®) 100–120 mg; two others were given an intravenous infusion of 20 mg propranolol. In the oral studies, heart rate responses to one of the four stimuli were recorded and a blood sample taken at 9.00 a.m. Further measurements were made at 2, 3, 5¼ and 6¾ hours after propranolol. Heart rate was measured with a digital ratemeter (Emons & Conolly, 1971) triggered by the R wave of the ECG. Exercise was performed on a bicycle ergometer for 3 min at 960 KPM/min by the male subjects and at 800 KPM/min by the female. Isoprenaline dose response curves were performed according to the method described by Conolly, Davies, Dollery & George (1971). Tilt and glyceryl trinitrate tachycardia were studied on the same day, a 0·5 mg tablet being chewed when the response to tilting to 80° head up had been obtained. Propranolol levels were measured by the fluorometric method (Black *et al.*, 1965) as modified by Shand *et al.* (1970).

## Results

Since in each subject measurements of pharmacological effect and plasma propranolol were made at the same four time intervals after oral dosing, it was possible to construct a log plasma propranolol–heart rate response curve for each individual and to analyse these curves for: (i) a relationship between the two measurements and (ii) individual differences in response to the same plasma levels of propranolol.

(a) *Exercise*

The results are summarised in Figure 1 and Table 1. In three subjects there was a close correlation between the percentage inhibition of exercise tachycardia and the log plasma concentration throughout the range studied (40–465 ng/ml.). In the other two subjects this relationship was shown at low plasma levels only. In subject 5 there was little further increase in the blockade of exercise tachycardia at propranolol levels above 50 ng/ml. An analysis of co-variance showed that the difference in response between subjects was highly significant, $F_{4,\ 11} = 8{\cdot}93$, $P<0{\cdot}01$. Thus at a 30% inhibition of exercise tachycardia, there was almost a five-

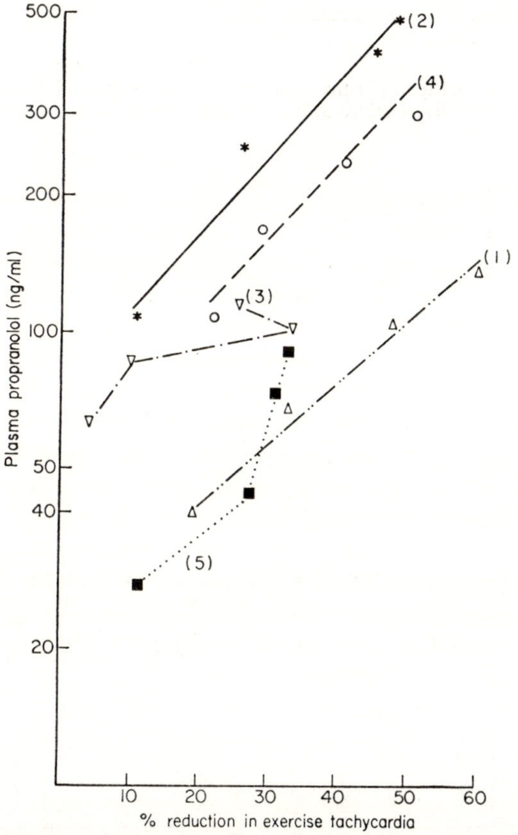


FIG. 1. Relationship between plasma level of propranolol and percentage inhibition of exercise tachycardia. The subject number is indicated in brackets.

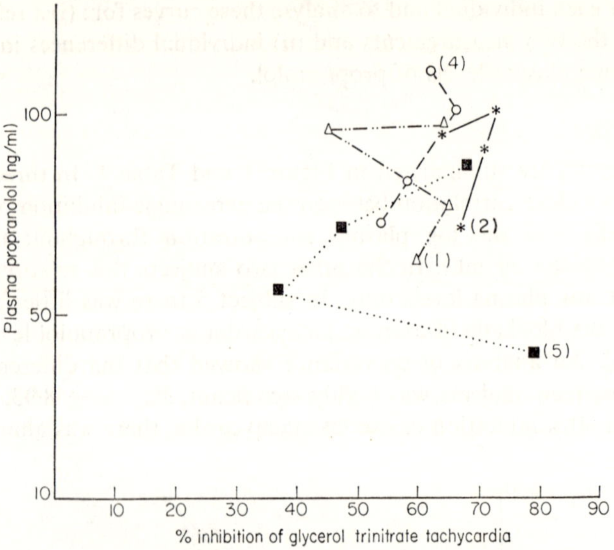


FIG. 2. Relationship between plasma concentration of propranolol and percentage inhibition of glyceryl trinitrate tachycardia. The subject number is in brackets.

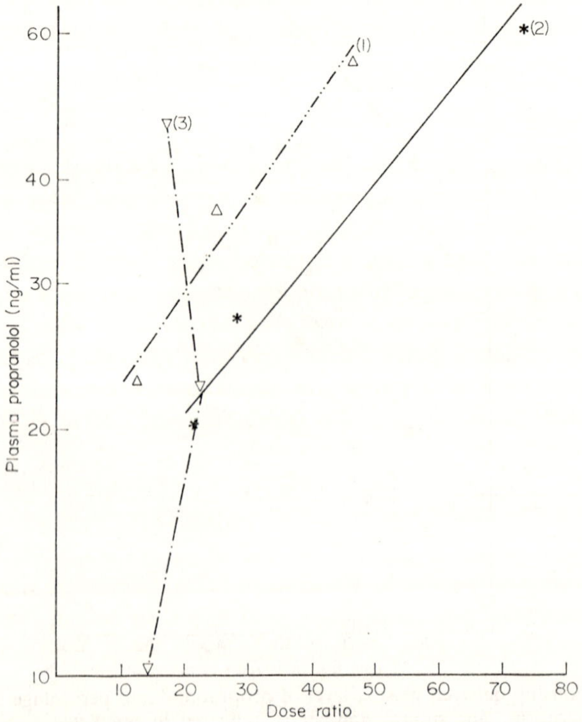


FIG. 3. Relationship between plasma level of propranolol and inhibition of isoprenaline tachycardia after oral propranolol. (The timing of each point differs slightly from that of the other studies.) The subject number is in brackets.

TABLE 1

| Subject No. | Plasma level at a given inhibition of exercise tachycardia | | | | | % inhibition of exercise tachycardia at given plasma propranolol (ng/ml) | | | | |
|---|---|---|---|---|---|---|---|---|---|---|
| | 10% | 20% | 30% | 40% | 50% | 50 | 100 | 200 | 300 | 400 |
| 1 | 23* | 42 | 66 | 91 | 117 | 24 | 44 | 78* | — | — |
| 2 | 95 | 196 | 300 | 420 | — | <10 | 10 | 21 | 30 | 39 |
| 3 | 66 | 86 | 98 | — | — | <10 | 31 | — | — | — |
| 4 | 48* | 102 | 167 | 236 | 303 | 10 | 21 | 35 | 50 | — |
| 5 | 26* | 37 | 64 | — | — | 28 | 34 | 38* | — | — |

* By extrapolation.

fold variation in plasma propranolol. However, the results of this test were repeatable from day to day in the same individual, the plasma level at a 30% inhibition varying from 66–76 ng/ml in subject 1.

(b) *Glyceryl trinitrate*

Before administration of propranolol, glyceryl trinitrate 0·5 mg given sublingually produced an increase in heart rate of 16 to 44 beats per minute (average = 27). After oral propranolol there was a 36–80% reduction in the tachycardia, but no correlation was demonstrated between the percentage inhibition and the plasma level of propranolol in either individual subjects or the group as a whole. See Figure 2.

(c) *Isoprenaline*

In each instance, heart rate responses were obtained to a minimum of four doses of intravenous isoprenaline. A regression of heart rate response on log isoprenaline dose was then calculated, the slopes of the series of curves tested for parallelism, a common slope formed and a dose-ratio computed. The blockade of isoprenaline tachycardia (expressed as the dose ratio) was closely related to plasma propranolol levels after both oral and intravenous dosing (Figures 3 and 4). A dose ratio of 12·5 was achieved with a plasma level of 37 ng/ml after intravenous propranolol, whereas in different individuals this shift was produced with a level of 18–23 ng/ml after oral dosing.

(d) *Tilting to 80° head up*

Propranolol produced a significant reduction in the tachycardia evoked by this manœuvre (Figure 5). In subjects 1–3 a correlation was found between plasma level and pharmacological effect. In two of these subjects, the tachycardia was totally abolished at plasma levels of 80 and 92 ng/ml respectively. In subject 5, plasma levels in excess of 50 ng/ml were not associated with any further reduction of tilt tachycardia. The results of this

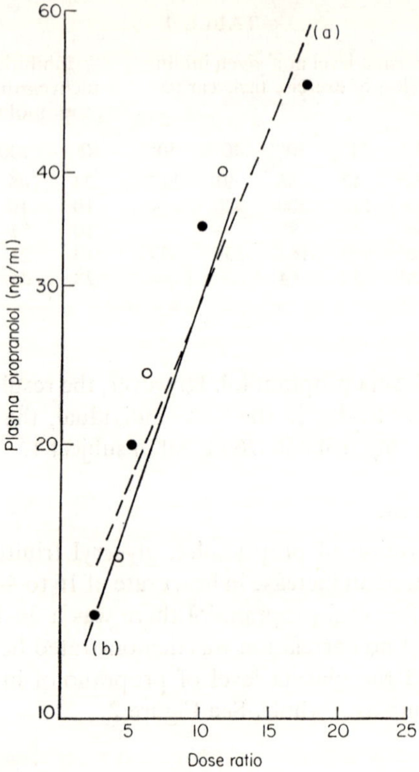


FIG. 4. Relationship between plasma level of propranolol and inhibition of isoprenaline tachycardia after intravenous propranolol.

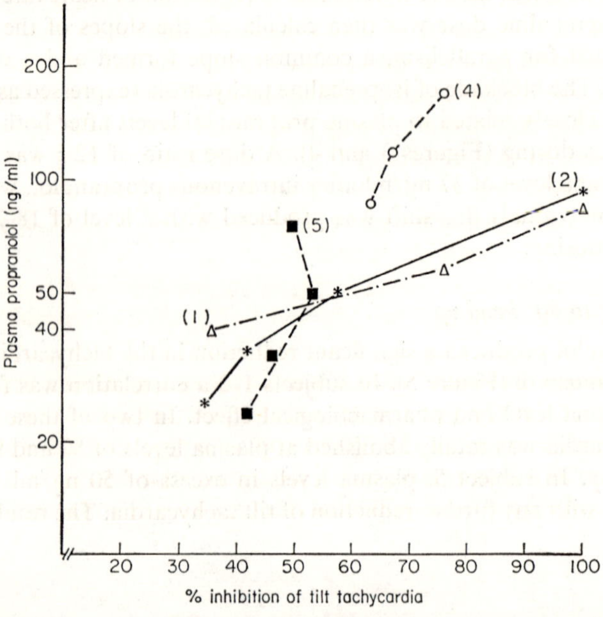


FIG. 5. Relationship between plasma level of propranolol and percentage inhibition of tilt tachycardia. The subject number is in brackets.

test were not repeatable in the same individual from day to day, a 60% inhibition of the response being produced by levels ranging from 42–94 ng/ml in subject 1.

## Discussion

The present study confirms that inhibition of tachycardia produced by exercise, glyceryl trinitrate, isoprenaline and tilting can be used as qualitative tests of β-adrenoceptor blockade, Glyceryl trinitrate is the simplest of these tests and does not require elaborate equipment to perform. Fitzgerald (1970) has reported a close relationship between the degree of inhibition of glyceryl trinitrate-induced tachycardia and the dose of propranolol given orally to the same subject. However, our results failed to demonstrate any quantitative relationship between the inhibition of glyceryl trinitrate-induced tachycardia and plasma propranolol. It is possible that the difference in results could have resulted for technical reasons since our studies were performed on a tilt table, whereas Fitzgerald's subjects stood on the floor. However, this explanation seems unlikely as a repeat study on one of our subjects using Fitzgerald's technique failed to show a close relationship between inhibition of tachycardia and plasma level. Leon *et al.* (1971) have reported that the tachycardia produced by nitrites is largely mediated by alterations in parasympathetic tone. However, in the light of the present study and Fitzgerald's findings it appears that the contribution played by the parasympathetic and sympathetic nervous systems may vary from one person to another.

Tilting to 80° head up is also a simple test of β-adrenoceptor blockade; our results suggest that this response is chiefly mediated by sympathetic reflexes. It is, however, a relatively weak stimulus since the response is totally abolished in some subjects to 100 mg oral propranolol. Furthermore, it is not a reliable quantitative test of β-adrenoceptor blockade as the day-to-day repeatability is poor and is profoundly affected by the level of hydration. In subject 1 the change in heart rate on tilting was normally $17{\cdot}8 \pm 0{\cdot}8$ beats per minute, but after 40 mg frusemide p.o. it rose to $25{\cdot}0 \pm 1{\cdot}0$, and following a rapid infusion of 500 ml saline the response was only $8{\cdot}0 \pm 2{\cdot}0$ beats per minute.

The response to intravenous isoprenaline has been widely used to test β-adrenoceptor function. The chief merit of this test is repeatability from day-to-day (George, Conolly, Fenyvesi, Briant & Dollery, 1972). However, the major drawback is that it is not a physiological stimulus. It is also inadvisable to apply this test to patients with ischaemic heart disease. Submaximal exercise, on the other hand, is a physiological stimulus and can be used as a quantitative test of β-adrenoceptor blockade. The results are repeatable in the same individual from day-to-day and reveal significant interperson differences in response. Although one of our subjects showed 'maximal' blockade of exercise tachycardia with a propranolol level of around 50 ng/ml as reported previously by Coltart *et al.* (1970), in another 'maximal' blockade was present at around 100 ng/ml and in the three others progressive inhibition of the heart rate response occurred with much higher levels.

The beneficial effect of $\beta$-adrenoceptor antagonists in angina pectoris derives from their action in reducing left ventricular work and appears to result mainly from a fall in heart rate (Robinson, 1971). Furthermore, the hypotensive effect of propranolol is thought to be due to a reduction in cardiac output (Frohlich, Tarazi, Dustan & Page, 1968) which is also the result of a change in heart rate. Thus, the present results have important therapeutic implications; individual differences in dosage required to produce a therapeutic response could result from variation in the plasma concentration achieved after oral dosing (Shand *et al.* 1970), and variability in response to the same level of propranolol. Thus a patient who achieves relatively high levels in blood after oral dosing and whose heart rate is maximally reduced by low levels should respond to quite small doses of propranolol. In contrast a person who requires high blood levels to produce the same reduction and who achieves low levels after oral propranolol would be expected to need relatively high doses to control angina or hypertension.

Whilst these explanations have not as yet been formally tested in a prospective trial there is some evidence in favour of them. Previous workers have demonstrated considerable differences in haemodynamic response to the same dose of intravenous propranolol (Epstein *et al.*, 1965; Cumming & Carr, 1966; Furberg & von Schmalensee, 1968), when there is little variation in plasma level achieved (Shand *et al*, 1970). More recently, McLean & Deane (1970) reported their findings on patients taking propranolol for angina pectoris in whom the daily dose varied from 80 to 520 mg (mean 218 mg). In these patients maximum relief of angina occurred at plasma levels ranging from 20 to 520 ng/ml. Furthermore, these authors showed that by giving propranolol every three hours instead of three or four times each day, higher blood levels were maintained and that in some patients these were associated with a further relief of symptoms.

There are two reservations which must be noted about measurements of propranolol in plasma. The first of these is that after oral administration some metabolism to 4-hydroxypropranolol takes place (Paterson *et al*, 1970) and this is pharmacologically active with much the same potency as a $\beta$-adrenoceptor antagonist as propranolol (Fitzgerald—personal communication). Thus after oral dosing the plasma level required to produce a given reduction in exercise tachycardia is between one-half and one-third of that required after intravenous administration. Although numerous attempts have been made to measure this metabolite it is extremely unstable so that most workers, including ourselves, have been unable to measure it without the use of carbon-14 labelled drug. It is, however, possible that there are interperson differences, in the amount of the metabolite formed. The second problem is that propranolol is normally given as a racemate and the $\beta$-adrenoceptor antagonism is due to the laevo isomer. Although both isomers fluoresce identically, the late half-life of the laevo isomer is longer than that of the dextro isomer (George, Fenyvesi, Conolly & Dollery, 1972). Thus, measurements of plasma propranolol may not give a reliable estimate of the amount of the laevo isomer as the proportion of the two may alter with time.

Routine measurements of plasma propranolol are of little value when taken in isolation since the therapeutic range is wide and the standard techniques do not estimate the active metabolite, 4-hydroxypropranolol. However, in those patients who fail to derive benefit from conventional doses the demonstration of a low plasma level should lead to either an increase in dose or a shorter dosing interval. Ideally, these measurements should be combined with assessments of the haemodynamic response to exercise.

**Summary**

The effect of propranolol has been studied on the tachycardia produced by exercise, glyceryl trinitrate, isoprenaline and tilting in five normal volunteers. After single oral doses of 100–120 mg, plasma propranolol and pharmacological responses were measured at 2, 3, $5\frac{1}{2}$ and $6\frac{3}{4}$ hours. A correlation was found between pharmacological response and plasma propranolol levels in the exercise, isoprenaline and tilt studies. Since the repeatability of the tilt tachycardia findings was unsatisfactory, it is concluded that only exercise and isoprenaline are reliable quantitative measures of $\beta$-adrenoceptor blockade. The exercise test revealed significant interperson differences in response to the same plasma concentration which, when taken in conjunction with the known variability in plasma propranolol achieved after oral dosing, could provide an explanation for the wide range in dose required to produce therapeutic benefit.

We wish to thank Dr. R. A. Wiseman of ICI Ltd. for supplies of propranolol and Miss A. Petrie for help with the statistical analysis.

## REFERENCES

BLACK, J. W., DUNCAN, W. A. M. & SHANKS, R. G. (1965). Comparison of some properties of pronethalol and propranolol. *Brit. J. Pharmacol.*, **25,** 577–591.

COLTART, D. J. & SHAND, D. G. (1970). Plasma propranolol levels in the quantitative assessment of $\beta$-adrenergic blockade in man. *Brit. med. J.*, **3,** 731–734.

CONOLLY, M. E., DAVIES, D. S., DOLLERY, C. T. & GEORGE, C. F. (1971). Resistance to $\beta$-adrenoceptor stimulants (a possible explanation for the rise in asthma deaths). *Brit. J. Pharmacol.*, **43,** 389–402.

CUMMING, G. R. & CARR, W. (1966). Haemodynamic response to exercise after propranolol in normal subjects. *Canad. J. Physiol.*, **44,** 465–474.

EMONS, E. & CONOLLY, M. E. (1971). Digital heart rate meter. *Cardiovasc. Res.*, **5,** 157–160.

EPSTEIN, S. E., ROBINSON, B. F., KAHLER, R. L. & BRAUNWALD, E. (1965). Effects of beta-adrenergic blockade on the cardiac response to maximal and sub-maximal exercise in man. *J. Clin. Invest.*, **44,** 1745–1753.

FITZGERALD, J. D. (1970). A new test of the degree of adrenergic beta receptor blockade. *Int. J. Clin. Pharmacol.*, **4,** 125–130.

FROHLICH, E. D., TARAZI, R. C., DUSTAN, H. P. & PAGE, I. H. (1968). The paradox of beta-adrenergic blockade in hypertension. *Circulation*, **37,** 417–423.

FURBERG, C. & VON SCHMALENSEE, G. (1968). Beta-adrenergic blockade and central circulation during exercise in sitting position in healthy subjects. *Acta. physiol. Scandinav.*, **73,** 435–466.

GEORGE, C. F., CONOLLY, M. E., FENYVESI, T., BRIANT, R. H. & DOLLERY, C. T. (1972). Intravenously administered isoproterenol sulfate dose-response curves in man. *Arch. int. Med.*, **130,** 361–364.

GEORGE, C. F., FENYVESI, T., CONOLLY, M. E. & DOLLERY, C. T. Pharmacokinetics of dextro, laevo and racemic propranolol in man. *Europ. J. Clin. Pharmacol.*, **4,** 74–76.

GILLAM, P. M. S. & PRICHARD, B. N. C. (1966). Propranolol in the therapy of angina pectoris. *Amer. J. Cardiol.*, **18,** 366–369.

GRANT, R. H. E., KEELAN, P., KERNOHAN, R. J., LEONARD, J. C., NANCE KIEVILL, L. & SINCLAIR, K. (1966). Multicenter trial of propranolol in angina pectoris. *Amer. J. Cardiol.*, **18,** 361–365.

LEON, D. F., SHAVER, J. A. & LEONARD, J. J. (1970). Reflex heart rate control in man. *Amer. Heart. J.*, **80,** 729–739.

MCLEAN, C. E. & DEANE, D. S. (1970). Propranolol dose determinants including blood level studies. *Angiology*, **21,** 536–545.

PATERSON, J. W., CONOLLY, M. E., DOLLERY, C. T., HAYES, A. and COOPER, R. G. (1970). The pharmacodynamics and metabolism of propranolol in man. *Europ. J. Clin. Pharmacol.*, **2,** 127–133.

ROBINSON, B. F. (1971). The mode of action of beta-antagonists in angina pectoris. *Postgrad. med. J.*, **47,** suppl., 41–43.

ROBINSON, B. F., EPSTEIN, S. E., BEISER, G. D. & BRAUNWALD, E. (1966). Control of heart rate by the autonomic nervous system. *Circulat. Res.*, **19,** 400–411.

SHAND, D. G., NUCKOLLS, E. M. & OATES, J. A. (1970). Plasma propranolol levels in adults. *Clin. Pharmacol. Ther.*, **11,** 112–120.

WOLFSON, S. & GORLIN, R. (1967). Physiological and clinical aspects of beta-adrenergic blockade. *Ann. N.Y. Acad. Sci.*, **139,** 1003–1009.

TEN

# Plasma Digoxin Concentrations as a Guide to Therapeutic Requirements

D. A. CHAMBERLAIN

*Royal Sussex County Hospital, Brighton*

**Introduction**

Digitalis has been used in clinical practice for nearly 200 years, yet there are still considerable problems in the selection of optimal dose requirements. As a result of these difficulties, many patients receive less than an adequate therapeutic dose; at the other end of the scale, many suffer from digitalis toxicity, more often than not unrecognized. Digitalis is thus responsible for an appreciable morbidity and mortality amongst patients with heart disease (Beller, Smith, Abelmann, Haber & Hood, 1971).

There are several reasons for the problems in dose selection: first, the correct maintenance dose varies from patient to patient; secondly, the therapeutic effects of the drug are difficult to measure in clinical practice; thirdly, the correct therapeutic dose is very close to that which will cause toxicity. Finally, the symptoms of toxicity are often non-specific and may be ascribed to a variety of causes including anxiety, depression or heart disease itself.

The recent development of assays capable of measuring therapeutic concentrations of cardiac glycosides in the blood has therefore aroused considerable interest. If it can be shown that these concentrations are related to clinical effect, then an important advance will have been made. Unfortunately, the very difficulties which make it important to have an assay also bedevil attempts to assess its value, for having determined concentrations, there is no satisfactory method for correlating them with therapeutic activity. There are no sensitive measures of contractility in clinical practice, and toxicity provides only a difficult and potentially dangerous end-point. The heart rate response in atrial fibrillation provides the only convenient yardstick. It is convenient, but imperfect, for some patients have slow rates without digitalis, and others have rapid rates despite treatment with glycosides to the very point of toxicity.

**Plasma Concentrations of Digoxin Related to Therapeutic Effect and Toxicity**

Chamberlain, White, Howard & Smith (1970) used a radioimmunoassay to measure plasma digoxin concentrations in 100 normokalaemic patients with atrial fibrillation who were on long-term oral treatment with the drug. An arbitrary division was made between those with resting heart rates ranging from 60 to 85 per min and those with rates exceeding 85 per min. For comparative purposes, digoxin levels were also measured in a group of 50 individuals who were not receiving digoxin and therefore acted as controls, and also in 22 patients with good clinical and electrocardiographic evidence of digoxin toxicity (Figure 1).

49 of the 50 control individuals had no detectable digoxin in the blood; a single sample gave a reading of 0·3 ng/ml, but repeated measurements

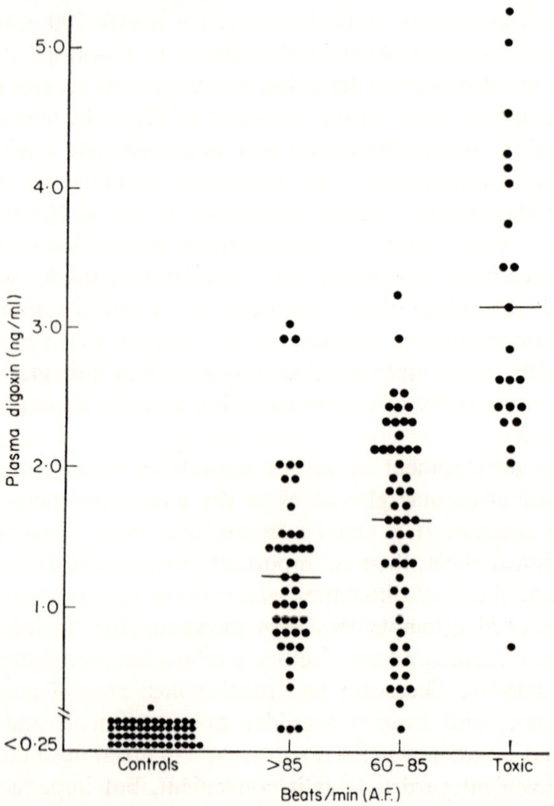


FIG. 1. Plasma digoxin concentrations in 44 patients with atrial fibrillation and relatively fast heart rates and in 56 patients with atrial fibrillation and slower heart rates. All subjects were normokalaemic. Concentrations in 22 patients with digoxin toxicity and in 50 control subjects are shown for comparison. The horizontal bars represent mean values. (Reproduced by permission of the Editor of the *British Medical Journal.*)

from the same subject were consistently negative. 21 of the 22 patients with digoxin toxicity had levels of 2 ng/ml or more. The other patient with a level of only 0·7 ng/ml was subsequently found to have been taking both digoxin and digitalis folia; glycosides other than digoxin would therefore have been present in the plasma and would not have been measured by the assay.

The patients with atrial fibrillation had digoxin concentrations ranging from less than 0·25 ng/ml (below the limit of the sensitivity of the assay) to 3·2 ng/ml. Thus there was an appreciable overlap between therapeutic and toxic groups particularly in the range 2 to 3 ng/ml. The overlap was not unexpected. The therapeutic dose is known to be very close to that which will cause toxicity. Furthermore, susceptibility to toxicity depends upon many factors other than digoxin concentration. These factors include serum potassium, sodium, calcium and magnesium concentrations, acid-base balance, and thyroid function (Surawicz & Mortelmans, 1969), and may act in part by influencing digoxin binding at the active receptor sites. They will vary from patient to patient, and also from one occasion to another in each individual. It should also be added that fibrillation itself can mask some aspects of toxicity, for coupled ventricular beats tend not to occur with an irregular rhythm, and there can be no prolongation of PR interval. The overlap in concentrations may be regarded as having a clinical counterpart; for just as no arbitrary figure divides therapeutic from toxic blood levels, so therapeutic effect and toxicity themselves merge without clear demarcation one into the other. However, the majority of estimations fall outside the doubtful range, and in practice plasma estimations can be of considerable help in the diagnosis of toxicity.

A poor correlation was found between plasma concentration of digoxin and the ventricular response to atrial fibrillation. The subjects in the slower rate group had a mean plasma digoxin level of 1·6 ± S.D. 0·7 ng/ml compared with a mean of 1·2 ± 0·7 ng/ml for the patients with the faster rates, but the ranges were similar. However, patients with atrial fibrillation do not comprise a homogeneous group, and the conductivity of the A-V junctional pathways varies widely from patient to patient independently of drugs. Thus their requirement for digoxin will vary, for in those with relatively slow rates undigitalized, the effect of the drug summates with the effect of impaired conductivity; such patients will usually be controlled at lower plasma concentrations than are required for those whose ventricular response tends to be rapid. The summation may be responsible not only for undue slowing in atrial fibrillation, but also for varying degrees of A-V block, and may be interpreted as undue sensitivity to digoxin.

Having regard to this difficulty, we re-examined our data, and selected 44 patients in whom we had electrocardiographic evidence of rapid heart rates (120 beats per minute or faster) either at rest or during exercise during the 12-month period before digoxin levels were measured. In this group we had evidence that conductivity through the junctional pathways was not seriously impaired, and that the slowed ventricular response was likely to be related in large degree to the drug and not to disease of the A-V node. Plasma digoxin concentration was plotted against heart rate (Figure 2) and a clear tendency was observed within the group for those with slower rates to have higher plasma digoxin levels.

The therapeutic range of values for plasma digoxin concentrations

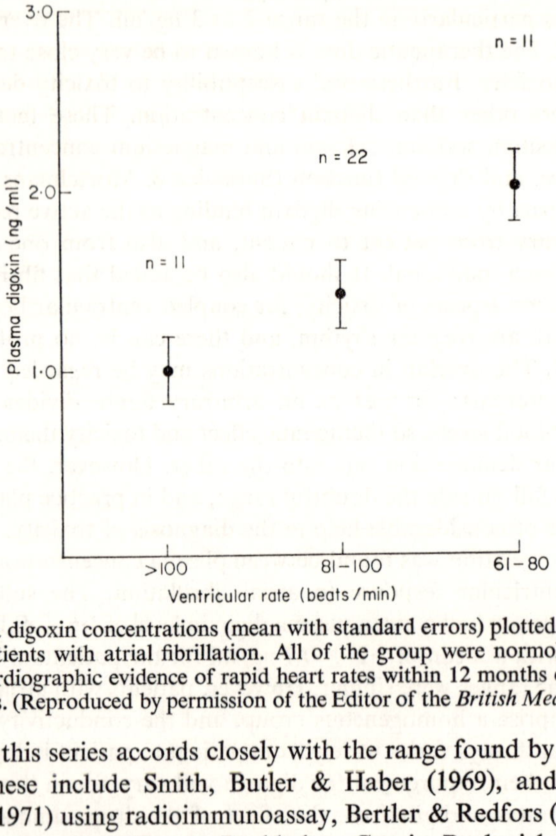


FIG. 2. Plasma digoxin concentrations (mean with standard errors) plotted against heart rate in 44 patients with atrial fibrillation. All of the group were normokalaemic and had electrocardiographic evidence of rapid heart rates within 12 months of the plasma measurements. (Reproduced by permission of the Editor of the *British Medical Journal*.)

reported in this series accords closely with the range found by most other workers; these include Smith, Butler & Haber (1969), and Evered & Chapman (1971) using radioimmunoassay, Bertler & Redfors (1971) using a rubidium assay, and Marcus, Burkhalter, Cuccia, Pavlovich & Kapadia (1966), who administered tritiated digoxin to patients and subsequently measured directly the radioactivity in their serum.

A wide measure of agreement also exists on the levels associated with digoxin toxicity. However, the extent of the overlap in concentrations between patients regarded as having toxicity and those without toxicity was greater in the series reported by Beller *et al.* (1971). These workers conducted a prospective study of 135 patients taking cardiac glycosides:

the diagnosis of toxicity depended upon ECG criteria evaluated by an investigator who was unaware of the corresponding plasma concentrations. The mean serum digoxin concentration in patients with 'definite' toxicity was 2·3 ± 1·6 ng/ml, compared with 1·0 ± 0·5 ng/ml in the non-toxic patients. Although the difference for the groups has highly significant ($p < 0{\cdot}005$), 29% of those classified as toxic had serum digoxin levels less than 1·7 ng/ml (or serum digitoxin levels correspondingly low). Two reasons were advanced for the unexpectedly large overlap: first, the prospective design of the study removed a tendency to include only the most floridly toxic patients; and second, some patients who still showed arrhythmias had omitted digitalis for as long as 48 hours before inclusion into the trial. To these may be added a third unavoidable criticism: no arrhythmia is pathognomonic of digitalis toxicity, and a diagnosis of 'definite' digitalis toxicity on ECG evidence alone is strictly untenable. Furthermore, some of the listed criteria cannot be regarded as stringent.

**Tissue Concentrations of Digoxin**

The assumption has usually been made that tissue rather than plasma concentrations determine the activity of digitalis, and it may be questioned how closely plasma digoxin levels reflect concentrations in the myocardium. Coltart, Howard & Chamberlain (1972) obtained samples of plasma and of papillary muscle from eight patients undergoing mitral valve replacement. The ratio of myocardial to plasma levels varied between individuals from 39:1 to 155:1. Doherty, Perkins & Flanigan (1967) found lower ratios using short-term experiments with tritiated digoxin, but the degree of variation in their series was similar. The relationship between plasma and myocardial concentrations is therefore inconsistent. However, it has been suggested that only about 10% of digoxin is bound to active sites (Kuschinsky, Lahrtz, Lüllman & van Zwieten, 1967) where it can exert a therapeutic effect; the greater part may be fixed to tissue in a non-specific manner. Whether or not the actively bound glycoside comprises a constant proportion remains to be shown. Meanwhile, it cannot be assumed that total myocardial concentrations would provide a better index of therapeutic effect than plasma concentrations.

**Dosage and Plasma Concentrations**

Digoxin is excreted in the urine, principally in an unchanged form (Marcus, Kapadia & Kapadia, 1964). In the presence of normal, or near-normal, renal function it would therefore be expected that dose should be the most important determinant of plasma concentration. Such is usually the case. Figure 3 shows plasma digoxin plotted against daily maintenance dose in 68 patients who had blood urea levels less than 40 mg/100 ml.

Patients receiving 0·125 mg daily had a mean level of 0·5 ± 0·2 ng/ml; with 0·25 to 0·375 mg daily, the level was 0·9 ± 0·4 ng/ml; with 0·5 mg, it was 1·5 ± 0·4 ng/ml; and with 0·625 to 0·75 mg, it was 2·1 ± 0·6 ng/ml. ($r = 0{\cdot}783$; $p < 0{\cdot}001$). It will be noted that 0·5 mg daily given to subjects without evidence of renal impairment provides concentrations below those

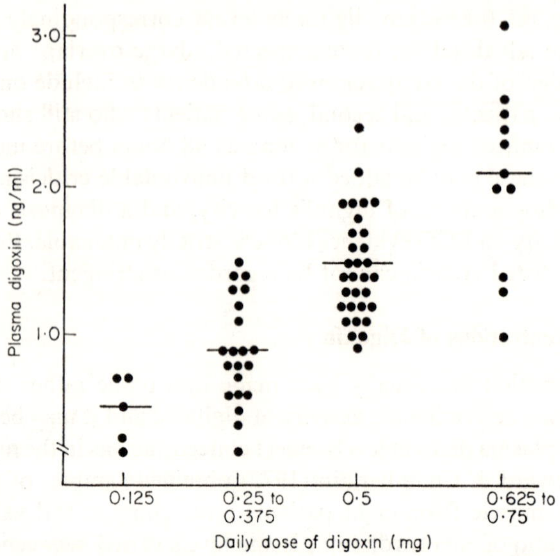


FIG. 3. Plasma digoxin concentrations plotted against oral dose of digoxin in 68 patients. All had normal or near-normal renal function. The horizontal bars represent mean values. (Reproduced by permission of the Editor of the *British Medical Journal*.)

usually associated with toxicity. Under these conditions it is therefore a safe dose, but not infrequently a dose of 0·75 mg daily is required especially in the control of atrial fibrillation. It can be seen from Figure 3 that some subjects who require this relatively large dose did not attain the expected high plasma concentrations.

### Uncontrolled Atrial Fibrillation at Usual Doses

Patients in atrial fibrillation who have a rapid ventricular response despite apparently adequate doses of digoxin do pose a problem in clinical practice. The problem is illustrated by an example (Figure 4) which shows electrocardiograms from two patients, both of whom were symptomatic with heart rates of 120 per minute. Patient A.S. (upper strip) had impaired renal function, and was on a maintenance dose of 0·25 mg daily. The plasma concentration was 2·9 ng/ml. Within two days of the recording, and before the digoxin level was known, he had developed manifest toxicity. Patient M.I. (lower strip) was receiving 0·75 mg digoxin daily, but despite this large dose the concentration was only 0·7 ng/ml. The dose was therefore increased to 1·0 mg per day. He has no manifestations of toxicity, and his rate has slowed on the larger dose. Thus one patient had

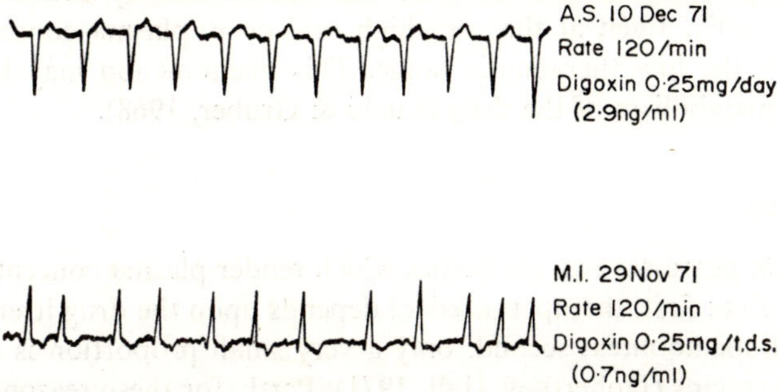


FIG. 4. The electrocardiograms of two patients with atrial fibrillation and a rapid ventricular response (120/min). The upper patient was taking 0·25 mg digoxin per day and had a high plasma concentration. The lower patient was taking 0·75 mg digoxin per day and had a low plasma concentration. See text for details.

true refractory rapid atrial fibrillation; the other failed to achieve an adequate blood level despite a large maintenance dose. In both, plasma digoxin concentrations provided a valuable guide to optimal dose requirements.

It is becoming increasingly evident that a small minority of subjects do require unusually large doses. This occurs in malabsorption syndromes

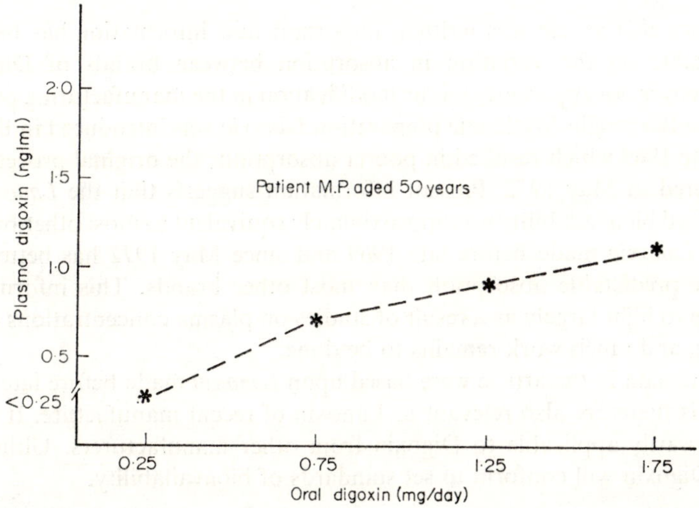


FIG. 5. Plasma concentrations plotted against daily maintenance dose of digoxin in patient M.P. See text for details. (The data were kindly supplied by Dr. T. R. D. Shaw.)

(Heizer, Smith & Goldfinger, 1970), and rarely in patients without evidence of malabsorption. An example of a patient who did not respond adequately to conventional doses of digoxin is shown in Figure 5; she had no evidence of gastrointestinal disease. The figure shows plasma concentrations plotted against maintenance dose which was incremented slowly from 0·25 mg to 1·75 mg daily. Even at the very high oral dose, plasma concentrations remain in the low therapeutic range. This phenomenon may be due to unusual metabolism of the drug (Luchi & Gruber, 1968).

**Conclusion**

Digoxin possesses two properties which render plasma concentration of special value: first, therapeutic effect depends upon the drug itself and not on active metabolites; second, only a very small proportion is bound to plasma proteins (Doherty & Hall, 1971). Partly for these reasons, plasma concentrations have provided an invaluable tool in recent years for research into the clinical pharmacology of digoxin. They can also provide a measure of therapeutic activity useful in clinical practice, especially as an aid for determining optimal doses in malabsorption syndromes and renal failure, in the diagnosis of toxicity, and as a guide to the treatment of refractory fast atrial fibrillation. However, one cannot emphasize too strongly that the measurements must be considered in the full clinical context, and not taken as the sole arbiter of dosage.

**Addendum**

Since this article was written, important new information has become available on the variation in absorption between brands of Digoxin. Moreover, an apparently minor modification in the manufacturing process of the Burroughs Wellcome preparation *Lanoxin* was introduced in Britain in late 1969 which resulted in poorer absorption; the original process was restored in May 1972. Present information suggests that the *Lanoxin* of reduced bioavailability was approximately equivalent to most other brands. The *Lanoxin* made before late 1969 and since May 1972 has better and more predictable absorption than most other brands. This information came to light largely as a result of studies on plasma concentrations of the drug, and much work remains to be done.

The data in the article were based upon *Lanoxin* made before late 1969, and is therefore also relevant to Lanoxin of recent manufacture. It is not necessarily applicable to Digoxin from other manufacturers. Ultimately all Digoxin will conform to set standards of bioavailability.

## REFERENCES

BELLER, G. A., SMITH, T. W., ABELMANN, W. H., HABER, E., & HOOD, W. B. (1971). Digitalis intoxication. A prospective clinical study with serum level correlations. *New Eng. J. Med.*, **284**, 989–997.

BERTLER, A. & REDFORS, A. (1971), Plasma levels of digoxin in relation to toxicity. *Acta Pharm. Tox.*, **29**, Suppl. 3, 281–287.

CHAMBERLAIN, D. A., WHITE, R. J., HOWARD, M. R. & SMITH, T. W. (1970). Plasma digoxin concentrations in patients with atrial fibrillation. *Brit. med. J.*, **3**, 429–432.

COLTART, D. J., HOWARD, M. R. & CHAMBERLAIN, D. A. (1972). Myocardial and skeletal muscle concentrations of digoxin in patients on long-term therapy. *Brit. med. J.*, **2**, 318–319.

DOHERTY, J. E. & HALL, W. H. (1971). Tritiated digoxin XV. Serum protein binding in human subjects. *Amer. J. Cardiol.*, **28**, 326–330.

DOHERTY, J. E., PERKINS, W. H. & FLANIGAN, W. J. (1967). The distribution and concentration of tritiated digoxin in human tissues. *Ann. intern. Med.*, **66**, 116–124.

EVERED, D. C. & CHAPMAN, C. (1971). Plasma digoxin concentrations and digoxin toxicity in hospital patients. *Brit. Heart J.*, **33**, 540–545.

HEIZER, W. D., SMITH, T. W., & GOLDFINGER, S. E. (1970). Absorption of digoxin in patients with malabsorption syndromes. *New Eng. J. Med.*, **285**, 257–259.

KUSCHINSKY, K., LAHRTZ, H., LÜLLMAN, H. & VAN ZWIETEN, P. A. (1967). Accumulation and release of $^3$H-digoxin by guinea-pig heart muscle. *Brit. J. Pharmacol.*, **30**, 317–328.

LUCHI, R. J. & GRUBER, J. W. (1968). Unusually large digitalis requirements. A study of altered digoxin metabolism. *Amer. J. Med.*, **45**, 322–328.

MARCUS, F. I., BURKHALTER, L., CUCCIA, C., PAVLOVICH, J. & KAPADIA, G. G. (1966). Administration of tritiated digoxin with and without a loading dose: a metabolic study. *Circulation*, **34**, 865–874.

MARCUS, F. I., KAPADIA, G. J. & KAPADIA, G. G. (1964). The metabolism of digoxin in normal subjects. *J. Pharmacol.*, **145**, 203–209.

SMITH, T. W., BUTLER, V. P. & HABER, E. (1969). Determination of therapeutic and toxic serum digoxin concentrations by radioimmunoassay *New Eng. J. Med.*, **281**, 1212–1216.

SURAWICZ, B. & MORTELMANS, S. (1969). Factors affecting individual tolerance to digitalis. In: *Digitalis*, ed. by Surawicz, B. & Fisch, C., p. 127. New York: Grune and Stratton.

ELEVEN

# Measurement of Plasma Warfarin Concentrations in Clinical Practice

A. BRECKENRIDGE AND M. L'E. ORME

*Department of Clinical Pharmacology &*
*MRC Clinical Pharmacology Research Group,*
*Royal Postgraduate Medical School, DuCane Road, London, W12*

**Introduction**

The rationale for anticoagulant therapy is that interference with haemostasis decreases the morbidity and mortality of thromboembolic disorders. In 1972, 20 years after the introduction of oral anticoagulants, their mode of action, the relationship between plasma concentration and pharmacological effect and even their therapeutic efficacy are still subjects of controversy.

Oral anticoagulants fall into two chemical groups: coumarins, of which warfarin is the most widely used, and indanediones, for example, phenindione. Because of its slower rate of elimination, allowing once daily administration, and the lower incidence of toxic effects (apart from haemorrhage) warfarin is more frequently used.

Three aspects of warfarin therapy are reviewed in this paper: (1) The basis of inter-individual differences in the response to warfarin. (2) Clinical situations where measurement of plasma warfarin concentrations are of value are considered. (3) Animal data are presented on the pharmacokinetics and pharmacodynamics of two enantiomers of warfarin, and implications of these are discussed. Two initial points must be made, however. The pharmacological response to warfarin, as measured by the prothrombin time or a variant of this, is an indirect index of its action, reflecting both the decay of clotting factors already present in the liver and plasma and the repression of the synthesis of these clotting factors which is considered to be the direct action of oral anticoagulants (O'Reilly & Aggeler, 1970). Measurement of plasma concentration of warfarin also presents problems. Two widely used methods (O'Reilly *et al.*, 1963; Corn & Berberich, (1967) measure not only warfarin but also warfarin metabolites. In the studies reported in this paper, unchanged warfarin was measured according to the method of Lewis, Ilnicki & Carlstrom (1970) and anticoagulant control by the thrombotest method of Owren (1959).

## I. Inter-individual Differences in the Response to Warfarin

### (a) *Differences in the Pharmacological Response*

If a drug acts by a reversible mechanism, differences in drug plasma concentration producing the same pharmacological response may be equated with differences in receptor sensitivity, irrespective of the dose of drug or the rate of its metabolism, provided that there are no marked inter-individual differences in the liver-plasma warfarin ratio.

The steady-state plasma concentration of warfarin was measured in

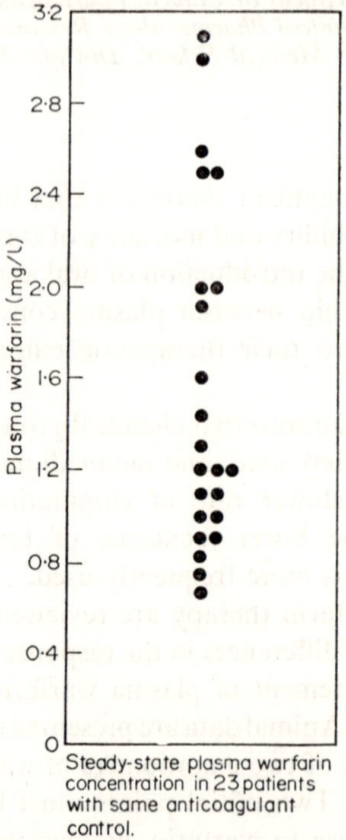


FIG. 1. Steady-state plasma warfarin concentration in 23 patients with the same anticoagulant control (thrombotest 5–8%).

23 patients, each of whom had been taking the drug for at least three months, and each of whom had the same degree of anticoagulant control (thrombotest 5–8%). Twice-weekly blood samples were taken into plastic syringes and collected in sodium citrate. The results shown in Figure 1 are the mean plasma warfarin concentrations in eight such samples taken from each patient. No patient was taking any drug which would interfere either with anticoagulant control or plasma warfarin concentration. Plasma warfarin concentrations range from 0·6 to 3·1 mg/l, representing a five-fold inter-individual difference.

(b) *Differences in Warfarin Kinetics*

(1) *Relationship between the dose of warfarin and the steady-state plasma warfarin concentration.* The steady-state plasma concentration of a drug ($C_{ss}$) is related to the dose (D), the fraction of the dose absorbed (F), the half-life of drug elimination ($t\frac{1}{2}$), the apparent volume of distribution (VD) and the dosing interval ($\Delta_t$) according to the following equation (Wagner *et al.*, 1965).

$$C_{ss} = \frac{1 \cdot 44 \times F \times D \times t\frac{1}{2}}{VD \times \Delta_t}$$

In the 23 patients, the relationship between the steady state plasma warfarin concentration and the dose of warfarin was examined. Figure 2 shows

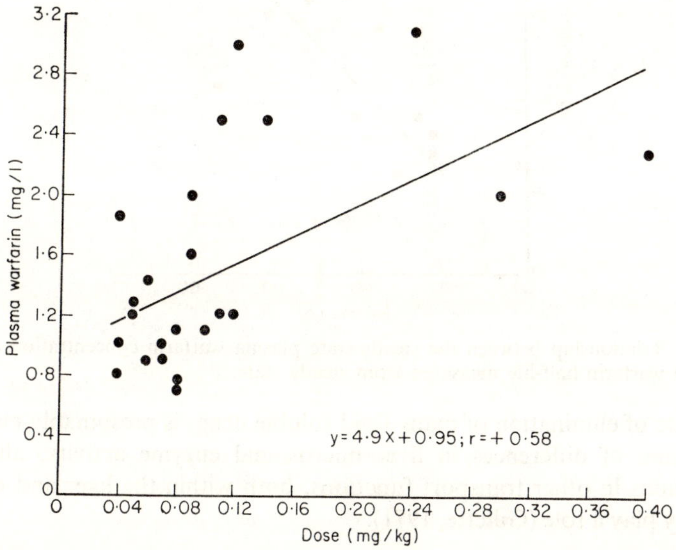


FIG. 2. Relationship between the steady-state plasma warfarin concentration and the dose of warfarin in 23 patients.

a poor correlation between these two parameters (r = + 0·58). Since warfarin is well absorbed in man, (O'Reilly *et al.*, 1962) and the dosing interval is the same in each patient, this implies inter-individual differences in the rate of warfarin elimination, or in the apparent volume of distribution of warfarin, or in both.

(2) *Relationship between the steady state plasma warfarin concentration, the plasma half-life and the apparent volume of distribution.* In 12 of these 23 patients the plasma warfarin half-life was measured from steady state by stopping warfarin for 96 h and obtaining 5 or 6 blood samples over this time. The half-life was calculated by a least squares method using a computer programme.

Figure 3 shows a better correlation between steady state plasma warfarin concentration and plasma warfarin half-life ($r = +0{\cdot}78$) than between the plasma concentration and dose. Interindividual variations in

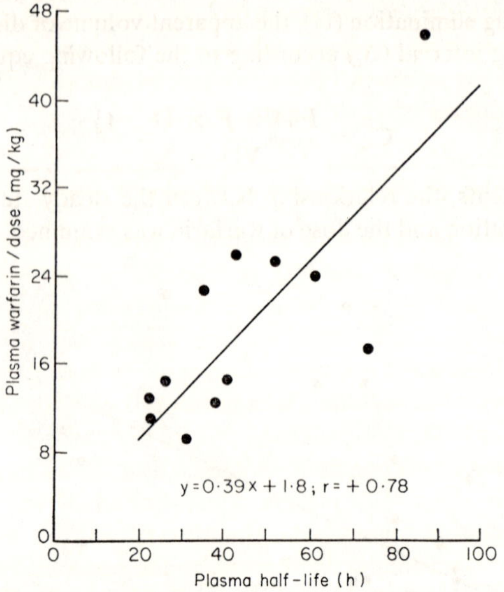


FIG. 3. Relationship between the steady-state plasma warfarin concentration and the plasma warfarin half-life measured from steady state.

the rate of elimination of many lipid soluble drugs is presumably mainly a reflection of differences in liver microsomal enzyme activity, although variations in other transport functions, both within the liver and outside it, may play a role (Gillette, 1971).

TABLE 1. *Kinetics of warfarin in 12 patients*

| Patient | Plasma half-life (h) | Dose of warfarin (mg/kg/day) | Steady state concentration (mg/l) | Apparent VD (l) | % body weight |
|---|---|---|---|---|---|
| 1 | 42·8 | 0·22 | 3·1 | 8·0 | 13·9 |
| 2 | 60·7 | 0·05 | 0·9 | 11·2 | 18·2 |
| 3 | 87·3 | 0·04 | 1·1 | 9·7 | 14·5 |
| 4 | 70·5 | 0·14 | 3·4 | 10·5 | 12·3 |
| 5 | 67·3 | 0·11 | 2·5 | 9·1 | 12·3 |
| 6 | 53·1 | 0·12 | 3·1 | 7·1 | 8·5 |
| 7 | 49·3 | 0·09 | 1·1 | 8·7 | 17·0 |
| 8 | 32·6 | 0·15 | 1·1 | 17·7 | 18·7 |
| 9 | 42·3 | 0·04 | 0·7 | 10·6 | 14·8 |
| 10 | 20·2 | 0·08 | 1·0 | 6·7 | 6·4 |
| 11 | 21·2 | 0·09 | 1·1 | 3·2 | 7·2 |
| 12 | 29·6 | 0·07 | 1·1 | 4·8 | 8·0 |

From a knowledge of the steady-state plasma warfarin concentration and the plasma warfarin half-life measured from that steady state, the apparent volume of distribution of warfarin can be calculated. The results in Table 1 show a variation in this parameter from 6·4% to 18·7% of body weight. Reasons for this variation are at present under study. In this context, it should be remembered that all subjects studied here were patients requiring warfarin for cardiovascular disease; little is known of the effects of disease on distribution of drugs.

## II. Clinical Value of Measurement of Plasma Warfarin Concentrations

In view of the precision with which the pharmacological effect of warfarin can be measured, and the inter-individual kinetic and dynamic variations outlined above, there are few clinical situations in which measurement of plasma levels of warfarin are useful.

The first of these is the documentation of warfarin resistance. Hereditary resistance to oral anticoagulants in man was first described by O'Reilly and his colleagues in 1964. This patient was found to require 145 mg of warfarin per day to achieve anticoagulant control, a dose 25–30 times greater than the usual daily dose. The plasma concentration of warfarin was high (55 mg/l), suggesting there was no alteration of warfarin metabolism. The patient, however, was markedly sensitive to the antidotal action of vitamin K. Prior to anticoagulant therapy, the level of factors II, VII, IX and X in this patient were low. Studies of the family showed that the trait was inherited. In 1969, O'Reilly described a second family showing warfarin resistance. 18 of 40 family members were resistant to a large dose of warfarin, and since male-to-male transmission of the gene was shown, a gene location on the X chromosome was ruled out, confirming an autosomal dominant mode of inheritance. Studies in rats, where a similar type of resistence has been demonstrated, suggest that the biochemical basis for this resistance is a genetic mutation in the vitamin K–warfarin receptor site (Pool *et al.*, 1968).

There are other causes of resistance to warfarin. If the rate of warfarin metabolism is increased by microsomal enzyme inducing agents, such as barbiturates, or the level of vitamin K dependent clotting factors is increased, as found in pregnancy or after administration of oral contraceptives, a large dose of warfarin may be required to achieve anticoagulant control. To distinguish such patients from those with hereditary resistance, in these situations, measurement of plasma warfarin concentrations may be helpful.

Figure 4 shows details of such a patient who required between 180 and 200 mg warfarin/day to achieve anticoagulant control. This lady of 55 years was found to have a plasma warfarin concentration of between

2·0 and 2·5 mg/l while taking 180 mg warfarin/day. Her prothrombin time varied between 20 and 25 s. It is worth comparing this data from one of the patients with hereditary resistance to warfarin (Table 2). Further questioning of this patient revealed that for many months she had been in the habit of taking nightly tuinal, a mixture of quinalbarbitone and amylobarbitone. When this was withdrawn, her warfarin requirements steadily fell from 180 mg to 25 mg/day, although there was no significant change in either anticoagulant control or in plasma warfarin concentration. The plasma warfarin half-life in this patient six months after withdrawal of barbiturates was 17·5 h. Since the steady-state plasma warfarin

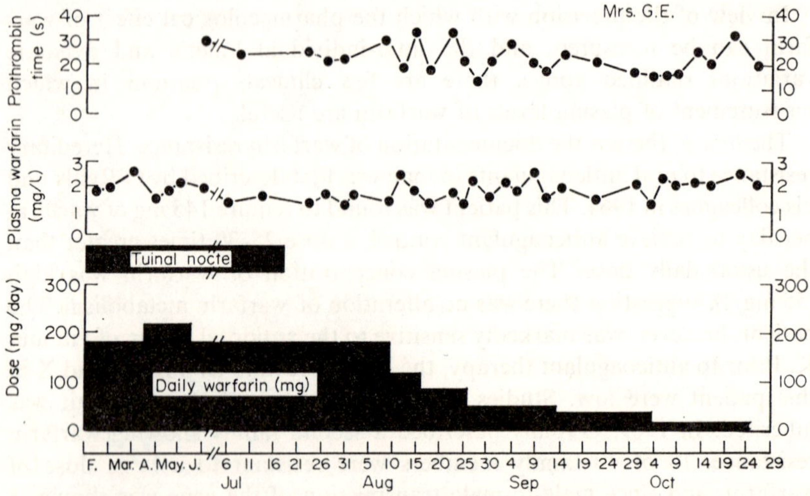


FIG. 4. Patient with resistance to warfarin, showing change in warfarin dose on stopping inducing agent.

concentration was 2·2 mg/l and the required dose of warfarin 29 mg/kg/day, this data falls very close to the line of identity in Figure 3.

The second situation where measurement of plasma warfarin concentrations is of practical value is in the understanding of drug interactions with warfarin. An example of the administration of an enzyme inducing agent altering warfarin metabolism is given above. If the dose of warfarin is kept constant throughout the time that the inducing agent is given, there will be a fall in both steady-state warfarin concentration and in the degree of anticoagulant control. If the steady-state plasma concentration of warfarin has been measured prior to and during administration of the hypnotic agent, the fall in steady-state warfarin concentration provides indirect evidence of an increased rate of warfarin metabolism. This should be complemented with other measurements of change in warfarin metabolism, such as an increase in the rate of formation of warfarin metabolites, as we have shown when antipyrine is given to patients taking warfarin (Breckenridge, Orme, Thorgeirsson, Davies & Brooks, 1971).

Measurement of plasma warfarin concentrations is important in studying the effect of an agent which displaces warfarin from sites of protein binding. Displaced warfarin gives rise to an enhanced pharmacological effect, but is also more available for metabolism within the liver. This gives rise to discrepancy between the prothrombin time and the plasma warfarin concentration. In such studies it is important to measure both these parameters regularly over the first few days of administration of the displacing agent, as a new (lower) steady state warfarin concentration is

TABLE 2. *Warfarin resistance*

| | Patient 1* | Patient 2 |
|---|---|---|
| Dose (mg/day) | 145 | 180 |
| Prothrombin time (s) | 23 | 25 |
| Plasma warfarin concentration (mg/l) | 55 | 2·2 |

* O'Reilly *et al.* (1964)

soon achieved. One of the best examples of warfarin displacement is when chloral hydrate is administered (Sellers & Koch-Weser, 1970). Chloral hydrate is metabolized to trichloracetic acid which is strongly bound to plasma albumin, displacing the warfarin, resulting in a lower level of warfarin in plasma but an augmentation of the prothrombin time.

The third situation where measurement of plasma warfarin concentrations is of clinical value, is in patients who have surreptitiously taken the anticoagulant to produce haemorrhagic manifestations. A few such patients have been described (O'Reilly & Aggeler, 1970), and if warfarin is found in measureable quantities in the plasma, more complex haematological analysis of the haemorrhagic problem becomes unnecessary.

## III. Pharmacokinetics and Pharmacodynamics of the Enantiomers of Warfarin

Commercially available warfarin is a racemic mixture of two enantiomers: R (+) and S (—) warfarin. These enantiomers were resolved in 1966 by Eble, West & Link. It was also shown by these workers that (—) warfarin was five to six times more potent than (+) warfarin. Recently we have investigated the reason for this difference in anticoagulant potency (Breckenridge & Orme, 1972). Firstly, we measured the rate of elimination of these enantiomers in male rats given the drugs by tail vein injection. The plasma half-life of (+) warfarin was found to be 8·6 h and of (—) warfarin 15·2 h. Further, there was no difference in the apparent volume of distribution of the warfarins, which is in keeping with the recent observation of O'Reilly (1971) that the albumin-binding of the two enantiomers does not differ. Secondly, we examined the relative anticoagulant potency of the two enantiomers using the pharmacokinetic approach outlined by Nagashima, O'Reilly & Levy (1969) which is described by Dr. Levy elsewhere in this volume. By this technique, the effect of warfarin on the rate of clotting factor synthesis can be calculated. (—) warfarin was shown to

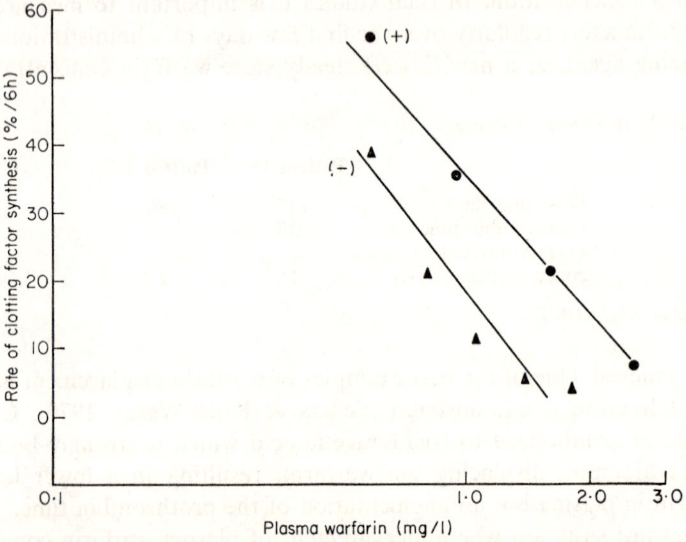


FIG. 5. Effect of (+) and (—) warfarin on prothrombin complex synthesis in male rats.*

be 1·9 more potent than (+) warfarin at similar plasma warfarin concentrations (Figure 5). Thus there are two causes for the difference in anticoagulant potency of the warfarin isomers. These differences have interesting implications for the pharmacokinetic and pharmacodynamics of warfarin in man.

## Conclusions

(1) There are wide inter-individual variations in the sensitivity to warfarin, in the rate of warfarin elimination and in the apparent volume of distribution of warfarin.

(2) Because of these differences and because the pharmacological effect of warfarin can be easily measured, there are few situations where measurement of plasma warfarin concentrations are of value. There are in the study of resistance to warfarin, in documentation of drug interactions involving warfarin and in the detection of patients who take warfarin surreptitiously.

* Reproduced by permission of *Life Sciences*.

(3) In the rat, the enantiomers of warfarin have a different anticoagulant potency which depends partly on a different rate of elimination and partly on a different effect on clotting factor synthesis.

We are grateful to Dr. Paul Turner and Dr. Peter Storey of St. Bartholomew's Hospital for permission to publish details of their patient with warfarin resistance.

We thank Mrs. Wendy Watts for technical assistance. This work was supported by the Medical Research Council.

## REFERENCES

BRECKENRIDGE, A. & ORME, M. L'E. (1972). The plasma half-lives and the pharmacological effect of the enantiomers of warfarin in rats. *Life Sciences*, **2,** Part 2, 337–345.

BRECKENRIDGE, A., ORME, M. L'E., THORGEIRSSON, S., DAVIES, D. S. & BROOKS, R. V. (1971). Drug interactions with warfarin. *Clinical Science*, **40,** 351–364.

CORN, M. & BERBERICH, R. (1967). Rapid fluorometric assay for warfarin. *Clin. Chemistry*, **13,** 126–131.

EBLE, J. N., WEST, B. D. & LINK, K. P. (1966). A comparison of the isomers of warfarin. *Biochemical Pharmacology*, **15,** 1003–1006.

GILLETTE, J. R. (1971). Factors affecting drug metabolism. *Ann. N.Y. Acad. Sci.*, **179,** 43–66.

LEWIS, R. J., ILNICKI, L. P. & CARLSTROM, M. (1970). The assay of warfarin in plasma or stool. *Biochem. Medicine*, **4,** 376–382.

NAGASHIMA, R., O'REILLY, R. A. & LEVY, G. (1969). Kinetics of pharmacological effects in man: the anticoagulant action of warfarin. *Clin. Pharm. Ther.*, **10,** 22–35.

O'REILLY, R. A. (1971). Interaction of several coumarin compounds with human and canine plasma albumin. *Molecular Pharmacology*, **7,** 209–212.

O'REILLY, R. A. & AGGELER, P. M. (1970). Determinants of the response to oral anticoagulants in man. *Pharmacological Reviews*, **22,** 35–96.

O'REILLY, R. A., AGGELER, P. M., HOAG, M. S. & LEONG, L. (1962). Studies on the coumarin anticoagulants: the assay of warfarin and its biological application. *Thrombosis et Diathesis Haemorrhagica*, **8,** 82–95.

O'REILLY, R. A., AGGELER, P. M., HOAG, M. S. & LEONG, L. (1964). Hereditary transmission of exceptional resistance to coumarin anticoagulant drugs. *New Eng. J. Med.*, **271,** 809–815.

OWREN, P. A. (1959). Thrombotest, a new method for controlling anticoagulant therapy. *Lancet*, **2,** 754–758.

POOL, J. G., O'REILLY, R. A., SCHNEIDERMAN, L. J. & ALEXANDER, M. (1968). Warfarin resistance in the rat. *Amer. J. Physiol.*, **215,** 627–631.

SELLERS, E. M. & KOCH-WESER, J. (1970). Displacement from albumin and potentiation of warfarin by five acidic drugs. *Clinical Research*, **18**, 344.

WAGNER, J. G., NORTHAM, J. I., ALWAY, C. D. & CARPENTER, D. S. (1965). Blood levels of drug at equilibrium state after multiple dosing. *Nature*, **207**, 1301–1302.

# Discussion: Therapeutic Use of Cardiovascular Drugs

PROFESSOR OATES You said that patients with heart failure have a smaller volume of distribution of lignocaine. This implies that there is less drug in tissues outside the plasma compartment. Some of these tissues may be those where the drug has its action, like the brain and the heart, so that there might be poor distribution to the site of action of the drug. Could you comment on that?

PROFESSOR MELMON In all probability organs such as heart and brain are preferentially perfused in congestive heart failure. Therefore with a raised concentration of the drug in plasma one would expect to see an increased therapeutic effect.

PROFESSOR CROOKS (DUNDEE) I have a question about digitalis toxicity. There is a rumour that the elderly are much more sensitive to digitalis and possibly to drugs in general. The practice of giving elderly patients paediatric doses—very small doses—has begun. I would like to ask Dr. Chamberlain if there is any evidence that the elderly are more sensitive to this drug.

DR. CHAMBERLAIN We took two groups of patients who had been in rapid atrial fibrillation and who were adequately controlled with digoxin. A group aged 32 to 59, and a group aged 60 to 84. In these two groups, the slowing of atrial fibrillation was very well matched at very similar mean plasma levels. However, I want to stress one point: although the elderly had the same plasma levels as the younger patients these were achieved with lower doses. The elderly had lower doses because, on average, they had less good renal function, so that the most important cause of their apparent sensitivity is that the elderly tend to have poor renal function. There is one other factor which plays a part. It is very common in the elderly to have disorders of the conducting system, either sino-atrial or atrioventricular. A patient who has a heart rate of 110, without any glycoside, will come under control with a plasma level of 0·5, 0·6, or 0·7 ng/ml, a much lower level than in somebody whose heart rate is 150 or 160, because the effect of digoxin is summating with the disease.

Session 3

Chairman: Professor D. A. Price Evans

Therapeutic Use of Antibacterial Drugs

TWELVE

# Dosage Regimens of Sulphonamides Based on Pharmacokinetic Parameters: Principles and Experimental Results

L. DETTLI AND P. SPRING

*Department of Internal Medicine, Buergerspital, 4000 Basel, Switzerland*

## Krueger-Thiemer's Theory on Drug Dosage: a Simplified Presentation

Krueger-Thiemer's theory on the dosage regimen of bacteriostatic agents published 12 years ago (Krueger-Thiemer 1960; 1966) is a milestone in pharmacotherapeutics because it contains the first rational theory on the dosage of reversibly acting drugs. However, most clinicians and even many pharmacologists feel that its mathematical background is too complex to be readily understood. In the following report Krueger-Thiemer's theory is therefore presented in such a way that even the mathematically untrained should be able to understand its principles. For this purpose some of the clinically unimportant complexities which are not necessary for an understanding are replaced by approximations. Furthermore, some experimental results in the field of sulphonamide pharmacokinetics will be discussed. A selective list of the abundant literature is given.

*Assumptions and Postulates*

*The assumptions* are as follows:

1. Except for the transcellular water (e.g. urine, bile) the drug's concentration in the tissue water ($c_t$) after reaching diffusion equilibrium is

identical with the concentration of freely dissolved drug molecules ($c$) in the plasma water (Dettli, 1961):

$$c_t = c \tag{1}$$

2. The rate of drug elimination ($-dm/dt$) is proportional to the amount of drug in the organism ($m$):

$$-dm/dt = k_2' \cdot m \tag{2}$$

$k_2'$ being the overall rate constant of drug elimination.

3. At any time the drug's total concentration in the plasma ($c'$) is proportional to the amount of drug in the organism ($m$):

$$\mathrm{D}/c_0' = m/c' = \mathrm{V}' = \Delta' \cdot \mathrm{G} \tag{3}$$

D is the dose, $c_0'$ the 'apparent initial concentration' at $t = \mathrm{O}$, and V′ a dose-independent constant, the so-called 'absolute distribution volume'. The 'relative distribution volume' $\Delta' = \mathrm{V}'/\mathrm{G}$ relates V′ to the body weight (G).

4. The drug is partly bound to the plasma albumin. A certain fraction ($f$) of its total concentration ($c'$) is unbound:

$$f = c/c' \quad \text{or} \quad c' \cdot f = c \tag{4}$$

5. Only the unbound drug molecules are chemotherapeutically active (Davis & Wood, 1942; Anton, 1960; Newbould & Kilpatrick, 1960; Dettli, 1961)

6. The minimum therapeutically effective concentration of unbound drug molecules ($c_{\min}$) in the tissue water is proportional to its minimum inhibitory concentration ($\mu$) against the infectious agent *in vitro* when a medium free of binding macro-molecules and free of antagonists is used:

$$c_{\min} = \sigma \cdot \mu \tag{5}$$

*The therapeutic postulate* formulates two requirements:

1. $c_{\min}$ should be maintained in the tissue-water during the entire period of therapy.

2. $c_{\min}$ should be reached immediately after starting therapy.

*Continuous drug administration*

*The maintenance dose.* When a drug which is eliminated according to eqn. (2) is administered by continuous infusion, it will accumulate in the organism and eventually approach a final steady-state amount ($m_\infty$). It follows from eqn. (2) (as well as from intuitive reasoning) that $m_\infty$ will be proportional to the dose administered per unit of time ($\mathrm{D}/t$) and inversely proportional to the elimination rate constant ($k_2'$) of the drug (Dost, 1968; Dettli, Spring & Ryter, 1971; Wagner, 1971):

$$m_\infty = \frac{\mathrm{D}/t}{k_2'} \tag{6}$$

The corresponding steady-state concentration in the plasma ($c'_\infty$) is found according to eqn.(3):

$$c'_\infty = \frac{m_\infty}{\Delta' \cdot \mathrm{G}} = \frac{\mathrm{D}/t}{\Delta' \cdot \mathrm{G} \cdot k'_2} \tag{7}$$

It follows from eqn. (1) and eqn. (4) that the steady-state concentration of unbound drug molecules ($c_\infty$) will be:

$$c_\infty = c'_\infty \cdot f = \frac{\mathrm{D}/t \cdot f}{\Delta' \cdot \mathrm{G} \cdot k'_2} \tag{8}$$

According to eqn. (5) the first requirement of the therapeutic postulate is fulfilled when $c_\infty = c_{\min} = \sigma \cdot \mu$. Introducing eqn. (5) into eqn. (8) yields

$$\sigma \cdot \mu = \frac{\mathrm{D}/t \cdot f}{\Delta' \cdot \mathrm{G} \cdot k'_2} \tag{9}$$

The maintenance dose is found by solving eqn. (9) for $\mathrm{D}/t$:

$$\mathrm{D}/t = \sigma \cdot \left( \frac{\mu \cdot \Delta' \cdot \mathrm{G} \cdot k'_2}{f} \right) \tag{10}$$

*The loading dose.* According to the second requirement of the therapeutic postulate the steady-state drug concentration should be reached immediately, rather than after a period of drug accumulation. This is accomplished by the administration of an additional loading dose (D*) at the start of the infusion. It is evident that D* should be equal to the drug amount in the organism after reaching the steady state ($m_\infty$). From $\mathrm{D}^* = m_\infty$ it follows from eqn. (6) (Dettli, Spring & Ryter, 1971):

$$\mathrm{D}^* = m_\infty = \frac{\mathrm{D}/t}{k'_2} \tag{11}$$

*Intermittent Drug Administration*

The equations for intermittent drug administration are much less complex (Dettli, 1970) when the discussion is restricted to completely absorbed drugs (i.e. the absorbed fraction of the dose $\delta = 1{\cdot}0$) and when the absorption rate ($k_1$) is much greater than the elimination rate (i.e. $k_1 \gg k_2$ or $k_1 \rightarrow \infty$ as in the case of i.v. administration). Immediately after the administration of the first dose (D) the amount of drug in the organism ($m_{0,1}$) will be

$$m_{0,1} = \mathrm{D} \tag{12}$$

During the dosage interval ($\tau$) the dose will be partly eliminated; a certain fraction (p) will remain in the organism (Augsberger, 1954). Consequently, the drug amount at the end of the first dosage interval ($m_{\tau,1}$) will be:

$$m_{\tau,1} = \mathrm{D} \cdot p \tag{13}$$

Since $0 < p < 1$ algebraic theory predicts that the drug amount in the organism at the beginning of the dosage intervals ($m_{0,n}$) will increase with each additional dose in the form of a geometric series and eventually approach the following finite steady-state value ($m_{0,\infty}$):

$$m_{0,\infty} = D \cdot \frac{1}{1-p} \tag{14}$$

Evidently the amount of drug at the end of the dosage intervals ($m_{\tau,\infty}$) must be p times smaller (see eqn. (12) and eqn. (13)). The corresponding drug concentration in the plasma water ($c_{\tau,\infty}$) is found by introducing eqn. (3) and (4). It follows

$$c_{\tau,\infty} = \frac{D \cdot f}{\Delta' \cdot G} \cdot \frac{p}{1-p} \tag{15}$$

$c_{\tau,\infty}$ should be equal to the minimal therapeutically effective concentration described by eqn. (5):

$$c_{\tau,\infty} = c_{\min} = \sigma \cdot \mu \tag{16}$$

When $t = \tau$ it follows from eqn. (2):

$$p = e^{-k_2' \cdot \tau} \tag{17}$$

The maintenance dose is found by solving eqn. (15) for D after introducing eqn. (16) and eqn. (17):

$$D = \sigma \cdot \left(\frac{\mu}{f} \cdot \Delta' \cdot G \cdot \frac{1 - e^{-k_2' \cdot \tau}}{e^{-k_2' \cdot \tau}}\right) \tag{18}$$

The correct loading dose must be equal to $m_{0,\infty}$ and is thus found from eqns. (14) and (17):

$$D^* = m_{0,\infty} = D \cdot \frac{1}{1 - e^{-k_2' \cdot \tau}} \tag{19}$$

## Krueger-Thiemer's Original Equations

Krueger-Thiemer's dosage equations appear somewhat more complex for the case of continuous drug administration:

$$D/t = \sigma \cdot \left[\frac{\mu \cdot M}{1000}\left(w + \frac{\beta \cdot p}{K'' + c_{\min}}\right)\frac{\Delta' \cdot G \cdot k_2'}{\delta}\right] \tag{20}$$

$$D^* = \frac{D/t}{k_2'} \tag{21}$$

and still more complex for the case of intermittent administration:

$$D = \sigma \cdot \left[\frac{\mu . M}{1000} \cdot \left(w + \frac{\beta \cdot p}{K'' + c_{\min}}\right) \cdot \frac{\Delta' \cdot G}{\delta} \cdot \frac{\left(1 - \frac{k_2'}{k_1'}\right) \cdot (1 - e^{-k_1' \cdot \tau}) \cdot (1 - e^{-k_2' \cdot \tau})}{e^{-k_2' \cdot \tau} - e^{-k_1' \cdot \tau}}\right] \tag{22}$$

$$D^* = D \cdot \frac{1}{(1 - e^{-k_2' \cdot \tau})(1 - e^{-k_1' \cdot \tau})} \tag{23}$$

However, the difference in complexity is more apparent than real when the following approximation is introduced: Krueger-Thiemer considers the fact that the fraction of unbound drug molecules ($f$) is not a true concentration-independent constant. Instead, $f$ depends on the law of mass action as follows:

$$f = \frac{c}{c'} = \frac{1}{w + \dfrac{\beta \cdot p}{K'' + c_{min}}} \tag{24}$$

$\beta$ is the apparent maximum binding capacity of albumin for the drug, K″ is the dissociation constant of the drug-albumin complex, $p$ is the plasma albumin concentration and $w$ is the water content of plasma. However, the error introduced by substituting eqn. (24) by the much simpler approximation '$f$ = constant' is small because for most sulphonamides the statement $K'' \gg c_{min}$ holds true. Under this condition it follows from eqn. (24) that $f$ is nearly constant at least in the therapeutic concentration range (Dettli & Spring, 1968a). As a consequence, the expression M/1000 in Krueger-Thiemer's equations which converts common weight units into molar units can also be omitted. Furthermore, when the restrictions mentioned above —namely $k_1 \to \infty$ and $\delta = 1{\cdot}0$—are introduced Krueger-Thiemer's eqns (20)–(23) will be reduced to the simplified form of our eqns (10), (11), (18) and (19).

*The Pharmacological Significance of the Dosage Equations*

The parameters between brackets in eqn. (10) and eqn. (18) can be determined *in vitro* ($\mu, f$) or in the pharmacokinetic experiment in vivo ($k'_2, \Delta'$, G) and $\tau$ may be freely choosen according to practical considerations. Consequently there remains $\sigma$ as the only unknown to be determined in the therapeutic or toxicological experiment. This is accomplished by varying $\sigma$ until the optimum therapeutic result is reached or signs of toxicity appear. This means that the therapeutic efficacy, or the toxicity of two compounds, can be compared based on a true quantitative null-hypothesis which considers the fact that efficacy and toxicity depend not only on the drug itself but also on its concentration in the biophase, i.e. on the dosage regimen.

## Experimental Results

*Calculated and Conventional Dosage Regimens of Sulphonamides*

The relevant kinetic parameters of all commonly used sulphonamides (Krueger-Thiemer 1961; Scholtan, 1961, 1962; Spring, 1966; Dettli &

Spring, 1966, 1968) and of several experimental compounds (Krueger-Thiemer *et al.*, 1969) have been determined. A few characteristic examples are given in Table 1. In summarizing these results it can be said, that $\Delta'$, $\beta$ and $\mu$ (Kutzche, 1964) are almost identical for all compounds. In contrast K″ and $k_2$ may differ by two orders of magnitude. Buenger *et al.* evaluated several sulphonamides according to Krueger-Thiemer's principles in therapeutic trials (Buenger, 1960, 1963, 1964; Buenger & Koch, 1961). For all compounds studied the authors found a value of $\sigma \sim 10$, indicating that $\sigma$ has possibly the same value for all sulphonamides. The dosage regimens in Table 1 are calculated based on this assumption.

*Factors Influencing Sulphonamide Kinetics*

During recent years the following factors have been shown to influence the pharmacokinetic parameters of sulphonamides (Dettli & Spring, 1968a):

*Non-ionic diffusion.* Since sulphonamides are weak acids they undergo 'non-ionic tubular reabsorption' (Milne, Scribner & Crawford, 1958) in the kidney. Reabsorption decreases and the rate of renal elimination may increase by several hundred per cent under the influence of alkali administration (Kostenbauder, Portnoff & Swintowsky, 1962; Dettli & Spring, 1964, 1968a; Dettli, Spring & Raeber, 1967). In addition alkalinization of the organism results in a decrease of the distribution volume (Krauer, 1971).

*Sleep and wakefulness.* The elimination rate and the distribution volume of many sulphonamides are smaller during sleep. The diurnal periodicity of elimination is absent in the new-born and develops during the first year of life in parallel with the transition of the sleeping behaviour from a polycyclic to a bicyclic pattern (Kleitman, 1963). Furthermore, the periodicity is more pronounced with compounds of a low *p*K*a*′ and can be abolished by alkali administration during sleep (Krauer, 1971; Dettli & Spring, 1966a; Krauer & Dettli, 1969). These facts indicate that the circadian rhythm is also caused by 'non-ionic partitioning' (Schanker, 1962) during the acidosis induced by sleep.

*Position of the body.* The elimination of several sulphonamides is markedly slower in the upright position. In addition the plasma concentration of highly albumin-bound sulphonamides shows a transitory increase when the body position is changed from lying to upright. The distribution volume remains uninfluenced (Dettli & Spring, 1966a; Krauer, 1971).

*Enzyme induction.* Experiments undertaken to demonstrate an increased metabolic transformation of sulphonamides caused by enzyme induction yielded controversial results (Gladtke, 1969; Krauer, 1971).

*Drug interactions.* The simultaneous administration of sulphonamides and other albumin-bound drugs involves the risk of mutual competitive

TABLE 1. Pharmacokinetic parameters (left) and calculated and conventional dosage regimens (right) of five sulphonamide compounds. $\mu$: minimum inhibitory concentration *in vitro* against mykobacterium smegmatis in a medium free of protein and antagonists; $\Delta'$: relative distribution volume; K″: dissociation constant of the sulphonamide-albumin complex in human plasma at 37°C; $\beta$: apparent maximum binding capacity of human plasma albumin for the sulphonamide; $f$: the fraction of non albumin-bound sulphonamide in human plasma when $c = c_{min} = 10.\sigma$; $k'_2$: overall rate constant of drug elimination; D: maintenance dose; D*: loading dose; $\tau$: dosage interval. The dosage regimens for intermittent administration have been calculated based on the following standard values: body weight G = 70 kg; concentration of albumin in the plasma $p = 40$ g/l; $\sigma = 10$. Conventional dosage regimens according to the suggestions of the producers

| Compound | Pharmacokinetic parameters | | | | | | Dosage regimens | | | | | |
|---|---|---|---|---|---|---|---|---|---|---|---|---|
| | | | | | | | Calculated | | | Conventional | | |
| | $\mu$ (mg/l) | $\Delta'$ l/kg) | K″ ($\mu$mol/l) | $\beta$ ($\mu$mol/g) | | $k_2$ ($h^{-1}$) | $\tau$ (h) | D (mg) | D*/D | $\tau$ (h) | D (mg) | D*/D |
| Sulphadiazine | 0·250 | 0·31 | 1193 | 31·50 | 0·501 | 0·058 | 12 | 111 | 1·9 | 4–6 | 1000 | 2 |
| Sulphamethoxy-pyrazine | 0·448 | 0·25 | 341 | 29·75 | 0·233 | 0·011 | 24 | 102 | 4·3 | 24 | 200 | 4 |
| Sulphamethoxy-pyridazine | 0·336 | 0·20 | 70 | 29·75 | 0·065 | 0·019 | 24 | 418 | 2·7 | 24 | 500 | 2 |
| Sulphamethoxy-diazine | 0·364 | 0·25 | 105 | 29·75 | 0·091 | 0·019 | 24 | 404 | 2·7 | 24 | 500 | 2 |
| Sulphadimethoxine | 0·279 | 0·15 | 11·5 | 31·50 | 0·016 | 0·019 | 24 | 1058 | 2·7 | 24 | 500 | 2 |

displacement from the binding sites (Anton, 1961, 1968). There is the additional possibility of competitive inhibition of metabolic elimination. The interaction between sulphaphenozole and tolbutamide may be taken as an example (Kristensen & Christensen, 1969). A sulphonamide may be displaced from the albumin-binding by its metabolites, and vice versa (Dettli (unpublished) 1971). This may increase the risk of side-effects in patients with renal failure.

*Pharmacogenetics.* Evans (1962) demonstrated the existence of genetically determined 'slow-acetylators' and 'fast-acetylators' of isoniazide. The same is true for the acetylation of sulphonamides (Evans, 1962; Frymoyer & Jacox, 1963).

*Hypoalbuminaemia.* The renal excretion of sulphisomidine is considerably faster in hypoalbuminaemic children (Krauer, 1971).

*Impaired renal function.* It follows from Bricker's 'intact nephron hypothesis' (Bricker, Morrin & Kime, 1960) that the elimination rate ($k_2'$) of drugs, which are eliminated partly or completely by the kidneys, is proportional to the glomerular filtration rate as measured by the endogenous creatinine clearance ($\dot{V}_{cr}$). The relationship may be described by the following equation (Dettli, Spring & Habersang, 1970; Dettli, Spring & Ryter, 1971; Wagner, 1970):

$$k_2 = k_{nr} + a \cdot \dot{V}_{cr} \tag{25}$$

where $k_{nr}$ is the rate constant of extrarenal elimination. The validity of eqn. (25) has been demonstrated for sulphadiazine (Dettli, 1971) and sulphamethoxazole (Baethke, 1972) in adults and for sulphisomidine (Krauer, 1971) in children. The elimination of sulphisomidine depends extremely on the degree of kidney impairment. The opposite is true for sulphamethoxazole. Sulphadiazine takes an intermediate position.

The unbound fraction ($f$) of sulphonamides in the plasma of uraemic patients is greater than normal (Buettner, Portwich, Manzke & Staudt, 1964). This may again increase the risk of side-effects in such patients.

*Age of the patient.* The elimination of sulphonamides in new-born children is much slower than in adults. During the first years of life the elimination rate increases sharply up to seven-fold and then decreases slowly with increasing age, until the 'normal' value of the adult is reached at about twenty years. The distribution volume decreases steadily during the same time period (Rind & Gladtke, 1964; Krauer, Spring & Dettli, 1968; Vest (unpublished) 1971; Krauer, 1972). A further decrease of the elimination rate during adult life has been reported for sulphamethoxazole (Otaya (unpublished) 1971). The empirically established and generally accepted rules of sulphonamide dosage in pediatrics are in accordance with these pharmacokinetic facts.

The albumin binding of sulphamethoxypyrazine in young children has shown to be somewhat less than in adults (Sereni, Perletti, Marubini & Mars, 1968).

**Conclusions**

For drugs which follow relatively simple pharmacokinetic patterns the dosage theory of Krueger-Thiemer clearly elucidates the functional relationships between the pharmacokinetic parameters and the dosage regimen on one hand and the resulting drug concentration at the site of action on the other. Furthermore, $\sigma$ directly relates the minimum inhibitory concentration of a bacteriostatic agent *in vitro* to the chemotherapeutic efficacy *in vivo*. As a consequence it should be possible to replace most of the extremely time-consuming 'trial-and-error' methods in the chemotherapeutic clinical experiment by a rational methodology based on quantitative null-hypotheses. When some of the less important complex relationships in Krueger-Thiemer's theory are substituted by reasonable approximations the dosage equations prove to be relatively simple. However, taking into consideration all sources of intrasubject and intersubject variability of pharmacokinetic 'constants' we have to realize that the quantitative therapeutic evaluation of chemotherapeutic agents still remains an arduous task.

Aided by Schweizerischer Nationalfonds zur Foerderung der wissenschaftlichen Forschung.

## REFERENCES

ANTON, A. H. (1960). The relation between the binding of sulphonamides to albumin and their antibacterial efficacy. *J. Pharmacol. exp. Ther.*, **129,** 282–290.

ANTON, A. H. (1961). A drug-induced change in the distribution and renal excretion of sulfonamides. *J. Pharmacol. exp. Ther.*, **134,** 291–303.

ANTON, A. H. (1968). The effect of disease, drugs and dilution on the binding of sulfonamides in human plasma. *Clin. Pharmacol. Ther.*, **9,** 561–567.

AUGSBERGER, A. (1954). Quantitatives zur Therapie mit Herzglykosiden II. Kumulation und Abklingen der Wirkung. *Klin. Wschr.*, **32,** 945–951.

BAETHKE, R. (1972). Personal communication.

BRICKER, N. S., MORRIN, P. A. F. & KIME, S. W. (1960). The pathologic physiology of chronic Bright's disease. *Amer. J. Med.*, **28,** 77–98.

BUENGER, P. (1960). Untersuchungen mit einem neuen Langzeitsulfonamid. *Aerztl. Forsch.*, **14,** 3–10.

BUENGER, P. (1963). Praktische Erfahrungen mit der Anwendung neuer Sulfonilamide. *Chemotherapia* (*Basel*), **6,** 237–242.

BUENGER, P. (1964). Die Bedeutung der Sulfonamide heute. *Hamburger Aerzteblatt*, **18,** 349–359.

BUENGER, P. & KOCH, G. (1961). Klinische Untersuchungen mit 2-Sulfanilamido-5-methoxy-pyrimidin. *Arzneimittel-Forsch.*, **11,** 726–736.

BUETTNER, H., PORTWICH, F., MANZKE, E. & STAUDT, N. (1964). Zur Pharmakokinetik von Sulfonamiden unter pathologischen Bedingungen. *Klin. Wschr.*, **42,** 103–108.

DAVIS, B. D. & WOOD, W. B. (1942). Studies on antibacterial action of sulfonamide drugs. III. Correlation of drug activity with binding to plasma. *Proc. Soc. exp. Biol.* (*N.Y.*), **51,** 283–285.

DETTLI, L. (1961). Der Konzentrationsbegriff in der Chemotherapie mit Sulfanilamiden. *Arzneimittel-Forsch.*, **11,** 861–866.

DETTLI, L. (1970). Multiple dose elimination kinetics and drug accumulation in patients with normal and with impaired kidney function. In *Advances in the Biosciences*, **5,** 39–54. Oxford, New York and Braunschweig: Pergamon Press & Vieweg.

DETTLI, L. & SPRING, P. (1964). Der Einfluss des Urin-pH auf die Eliminationsgeschwindigkeit einiger Sulfanilamid-Derivate. *Proc. 3rd Int. Congr. Chemother.*, **1,** 641–644. (Stuttgart: Thieme.)

DETTLI, L. & SPRING, P. (1966). Pharmakokinetik der Chemotherapeutica: Theorie und Praxis. *Regensburg. Jb. aerztl. Fortbild.*, **14,** 17–26.

DETTLI, L. & SPRING, P. (1966a). Diurnal variations in the elimination rate of a sulfonamide in man. *Helv. med. Acta*, **33,** 291–306.

DETTLI, L., SPRING, P. & RAEBER, I. (1967). The influence of alkali administration on the biological half-life of two sulfonamides in human blood serum. *J. clin. Pharmacol.* (*München*), **1,** 130–134.

DETTLI, L. & SPRING, P. (1968). Pharmacokinetics as a basic medical problem. In: *Physico-chemical Aspects of Drug Actions.* Oxford & New York: Pergamon Press.

DETTLI, L. & SPRING, P. (1968a). Factors influencing drug elimination in man. *Farmaco* (*Ed. sci.*), **23,** 795–812.

DETTLI, L., SPRING, P. & HABERSANG, R. (1970). Drug dosage in patients with impaired kidney function. *Postgrad. med. J.*, **46,** (Suppl.), 32–35.

DETTLI, L., SPRING, P. & RYTER, S. (1971). Multiple dose kinetics and drug dosage in patients with kidney disease. *Acta pharmacol.* (*Kbh*), **29,** (Suppl. 3), 211–224.

DOST, F. H. (1968). *Grundlagen der Pharmakokinetik*, 2nd ed. Stuttgart: Thieme.

EVANS, P. D. A. (1962). Pharmacogénétique. *Méd. et Hyg.* (*Génève*), **20,** 905–908.

FRYMOYER, J. W. & JACOX, R. (1963). Investigation of the genetic control of sulfadiazine and isoniazid metabolism in the rabbit. *J. Lab. clin. Med.*, **62,** 891–897.

GLADTKE, E. (1970). The systematic influence of elimination. In: *Advances in the Biosciences*, **5,** 168–183. Oxford, New York & Braunschweig: Pergamon Press & Vieweg.

KLEITMAN, N. (1963). *Sleep and Wakefulness*, 2nd ed. Chicago: University of Chicago Press.

KOSTENBAUDER, H. B., PORTNOFF, J. B. & SWINTOSKY, J. V. (1962). Control of urine pH and its effect on sulfaethidole excretion in humans. *J. pharm. Sci.*, **51,** 1084–1089.

KRAUER, B., SPRING, P. & DETTLI, L. (1968). Zür Pharmakokinetik der Sulfonamide in ersten Lebensjahr. *Pharmacologia Clinica* (*Berlin*), **1,** 47–53.

KRAUER, B. & DETTLI, L. (1969). Diurnal variations in the elimination rate of sulfisomidine in children during the first year of life. *Chemotherapy*, **14,** 1–6.

KRAUER, B. (1971). Zur Pharmakokinetik zweier Sulfonamide im Kindesalter (to be published).

KRISTENSEN, M. & CHRISTENSEN, L. K. (1969). Drug-induced changes of the blood glucose lowering effect of oral hypoglycemic agents. *Acta diabetol. latina*, **6,** (Suppl. 1), 116–136.

KRUEGER-THIEMER, E. (1960). Dosage schedule and pharmacokinetics in chemotherapy. *J. Amer. pharm. Ass.* (*sci. Ed.*), **49,** 311–313.

KRUEGER-THIEMER, E. (1961). Sulfanilamide und verwandte Chemotherapeutica. In: *Handbuch der Haut- und Geschlechtskrankheiten*, *Ergänzungs-Werk*, Vol. V/**1,** 962–1122. Berlin-Göttingen-Heidelberg: Springer.

KRUEGER-THIEMER, E. (1966). Formal theory of drug dosage regimens. *J. theoret. Biol.*, **13,** 212–235.

KRUEGER-THIEMER, E., BERLIN, H., BRANTE, P., BUENGER, P., DETTLI, L., SPRING, P. & WEMPE, E. (1969). Dosage calculation of chemotherapeutic agents. Part V: 2-sulfanilamido-3-methoxy-pyrazine. *Chemotherapy*, **14,** 273–302.

KRUEGER-THIEMER, E., WEMPE, E. & TOEPFER, M. (1965). Die antibakterielle Wirkung des nicht eiweissgebundenen Anteils der Sulfanilamide im menschlichen Plasmawasser. *Arzneimittel-Forsch.*, **15,** 1309–1317.

KUTZSCHE, A. (1964). Die Bedeutung der *in vitro*-Teste für die klinische Prüfung von Chemotherapeutica. *Antibiot. et Chemother.* (*Basel*), **12,** 315–333.

MILNE, M. D., SCRIBNER, B. H. & CRAWFORD, M. A. (1958). Non-ionic diffusion and the excretion of weak acids and bases. *Amer. J. Med.*, **24,** 709–729.

NEWBOULD, B. B. & KILPATRICK, R. (1960). Long-acting sulphonamides and protein-binding. *Lancet*, **1,** 887–891.

RIND, H. & GLADTKE, E. (1964). Pharmakokinetische Untersuchungen zur Sulfonamidtherapie bei Trimenonkindern. *Mschr. Kinderheilk.*, **112,** 239–240.

SCHANKER, L. S. (1962). Passage of drugs across body membranes. *Pharmacol. Rev.*, **14,** 501.

SCHOLTAN, W. (1961). Die Bindung der Langzeitsulfonamide an die Eiweisskörper des Serums. *Arzneimittel-Forsch.*, **11,** 707–720.

SCHOLTAN, W. (1962). Ueber die Bindung der Langzeitsulfonamide an die Serumeiweisskörper. *Makromol. Chem.*, **54,** 24–59.

SERENI, F., PERLETTI, L., MARUBINI, E. & MARS, G. (1968). Pharmacokinetic studies with a long-acting sulfonamide in subjects of different ages. *Pediat. Res.*, **2,** 29–37.

SPRING, P. (1966). Die Bindung einiger Sulfanilamide an die Bluteiweisskörper des Menschen. *Arzneimittel-Forsch.*, **16,** 346–354.

WAGNER, J. G. (1971). *Biopharmaceutics and Relevant Pharmacokinetics.* Hamilton: Drug Intelligence Publications.

# THIRTEEN

# Plasma Concentrations of Isoniazid in the Treatment of Tuberculosis

D. A. MITCHISON

*Medical Research Council Unit for Laboratory Studies of Tuberculosis, Royal Postgraduate Medical School, Ducane Road, London, W12 OHS*

**Introduction**

Isoniazid is the most widely used drug and one of the most active in the treatment of tuberculosis. Data have become available from a series of clinical trials at the Tuberculosis Chemotherapy Centre, Madras, making it possible to discover which of several parameters of the isoniazid concentration-time curve is best related to the incidence of toxicity and to the response to treatment of the patients. These relationships are presented here and are interpreted in terms of drug-microorganism interactions. They allow definition of optimal rhythms of drug dosage and provide a rationale for the development of regimens of intermittent chemotherapy.

**Assay**

Isoniazid and its metabolites can be measured by spectrophotometric and fluorimetric methods (Ellard, Gammon & Wallace, 1972). Microbiological assay (Lloyd & Mitchison, 1964) yields results closely similar to those obtained by chemical methods.

**Absorption and Metabolism**

Isoniazid is rapidly absorbed, peak plasma concentrations being obtained 1–2 h after an oral dose. Part of the dose is excreted unchanged or as acid-labile hydrazones in the urine. Most of the remainder is acetylated in the liver, but a small proportion is converted directly to isonicotinic acid (Ellard & Gammon 1973). All metabolites are microbiologically inactive.

The rate of acetylation (inactivation) is genetically controlled in a simple Mendelian manner. Homozygous slow inactivators are easily identifiable. However, it has only been possible so far to distinguish between heterozygous and homozygous rapid inactivators by genetic studies (Evans, Manley & McKusick, 1960; Scott, Wright & Weaver, 1971) and these two groups are usually classed together as rapid inactivators. About 40% of most populations examined are rapid inactivators (Evans, Manley & McKusick, 1960; Evans, 1969; Tiitinen, 1969; Tuberculosis Chemotherapy Centre, Madras, 1970), but the proportion rises to 80% or more in subjects of Mongolian origin (Armstrong & Peart, 1960; Sunahara, Urano & Ogawa, 1961; Tiitinen, Mattila & Eriksson, 1968).

Figure 1 shows examples of the serum concentrations of isoniazid attained in 20 slow inactivators and in 20 rapid inactivators after an oral

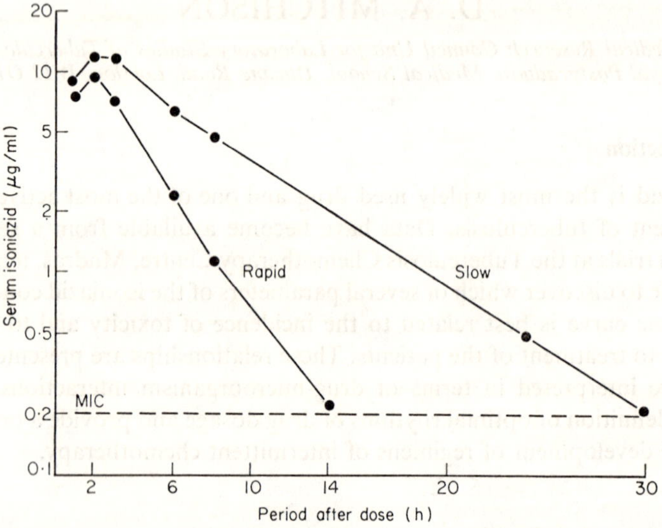


FIG. 1. Serum isoniazid concentrations in slow and rapid inactivators of isoniazid after an oral dose of 13–17 mg/kg.

dose of 13–17 mg/kg. Concentrations were measured chemically (Tuberculosis Chemotherapy Centre, Madras, 1973). It is evident that the peak concentrations were only slightly lower in rapid than in slow inactivators, the main difference in the curve being in the speed with which isoniazid disappeared. Both the half-life of the isoniazid and the integral of concentration × time (the area under the concentration–time curve) are 2·4 times greater in slower than in rapid inactivators.

## Toxicity

Acute toxicity to isoniazid is manifested as giddiness and sometimes convulsions occurring within a few hours after peak concentrations are attained. Convulsions occur rarely after a dose of about 15 mg/kg (Tuberculosis Chemotherapy Centre, Madras, 1964, 1970) but are more frequent if the dose is increased.

Peripheral neuropathy is the usual form of chronic toxicity. It can be prevented by the administration of as little as 6 mg pyridoxine with each dose of isoniazid (Tuberculosis Chemotherapy Centre, Madras, 1963b; Krishnamurphy *et al.*, 1967). The incidence of peripheral neuropathy in a number of studies at the Tuberculosis Chemotherapy Centre, Madras, in which patients were treated with isoniazid alone but without a supplement of pyridoxine, is set out in Table 1. Over the period concerned, there was

TABLE 1. *Incidence of peripheral neuropathy related to mean daily exposure to isoniazid*

| Dose of isoniazid (mg/kg) | Frequency of dosage (per week) | Inactivator status | Patients | | | Exposure* per day | Reference† |
|---|---|---|---|---|---|---|---|
| | | | Total | Peripheral neuropathy No. | % | | |
| 13·9 | 2 | rapid | 36 | 0 | *0* | 4·0 | (3), (4) |
| 2·2 | 14 | rapid | 36 | 0 | *0* | 4·5 | (1) |
| 4·4 | 14 | rapid | 28 | 0 | *0* | 8·7 | (1) |
| 8·7 | 7 | rapid | 32 | 2 | *6* | 8·7 | (1) |
| 13·9 | 2 | slow | 36 | 1 | *3* | 9·5 | (3), (4) |
| 2·2 | 14 | slow | 50 | 0 | *0* | 10·8 | (1) |
| 13·9 | 7 | rapid | 42 | 3 | *7* | 13·9 | (2) |
| 4·4 | 14 | slow | 44 | 6 | *14* | 20·9 | (1) |
| 8·7 | 7 | slow | 39 | 11 | *28* | 20·9 | (1) |
| 13·9 | 7 | slow | 37 | 17 | *46* | 33·4 | (2) |

* The dose of isoniazid in mg/kg body weight multiplied by 1·0 for rapid inactivators and by 2·4 for slow inactivators, i.e. a value proportional to the area under the serum concentration–time curve.
† *References*
(1) Devadatta *et al.* (1960).
(2) Tuberculosis Chemotherapy Centre, Madras (1963a, b).
(3) Tuberculosis Chemotherapy Centre, Madras (1964).
(4) Tuberculosis Chemotherapy Centre, Madras (1970).

no change in the diet of these patients, which was deficient in B group vitamins and in most other dietary components (Ramakrishnan *et al.*, 1961). They may therefore have been more prone to peripheral neuropathy than patients in other countries. For each group of patients, the 'exposure' to isoniazid has been calculated as the dose size, multiplied for slow inactivators by 2·4; it is therefore proportional to the integral of concentration × time. An association between the incidence of peripheral neuropathy and the mean exposure per day is evident. No association is present between the incidence of peripheral neuropathy and the number of doses per day, or the size of the individual dose of isoniazid. Thus, chronic toxicity appears to be best related to mean exposure to isoniazid.

**Response to Daily Treatment**

The response to treatment with one or two doses a day of isoniazid alone is related to various parameters of the concentration–time curve in

Table 2. The patients were again treated at the Tuberculosis Chemotherapy Centre, Madras (1960, 1963a, b). Those with bacteriologically quiescent disease at the end of one year of treatment were classified as having a favourable response. Serum concentrations of isoniazid were measured by microbiological assay (Gangadharam *et al.*, 1961), the values for the 13·9 mg/kg dose being obtained from later data of similar patients who received doses of 13 mg/kg (Tuberculosis Chemotherapy Centre, Madras, 1973). Coverage is defined as the period during which a concentration of at least 0·2 μg/ml isoniazid, the minimal inhibitory concentration for *Mycobacterium tuberculosis*, is present in the serum. The estimated coverage for rapid inactivators who receive 8·7 mg/kg once daily has been slightly altered from the value previously published (Gangadharam *et al.*, 1961) in the light of later estimates (Tuberculosis Chemotherapy Centre, Madras, 1973). It is evident from Table 2 that there is a good association between response and peak serum concentration up to a dose size of 6·7 mg/kg but that an increase in dose to 13·9 mg/kg did not confer any further benefit. Response was not related either to the period of coverage or to the mean exposure to isoniazid.

TABLE 2. *Response to treatment with isoniazid alone related to peak serum concentrations of isoniazid*

| Dosage of isoniazid (mg/kg) | Inactivator status | Patients: Total | Patients: Favourable response % | Peak concentration (μg/ml) | Coverage after 1 day's dose (h) | Exposure* per day |
|---|---|---|---|---|---|---|
| 2·2 | rapid | 36 | *44* | 0·7 | 4–12 | 4·5 |
| 2 × daily | slow | 46 | *48* | 1·2 | 26+ | 10·8 |
| 4·4 | rapid | 27 | *56* | 1·9 | 26+ | 8·7 |
| 2 × daily | slow | 39 | *59* | 2·6 | 26+ | 20·9 |
| 8·7 | rapid | 32 | *66* | 4·2 | 14 | 8·7 |
| 1 × daily | slow | 36 | *72* | 6·6 | 26+ | 20·9 |
| 13·9 | rapid | 62 | *66* | 8·4 | 15 | 13·9 |
| 1 × daily | slow | 81 | *69* | 9·2 | 26+ | 33·4 |

* See Table 1

An explanation for the association between response and peak serum concentrations has been given by Selkon *et al.*, (1964). In the suggested mechanism, as the dose of isoniazid was raised, isoniazid-resistant mutants with increasingly high degrees of resistance were inhibited. This mechanism is illustrated in Figure 2. The curve on the right-hand side shows the relationship between peak serum concentrations and the response of patients from the data of Table 2. The left-hand curve is the proportion of resistant mutants in sensitive strains of *M. tuberculosis* capable of forming colonies on medium containing various concentrations of isoniazid, from the data of Canetti & Grosset (1961). As the concentration of isoniazid was increased, the proportion of resistant mutants fell until, at about

5 μg/ml, all of the mutants were highly resistant. The curve relating response to peak serum concentrations also flattens at about 5 μg/ml, suggesting that any further increase in the peak serum concentration confers no additional benefit because all resistant mutants present were capable of growth in much higher concentrations. This relationship between *in vivo* and *in vitro* response not only provides additional evidence for the view that the dose response curve is largely dependent on the mutant structure

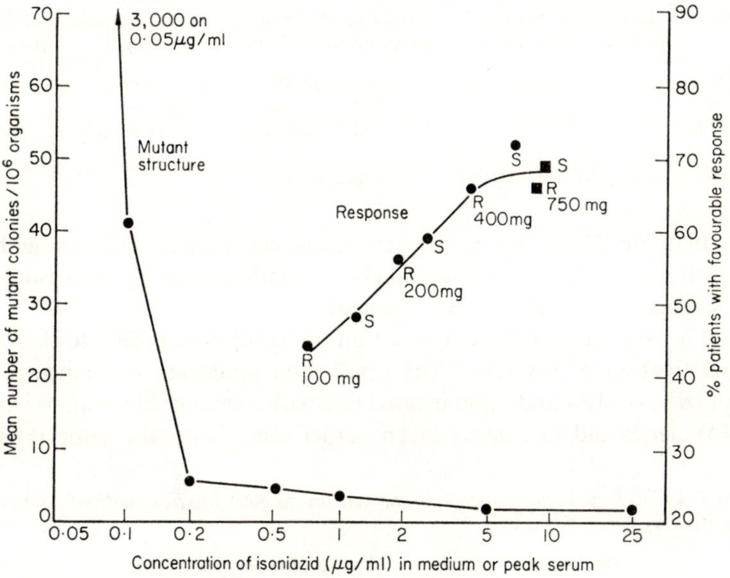


FIG. 2. Isoniazid resistant mutant structure and response of patients to treatment with isoniazid alone related to peak serum concentrations.

of the bacterial population, but also that growth of the mutants *in vivo* is determined by concentrations at or near the peak.

**Response to Once-weekly Intermittent Treatment**

The use of regimens in which drug doses are given at intervals of greater than one day has been explored for the primary reason that it enables full supervision of drug administration to be done by medical or other responsible personnel. When the doses are spaced at intervals of 7 days, new relationships between the response of the patients and the parameters of the serum concentrations–time curve become evident.

The first study of once-weekly chemotherapy was done at the Tuberculosis Chemotherapy Centre, Madras (1970). The regimens used are shown in Table 3. The SHTW regimen is a control as it was previously shown to be highly effective (Tuberculosis Chemotherapy Centre, Madras, 1964). In this regimen, isoniazid 15 mg/kg with streptomycin, given by random allocation in doses of 0·75 g or 1 g, were administered twice-weekly. In the SHOW regimen the same drug doses were given once-weekly. This basic once-weekly regimen was strengthened either by the addition of

TABLE 3. *Chemotherapy regimens in the first Madras study of intermittent (once weekly) chemotherapy*

| Regimen | Isoniazid 400 mg + streptomycin 0·75 or 1 g | Isoniazid 15 mg/kg + streptomycin 0·75 or 1 g | Pyrazinamide 90 mg/kg | Number of patients |
|---|---|---|---|---|
| SHTW | — | Twice weekly | — | 104 |
| SHOW | — | Once weekly | — | 79 |
| SHZOW | | Once weekly | Once weekly | 105 |
| SH/ SHOW | Daily for first month | Once weekly | — | 106 |

pyrazinamide 90 mg/kg, also given once-weekly (SHZOW regimen), or by giving a preliminary four weeks of daily treatment with isoniazid and streptomycin (SH/SHOW regimen).

The response of the patients is set out in Table 4 according to their rate of inactivation of isoniazid. The small, non-significant difference in the proportion of slow and rapid inactivators with a favourable response in the SHTW series did not occur in an earlier study with the same regimen

TABLE 4 *Classification of patients at one year in the first Madras study of intermittent (once-weekly) chemotherapy*

| Regimen | Total patients | Favourable response* (%) | | |
|---|---|---|---|---|
| | | Inactivation rate | | Total |
| | | slow | rapid | |
| SHTW | 96 | *97* | *91* | *94* |
| SHOW | 77 | *76* | *56*† | *68* |
| SHZOW | 101 | *87* | *53*† | *74* |
| SH/SHOW | 101 | *95* | *76*† | *88* |

* Bacteriologically quiescent disease at 1 year.
† The difference in response of slow and rapid inactivators in each of the three once weekly regimens is statistically significant ($P < 0{\cdot}05$).

(Tuberculosis Chemotherapy Centre, Madras, 1970). In the once-weekly regimens the response was much better in slow inactivators than in rapid inactivators, the difference for each of the three series being statistically significant. These results indicated that the factors limiting response became different as the interval between doses was spaced out from 3½ to 7 days.

A further study was designed which could, among its various aims, test whether response was related to peak concentrations or to some other parameter of the serum concentration curve (Tuberculosis Chemotherapy Centre, Madras, 1973). A total of 346 previously untreated patients were given the basic SH/SHOW regimen of the previous study. However, the following comparisons were added in a three-way factorial design. The first

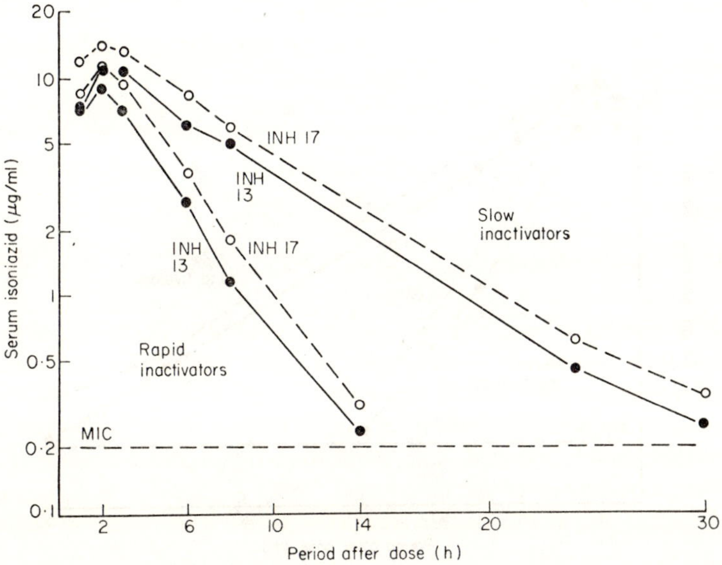


FIG. 3. Isoniazid serum concentrations in patients given 13 mg/kg or 17 mg/kg isoniazid by mouth.

comparison was between the basic regimen and the same regimen supplemented by sodium *p*-aminosalicylate (PAS) 6 g given with each dose of streptomycin and isoniazid. The second comparison was, as before, a comparison between streptomycin 0·75 g and 1 g. The third comparison was between isoniazid 13 mg/kg and 17 mg/kg during the once-weekly phase. Finally, patients were classified as slow or rapid inactivators of isoniazid.

The serum concentration–time curves are shown for the comparison

TABLE 5 *Response related to peak serum concentrations of isoniazid, coverage and mean exposure in the second Madras study of intermittent (once-weekly) chemotherapy (patients grouped by size of dose of isoniazid)*

| Dose of isoniazid (mg/kg) | Inactivator status | Peak serum concentration (μg/ml) | Coverage (h) | Exposure per day | Patients: Total | Patients: Favourable response (%) |
|---|---|---|---|---|---|---|
| 13 | rapid | 9·2 | 14 | 13 | 78 | *71* |
| 17 | rapid | 11·6 | 15 | 17 | 61 | *79* |
| 13 | slow | 11·3 | 29 | 31 | 100 | *93* |
| 17 | slow | 14·2 | 31 | 41 | 107 | *94* |

between the patients receiving 13 mg/kg or 17 mg/kg isoniazid in Figure 3. The mean exposure and period of coverage was calculated as before. The response of the patients, subdivided by isoniazid dose and inactivation rate, is related to parameters of the concentration–time curve in Table 5. It is now evident that there is an association between response and either

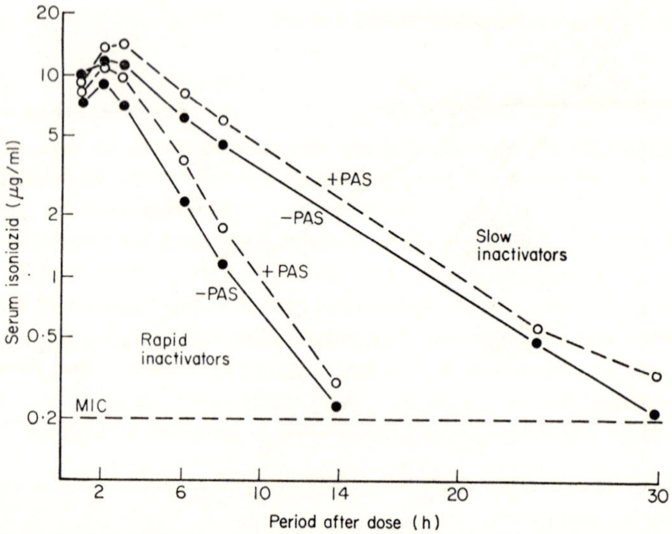


FIG. 4. Isoniazid serum concentrations in patients given 13–17 mg/kg isoniazid by mouth with or without sodium PAS 6 g.

the period of coverage or the mean exposure, but no association is present between response and the peak serum concentrations. The response in the slow inactivators receiving either 13 mg/kg or 17 mg/kg was almost as good as is possible since a few patients died, as is usual, in the early weeks of treatment before chemotherapy could influence their disease. Serum concentration–time curves for the patients receiving PAS and those not

TABLE 6. *Response related to peak serum concentrations of isoniazid, coverage and mean exposure in the second Madras study of intermittent (once-weekly) chemotherapy (patients grouped according to dosage with PAS)*

| Addition of sodium PAS 6 g | Inactivator status | Peak serum concentration (μg/ml) | Coverage (h) | Exposure per day | Patients: Total | Patients: Favourable response (%) |
|---|---|---|---|---|---|---|
| No | rapid | 9·4 | 14 | 15 | 67 | *72* |
| Yes | rapid | 11·5 | 15 | 19·6* | 72 | *76* |
| No | slow | 11·8 | 30 | 36·0 | 109 | *93* |
| Yes | slow | 13·7 | 31 | 44·9* | 101 | *95* |

* Calculated by measurement of area under concentration–time graph.

receiving PAS are shown in Figure 4. The increase in serum concentrations due to the addition of PAS is almost identical to the increase due to raising the dose of isoniazid from 13 mg/kg to 17 mg/kg (Figure 3). The response of the patients, grouped according to administration of PAS and inactivation rate, is set out in Table 6. Again there is an association between response and the period of coverage or the mean exposure but not between response and peak isoniazid concentration.

**Drug-organism Interactions**

Explanations for the associations between response to treatment and parameters of the concentration–time curve arise from experimental work on the interaction between the drug, isoniazid and the organism, *M. tuberculosis*. Two main methods have been used for investigating this interaction. First, cultures of *M. tuberculosis* were given pulsed exposures to isoniazid *in vitro* and the subsequent growth of the culture was measured in various ways. Second, experimental tuberculosis of the mouse or the guinea-pig was treated with isoniazid, varying the dose size and the rhythm of administration.

The main conclusions from the *in vitro* systems are as follows:

1. The antibacterial effect of a pulse is proportional to the exposure during the pulse, defined as the product of isoniazid concentration and exposure period (Bourgeois, Dubois-Verlière & Maël, 1958; Armstrong, 1960, 1965; Beggs & Jenne, 1969).
2. Small exposures, such as to 1 $\mu$g/ml for 2 h, usually have no detectable bactericidal activity and growth starts immediately after the pulse. Larger exposures are bactericidal; growth ceases for several days after the pulse but then recovers to a normal rate fairly abruptly (Dickinson & Mitchison, 1966a).
3. If a small pulse, which by itself has no detectable effect, is followed on successive days by further small pulses, the overall effect, measurable by bactericidal activity or lag in growth, is at least as great as a single large pulse producing the same total exposure (Awaness & Mitchison, 1973). Thus, recovery from a pulse is slow, and successive daily pulses are cumulative in their effect.
4. As the size of the pulse is increased, the subsequent lag in growth reaches a maximum of about 5–7 days (Dickinson & Mitchison, 1966a).

In daily chemotherapy, those resistant mutants which are just inhibited by peak concentrations will receive a series of short exposures. Even though one such exposure might have little effect, a succession of them would be cumulative so that, after a few doses, the mutants would begin to be killed.

The reason for the association between peak concentration and response is evident.

In once-weekly chemotherapy, it seems probable that sensitive organisms will often start to grow between doses since the maximum lag after an *in vitro* pulse was 5–7 days. Indeed, there was evidence of long-continued multiplication of sensitive organisms during once-weekly treatment in a few patients treated at the Tuberculosis Chemotherapy Centre, Madras (1970). The effect of the successive doses would not, therefore, be cumulative. The result of this break in continuity has been demonstrated in short-term treatment of experimental tuberculosis in the guinea-pig (Dickinson, Ellard & Mitchison, 1968). In groups of animals given the same mean dosage of isoniazid, the response was similar in those dosed at intervals of 1, 2 or 4 days, but much less good in those given doses at 8-day intervals. When dosage is not cumulative in effect, the overall antibacterial activity will be the summation of the effect of each dose. Since the *in vitro* findings indicated that the effect is proportional to exposure (concentration × exposure period), it is not surprising that the response to once-weekly chemotherapy in man is also best associated with the mean exposure during treatment. It is also evident that in the limiting situation of twice-weekly dosage, successive large pulses will have a cumulative effect on sensitive organisms, but the effect may not be cumulative on resistant mutants because they will receive much smaller exposures. Hence the importance of giving large doses of isoniazid in twice-weekly regimens.

**Applications to the Formulation of Regimens of Chemotherapy**

The most favourable schedule of dosage to provide high efficacy with a minimum of chronic toxicity would be high (15 mg/kg) doses of isoniazid given at intervals of greater than one day. Chronic toxicity can, however, be prevented by giving small doses of pyridoxine. Even more important, resistant mutants are not only inhibited by high peak concentrations but also by the second drug that is generally given with isonazid. Thus, no benefit would be expected from intermittent rhythms nor from an increase in the size of the dose during conventional combined chemotherapy. Nevertheless, improved response might occur if only one drug of low potency were given with isoniazid. In a cooperative study in the United States, a similar excellent response was obtained in patients treated with PAS and either isoniazid 100 mg three times daily or isoniazid 300 mg in a single daily dose (Hyde, 1966), but these patients had minimal disease. In the treatment of severe pulmonary tuberculosis in East Africa with isoniazid and thiacetazone 150 mg, given together in a single daily dose, the response was improved by increasing the dose of isoniazid from 200 mg to 300 mg (East African/British Medical Research Council, 1963), but no further improvement occurred as a result of an increase from 300 mg to 450 mg (East African/British Medical Research Council, 1966). A further example of the value of optimal schedules of dosage arose in the development of regimens of twice-weekly chemotherapy. In an early study in Britain, treatment with streptomycin 1 g twice-weekly and isoniazid in two doses of 100 mg (1–2 mg/kg) daily was unsatisfactory because of the early emergence of drug-resistant *M. tuberculosis* (Medical Research Council, 1955). However, when the same dosage of streptomycin with isoniazid 15 mg/kg, also twice-weekly, was given to patients with severe disease at Madras, their response was excellent (Tuberculosis Chemotherapy Centre, Madras, 1964). It seems probable that the improvement in response was due to the greater efficacy of isoniazid in high doses intermittently than in low doses twice daily.

Once-weekly chemotherapy with streptomycin and isoniazid, preceded by a month of daily administration of these drugs, has been shown to be an effective regimen of treatment in slow inactivators of isoniazid. The regimen could be made equally effective in rapid inactivators if the exposure of the organism to each dose of isoniazid could be increased by, at most, a factor of 2·4. A sufficiently large exposure cannot be obtained by a simple increase of dose size because of the risk of acute toxicity arising from the high peak concentrations. The exposure could theoretically be increased by giving compounds of isoniazid which slowly release the drug or by decreasing the acetylation of isoniazid by simultaneous administration of acetylisoniazid or sulphadimidine, which is acetylated by the same enzyme. These approaches have been disappointing so far. An effective and simple method is to give isoniazid as a slow-release preparation. Ellard *et al.* (1972) have described preliminary pharmacological studies on three such preparations, and the most promising, a matrix tablet, is now under clinical trial.

## REFERENCES

ARMSTRONG, A. R. (1960). Time-concentration relationships of isoniazid with tubercle bacilli *in vitro*. *Amer. Rev. resp. Dis.*, **81**, 498–503.

ARMSTRONG, A. R. (1965). Further studies on the time-concentration relationships of isoniazid and tubercle bacilli *in vitro*. *Amer. Rev. resp. Dis.*, **91**, 440–443.

ARMSTRONG, A. R. & PEART, H. E. (1960). A comparison between the behaviour of Eskimos and non-Eskimos to the administration of isoniazid. *Amer. Rev. resp. Dis.*, **81**, 588–594.

AWANESS, A. M. (1971). Laboratory studies on the suitability of isoniazid and rifampicin in intermittent chemotherapy of tuberculosis. *Thesis for PhD. degree*. University of London.

BEGGS, W. H. & JENNE, J. W. (1969). Isoniazid uptake and growth

inhibition of *Mycobacterium tuberculosis* in relation to time and concentration of pulsed drug exposures. *Tubercle*, **50,** 377–385.
BOURGEOIS, P., DUBOIS-VERLIÈRE, M. & MAÉL, M. (1958). Étude de l'action discontinué de l'isoniazide sur le bacilli de Koch par la méthode des cultures sur lames. *Rev. Tuberc.*, **22,** 108–111.
CANETTI, G. & GROSSET, J. (1961). Teneur des souches sauvages de *Mycobacteruim tuberculosis* en variants résistants à l' isoniazide et en variants résistants à la stréptomycine sur milieu de Löewenstein-Jensen. *Ann. Inst. Pasteur.*, **101,** 28–46.
DEVADATTA, S., GANGADHARAM, P. R. J., ANDREWS, R. H., FOX, W., RAMAKRISHNAN, C. V., SELKON, J. B. & VELU, S. (1960). Peripheral neuritis due to isoniazid. *Bull. Wld. Hlth. Org.*, **23,** 587–598.
DICKINSON, J. M., ELLARD, G. A. & MITCHISON, D. A. (1968). Suitability of isoniazid and ethambutal for intermittent administration in the treatment of tuberculosis. *Tubercle*, **49,** 351–366.
DICKINSON, J. M. & MITCHISON, D. A. (1966a). *In vitro* studies on the choice of drugs for intermittent chemotherapy of tuberculosis. *Tubercle*, **47,** 370–380.
DICKINSON, J. M. & MITCHISON, D. A. (1966b). Short-term intermittent chemotherapy of experimental tuberculosis in the guinea-pig. *Tubercle*, **37,** 381–393.
EAST AFRICAN/BRITISH MEDICAL RESEARCH COUNCIL (1963). Isoniazid with thiacetazone in the treatment of pulmonary tuberculosis in East Africa. Second Investigation. *Tubercle*, **44,** 301–333.
EAST AFRICAN/BRITISH MEDICAL RESEARCH COUNCIL (1966). Isoniazid with thiacetazone in the treatment of pulmonary tuberculosis in East Africa. Fourth Investigation. *Tubercle*, **47,** 315–449.
ELLARD, G. A., ABER, V. R., GAMMON, P. T., MITCHISON, D. A., LAKSHMINARAYAN, S., CITRON, K. M., FOX, W. & TALL, R. (1972). The pharmacology of some slow-release preparations of isoniazid of potential use in the intermittent treatment of tuberculosis. *Lancet*, **1,** 340–343.
ELLARD, G. A. & GAMMON, P. T. (1973). A kinetic study of the metabolic conversion of isoniazid to acetylisoniazid, isonicotinic acid, isonicotylglycine and diacetylhydrazine, and of the excretion of these compounds in the urine of man. (In preparation).
ELLARD, G. A., GAMMON, P. T. & WALLACE, S. M. (1972). The determination of isoniazid and its metabolites, acetylisoniazid, monoacetylhydrazine, diacetylhydrazine, isonicotinic acid and isonicotinylglycine in serum and urine. *Biochem. J.*, **126,** (In press).
EVANS, D. A. P. (1969). An improved and simplified method of detecting the acetylation phenotype. *J. Med. Genet.*, **6,** 405–407.
EVANS, D. A. P., MANLEY, K. A. & MCKUSICK, V. A. (1960). Genetic control of isoniazid metabolism in man. *Brit. med. J.*, **2,** 485–491.

GANGADHARAM, P. R. J., DEVADATTA, S., FOX, W., NAIR, C. N. & SELKON, J. B. (1961). Rate of inactivation of isoniazid in South Indian patients with pulmonary tuberculosis. 3. Serum concentrations of isoniazid produced by three regimens of isoniazid alone and one of isoniazid plus PAS. *Bull. Wld. Hlth. Org.*, **25**, 793–806.

HYDE, L. (1966). Comparison of single and divided daily doses of isoniazid in original treatment of minimal and noncavitary moderately advanced pulmonary tuberculosis. 18. *A report of the Veterans Administration–Armed Forces Cooperative Study on the Chemotherapy of Tuberculosis. Amer. Rev. resp. Dis.*, **96**, 204–208.

KRISHNAMURPHY, D. V., SELKON, J. B., RAMACHANDRAN, K., DEVADATTA, S., MITCHISON, D. A., RADHAKRISHNA, S. & STOTT, H. (1967). The effect of pyridoxine on vitamin $B_6$ concentrations and glutamic-oxalo-acetic transaminase activity in whole blood of tuberculous patients receiving high-dosage isoniazid. *Bull. Wld. Hlth. Org.*, **36**, 853–870.

LLOYD, J. & MITCHISON, D. A. (1964). A vertical diffusion method for the microbiological assay of isoniazid. *J. clin. Path.*, **17**, 622–626.

MEDICAL RESEARCH COUNCIL (1955). Various combinations of isoniazid with streptomycin or with P.A.S. in the treatment of pulmonary tuberculosis. *Brit. med. J.*, **1**, 435–445.

RAMAKRISHNAN, C. V., RAJENDRAN, K., JACOB, P. G., FOX, W. & RADHAKRISHNA, S. (1961). The role of diet in the treatment of pulmonary tuberculosis. An evaluation in a controlled chemotherapy study in home and sanatorium patients in South India. *Bull. Wld. Hlth. Org.*, **25**, 339–359.

SCOTT, E. M., WRIGHT, R. C. & WEAVER, D. D. (1969). The discrimination of phenotypes for rate of disappearance of isonicotinyl hydrazide from serum. *J. clin. Invest.*, **48**, 1173–1176.

SELKON, J. B., DEVADATTA, S., KULKARNI, K. G., MITCHISON, D. A., NARAYANA, A. S. L., NAIR, N. C. & RAMACHANDRAN, K. (1964). The emergence of isoniazid resistant cultures in patients with pulmonary tuberculosis during treatment with isoniazid alone or isoniazid plus PAS. *Bull. Wld. Hlth. Org.*, **31**, 273–294.

SUNAHARA, S., URANO, M. & OGAWA, M. (1961). Genetic and geographical studies in isoniazid inactivation. *Science*, **134**, 1530–1531.

TIITINEN, H. (1969). Isoniazid and ethionamide serum levels and inactivation in Finnish subjects. *Scand. J. resp. Dis.*, **50**, 110–124.

TIITINEN, H., MATTILA, M. J. & ERIKSSON, A. W. (1968). Comparison of the isoniazid inactivation in Finns and Lapps. *Annls. Med. intern. Fenn.* **57**, 161–165.

TUBERCULOSIS CHEMOTHERAPY CENTRE, MADRAS (1960). A concurrent comparison of isoniazid plus PAS with three regimens of isoniazid alone in the domiciliary treatment of pulmonary tuberculosis in South India. *Bull. Wld. Hlth. Org.*, **23,** 535–585.

Tuberculosis Chemotherapy Centre, Madras (1963a). The prevention and treatment of isoniazid toxicity in the therapy of pulmonary tuberculosis. 1. An assessment of two vitamin B preparations and glutamic acid. *Bull. Wld. Hlth. Org.* **28,** 455–475.

Tuberculosis Chemotherapy Centre, Madras (1963b). The prevention and treatment of isoniazix toxicity in the therapy of pulmonary tuberculosis. 2. An assessment of the prophylactic effect of pyridoxine in low dosage. *Bull. Wld. Hlth. Org.*, **29,** 457.

Tuberculosis Chemotherapy Centre, Madras (1964). A concurrent comparison of intermittent (twice-weekly) isoniazid plus streptomycin and daily isoniazid plus PAS in the domiciliary treatment of pulmonary tuberculosis. *Bull. Wld. Hlth. Org.*, **31,** 247–271.

Tuberculosis Chemotherapy Centre, Madras (1970). A controlled comparison of a twice-weekly and three once-weekly regimens in the initial treatment of pulmonary tuberculosis. *Bull. Wld. Hlth. Org.*, **43,** 143–206.

Tuberculosis Chemotherapy Centre, Madras (1973). A controlled comparison of two fully supervised once-weekly regimens in the treatment of newly diagnosed pulmonary tuberculosis. *Tubercle* (in press).

FOURTEEN

# Plasma Concentrations of Penicillin in Relation to the Antibacterial Effect

G. N. ROLINSON

*Beecham Research Laboratories, Brockham Park, Betchworth, Surrey*

When antibiotics are used in the treatment of bacterial infections the therapeutic effect is the result of a direct interaction between antibiotic molecules and bacterial cells. It follows, therefore, that a therapeutic effect will be dependent on an adequate concentration of drug being present at the site of infection. In this Symposium, however, the central theme is the relationship between plasma concentrations of drugs and biological action, and as far as bacterial infection is concerned the significance of plasma levels of antibiotic will depend on where the site of infection happens to be. If the infection is present within the vascular system itself, plasma levels can be expected to be directly related to antibacterial effect. On the other hand, if the infection is present in an extravascular compartment the plasma levels of antibiotic may only be of significance in so far as they may determine the levels of drug reached in such compartments when the distribution of the drug is governed by passive diffusion. Different antibiotics of course differ in the ease with which they diffuse from the plasma into extravascular spaces. The extravascular compartments themselves also differ in their relative accessibility; for example, plasma to tissue-fluid ratios may be very different from plasma to CSF ratios. Distribution of the antibiotic in the body may also be influenced by the extent of protein binding and the relationship between plasma levels and tissue levels of antibiotic therefore may be complex.

If the infection is present in a compartment of the body involving active secretion of drug for example in the urine, plasma levels of antibiotic may have little relevance because the levels of certain antibiotics in urine can be relatively high even though the plasma concentration may be negligible, or at least below an inhibitory level.

Clearly, plasma levels of antibiotic should not be thought of as being synonymous with levels at the site of infection, but in many instances the one is a function of the other. In order to assess the quantitative aspect of plasma concentration, however, it is necessary to consider not only drug distribution but also the dose response when bacteria are exposed to particular concentrations of antibiotic for certain periods of time.

In the experiments shown in Figure 1, benzylpenicillin was added to suspensions of resting cells of *Staphylococcus aureus* to give a range of concentrations and viable counts were made at intervals of time. It will be seen that the maximum rate of bactericidal action occurred with penicillin levels only slightly higher than the minimum inhibitory concentration, and as the antibiotic concentration increased, the rate of bactericidal action decreased, at least over the first 6 h. This paradoxical effect of

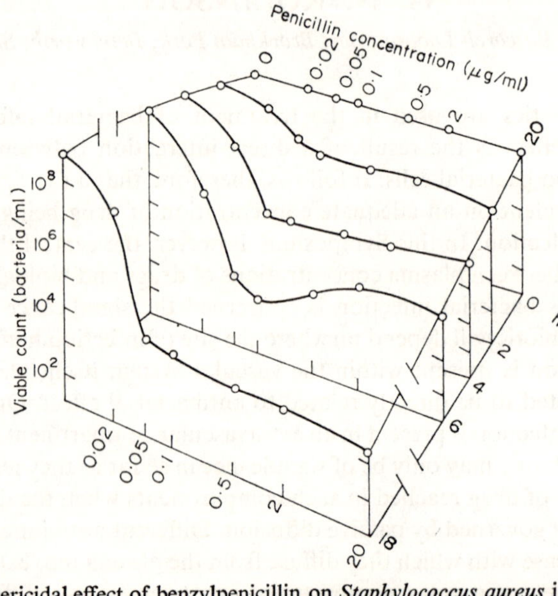


FIG. 1. Bactericidal effect of benzylpenicillin on *Staphylococcus aureus* in broth culture using an inoculum in the resting phase. [Elizabeth J. Russell and G. N. Rolinson, *unpublished results*.]

penicillin concentration was first reported in 1948 by Eagle and Musselman, and in our own laboratory using resting cells of *Staphylococcus aureus* and benzylpenicillin this is quite a reproducible phenomenon. However, when the experiment is carried out using cells in the logarithmic phase of growth, as distinct from resting cells, a very different dose response is obtained and results are shown in Figure 2. It will be seen that using an inoculum of actively growing cells the rate of bactericidal action increases directly with increasing concentration of drug until the maximum rate is reached and under these circumstances no zone phenomenon is seen. It will be noted, however, that penicillin levels at least twenty times the minimum inhibitory concentration were required in order to obtain the maximum rate of killing. The dose response seen with the dividing cells is thus quite different from that seen with resting cells. How far a zone phenomenon is seen with other bacteria, and with other penicillins, is at present not fully known.

In the experiments shown in Figures 1 and 2 the drug was present at a relatively uniform concentration for a considerable period of time. In the body this of course is not the case and with the penicillins in particular the drug is eliminated rapidly. Results are shown in Figure 3 in which *S. aureus* was exposed to benzylpenicillin for a period of 1½ h and the drug then removed by the addition of penicillinase. It will be seen that following removal

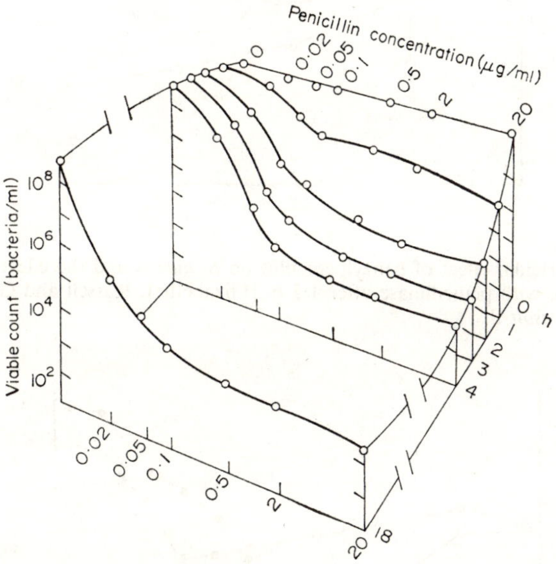


FIG. 2. Bactericidal effect of benzylpenicillin on *S. aureus* in broth culture using an inoculum in the logarithmic phase. [Elizabeth J. Russell and G. N. Rolinson, *unpublished results*.]

of the drug a period of some 2 h elapsed before an increase in the number of viable cells occurred. This recovery period with *S. aureus* and benzylpenicillin was described as long ago as 1946 by Parker and Marsh, and confirmed by Eagle in 1949 using streptococci and pneumococci. In our own laboratory a recovery period is clearly apparent, as can be seen from Figure 3, when benzylpenicillin and *S. aureus* are used, but a recovery period is not seen with carbenicillin and *Pseudomonas aeruginosa.*

In Figure 4 results of an experiment are shown in which *P. aeruginosa* was exposed to carbenicillin at a concentration of 50 and 200 μg/ml for 4 h and the drug then removed by the addition of *Escherichia coli* β-lactamase. It will be seen that following removal of the drug, resumption of rapid bacterial growth occurred almost immediately. Rapid growth of

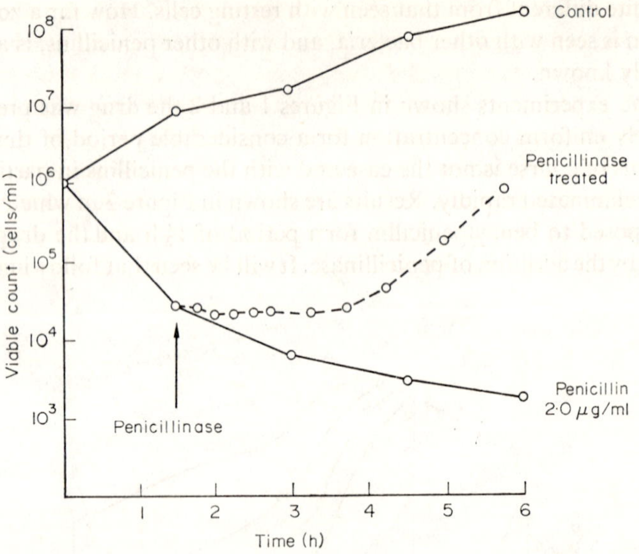


FIG. 3. Bactericidal effect of benzylpenicillin on *S. aureus* and the effect of removal of the antibiotic with penicillinase after 1·5 h. [Elizabeth J. Russell and G. N. Rolinson. *unpublished results*.]

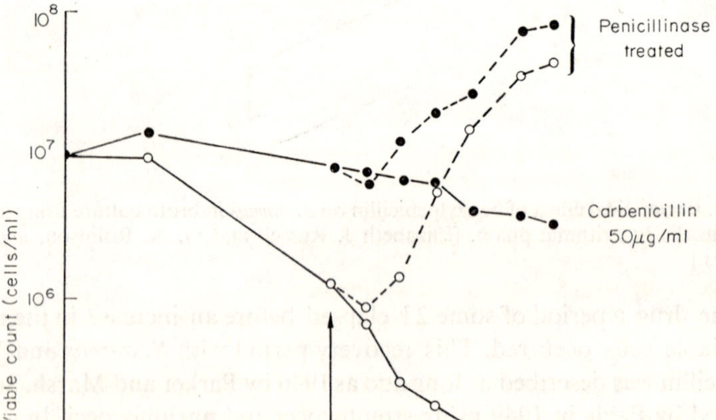


FIG. 4. Bactericidal effect of carbenicillin on *Pseudomonas aeruginosa* and the effect of removal of the antibiotic with penicillinase after 4 h. [Pamela A. Hunter, Doreen A. Witting and G. N. Rolinson, *unpublished results*.]

*P. aeruginosa* following elimination of carbenicillin from the body can also be seen in experiments *in vivo*. The experimental model used involved injection of a suspension of *P. aeruginosa* into the thigh muscle of mice followed by counts of the number of viable bacteria present in homogenates of the muscle. It will be seen from Figure 5 that in control untreated animals rapid bacterial growth occurred, whereas in animals in which carbenicillin was administered subcutaneously at a dose of 500 mg/kg at 0, 2, 4 and 6 h, bacterial numbers declined almost immediately and continued to fall over the following 48 h. Figure 6 shows the effect of a single

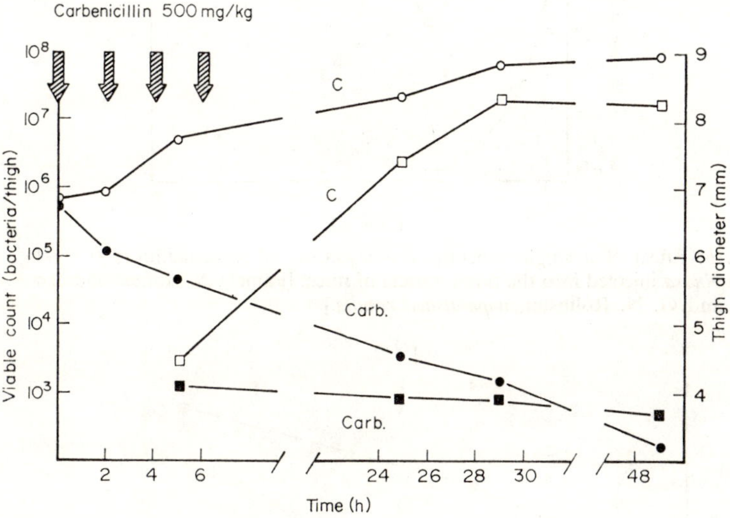


FIG. 5. Effect of repeated subcutaneous injection of carbenicillin on *P. aeruginosa* infection in the thigh muscle of mice. C = control; Carb. = carbenicillin.

○——○ viable count, control animals
●——● viable count, carbenicillin treated
□——□ thigh diameter, control animals
■——■ thigh diameter, carbenicillin treated.

[Pamela A. Hunter, Doreen A. Witting and G. N. Rolinson, *unpublished results*.

dose of 500 mg carbenicillin/kg at time 0. It will be seen that following an initial fall in the viable count while the drug was present, a resumption in growth occurred at a point corresponding to the elimination of the drug from the blood. The effect of subsequent dosage of carbenicillin during this resumption is shown in Figure 7. It will be seen that following each dose of carbenicillin a fall in the viable count occurred and this continued until the drug had been largely eliminated from the plasma. Rapid bacterial growth then occurred without any obvious recovery period. From this and the previous experiments it will be seen that in the case of *Pseudomonas* and carbenicillin the effect of a period of contact with the antibiotic

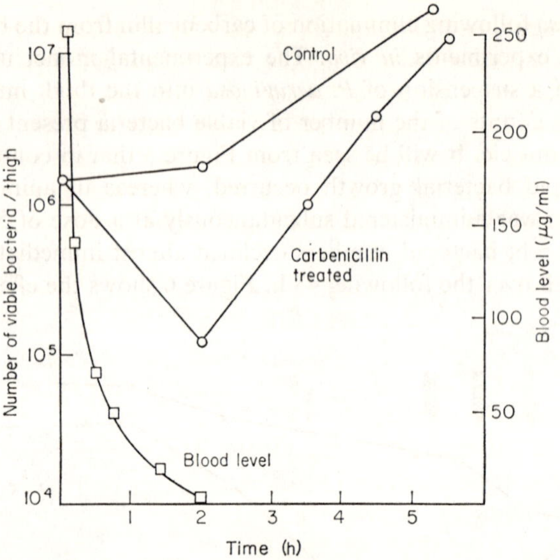


FIG. 6. Effect of a single subcutaneous injection of carbenicillin (500 mg/kg) on *P. aeruginosa* injected into the thigh muscle of mice. [Pamela A. Hunter, Doreen A. Witting and G. N. Rolinson, *unpublished results*.]

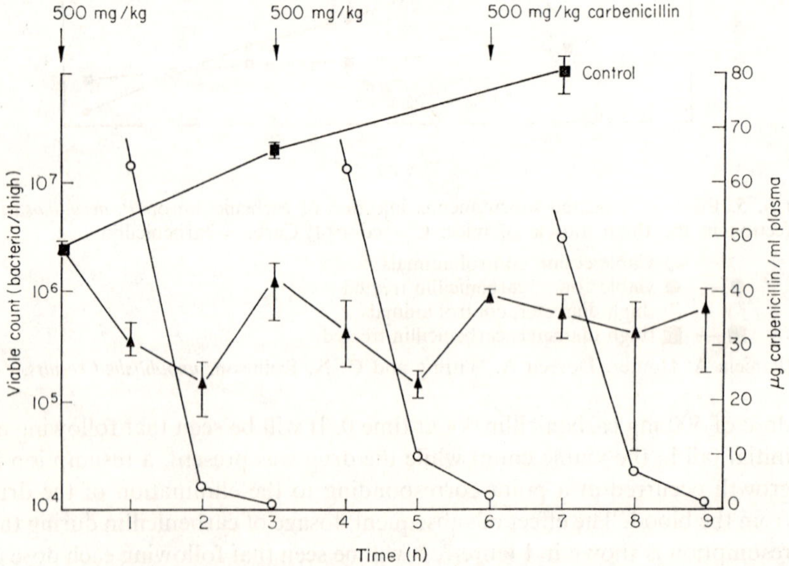


FIG. 7. Effect of repeated subcutaneous injection of carbenicillin on *P. aeruginosa* infection in the thigh muscle of mice.

■——■ viable count—control animals
▲——▲ viable count—carbenicillin treated
○——○ μg carbenicillin/ml plasma.

[Pamela A. Hunter, Doreen A. Witting and G. N. Rolinson, *unpublished results*.]

followed by removal of the drug appears to be different from that seen with *S. aureus* and benzylpenicillin, for which there is a significant recovery period. Returning to the main theme of this Symposium, namely the significance of plasma concentration, despite three decades of the medical use of antibiotics there would seem to be a need for further data both on distribution of penicillins and on the relationship between drug concentration and time of contact on the one hand, and antibacterial effect on the other.

## REFERENCES

EAGLE, H. (1949). The recovery of bacteria from the toxic effects of penicillin. *J. clin. Invest.*, **28**, 832–836.

EAGLE, H. & MUSSELMAN, A. D. (1948). The rate of bactericidal action of penicillin *in vitro* and as a function of its concentration, and its paradoxically reduced activity at high concentrations against certain organisms. *J. exp. Med.*, **88**, 99–131.

PARKER, R. F. & MARSH, H. C. (1946). The action of penicillin on *Staphylococcus*. *J. Bact.*, **51**, 181–186.

**Session 4**

Chairman: Professor F. Sjöqvist

Therapeutic Use of Drugs Acting on the Central Nervous System

FIFTEEN

# Relationship between the Steady-state Plasma Concentration of Nortriptyline and some of its Pharmacological Effects

BALZAR ALEXANDERSON, MARIE ÅSBERG AND DICK TUCK

*Department of Clinical Pharmacology, University of Linköping, 581 85 Linköping, the Karolinska Institute (Huddinge University Hospital) and the Department of Psychiatry, Karolinska Hospital, 104 01 Stockholm 60, Sweden*

Nortriptyline (NT), the desmethyl derivative of amitriptyline, is a tricyclic antidepressant drug which has been widely used in the treatment of depressive disorder for almost ten years.

After oral administration of a constant dose of NT thrice daily the drug level in plasma reaches a plateau, usually within 3–6 days of treatment, and then remains fairly constant (Figure 1). The steady-state level is a reproducible parameter (Sjöqvist *et al.*, 1968) provided that no concurrent drug therapy interferes (Alexanderson *et al.*, 1969). Early studies of the kinetics of desmethylimipramine and NT established that patients treated with similar doses of the respective drug developed markedly different (ten to thirty-fold ranges) steady-state plasma concentrations (Hammer & Sjöqvist, 1967; Sjöqvist *et al.*, 1968). These findings were reproduced in twin volunteers (Figure 2) (Alexanderson *et al.*, 1969) and in our own staff (Alexanderson, 1972) excluding unreliable drug intake as a significant factor in the variability.

These studies revealed that the steady-state plasma concentration of nortriptyline is a personal characteristic mainly determined by genetic factors. From a family study it was concluded that the mode of inheritance of the plasma kinetics of NT is likely to be polygenic (Åsberg *et al.*, 1971b).

How does the great variability in plasma levels affected the drug response? It is generally assumed that the therapeutic action of the tricyclic

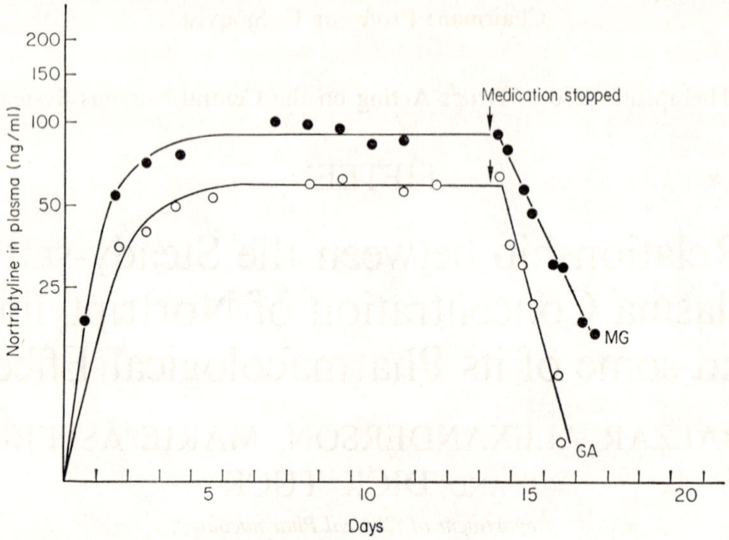


FIG. 1. Log NT concentration versus time after multiple oral doses (0·4 mg t.i.d.) in two subjects.

antidepressants is related to their ability to inhibit reuptake of transmitter substances in central monoaminergic neurons, thereby increasing the amount of monoamines available at the receptors.

Studies of the uptake of tritium-labelled noradrenaline in adrenergic neurons (rat's iris) have shown that at concentrations occurring under clinical conditions, the metabolites of NT are of minor importance for the

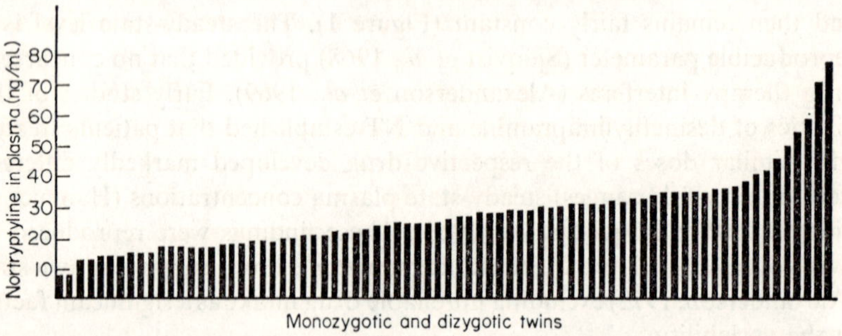


FIG. 2. Histogram of steady-state plasma levels of NT in 76 mono- and dizygotic twins. (From Alexanderson *et al.*, 1969.) Reproduced by permission of the *British Medical Journal*.

blockade of the uptake mechanisms as compared to the parent compound (Borgå *et al.*, 1970).

In the following studies steady-state levels of NT have been related to various effects, assuming that the free concentration of the drug in plasma is in equilibrium with the free concentration available at the receptors.

The first study was concerned with the blocking effect on the uptake of tyramine in the peripheral adrenergic neurons in patients on chronic treatment with NT. Normally, a small intravenous dose of tyramine causes a short lasting rise in blood pressure. This is probably because it

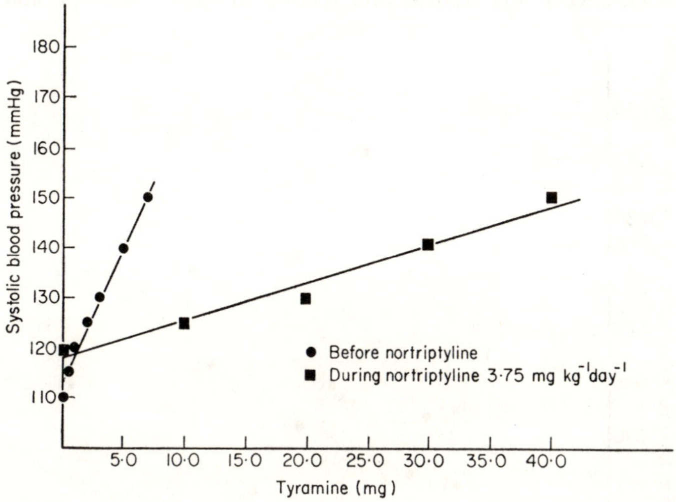


FIG. 3. Relation between systolic pressor effect and dose of tyramine in mg/kg before and during treatment with NT.

displaces noradrenaline from the nerve terminal. Tyramine enters the nerve terminal via the same route as the endogenous amines. Hence tyramine uptake can be blocked by the tricyclic antidepressants. The rationale behind the use of tyramine in our experiments has been discussed in detail in a previous paper (Freyschuss *et al.*, 1970).

Systolic blood pressure effects after i.v. injection of increasing doses of tyramine were recorded in 13 patients before and during treatment with NT in doses of 1·4–5 mg/kg/day for 3–4 weeks. During nortriptyline treatment, a several-fold decrease in the responsiveness to tyramine occurred (Figure 3). Patients treated with the same dose of NT showed markedly different decreases in the responsiveness to tyramine. There was no correlation between the blockade of the tyramine-pressor effects and the dose of NT given (Figure 4). By contrast a significant correlation between the blockade and the steady-state plasma concentration of NT (Figure 5) was obtained. These data suggest that the plasma level of NT seems to be more important for the pharmacological effect studied than individual differences in the sensitivity of receptor sites to the drug. Tyramine pressor effects were not changed in a small control group of depressed patients after electro-convulsive treatment (Freyschuss *et al.*, 1970). It should be noted that a few patients represented in Figure 5, such as W, do not fit the line. Other types of interindividual differences in the response to antidepressants may operate, but the only way to unravel these is to monitor the kinetics of the compounds.

In another investigation by Åsberg *et al.* (1970) the occurrence of subjective side-effects was studied and related to steady-state plasma levels

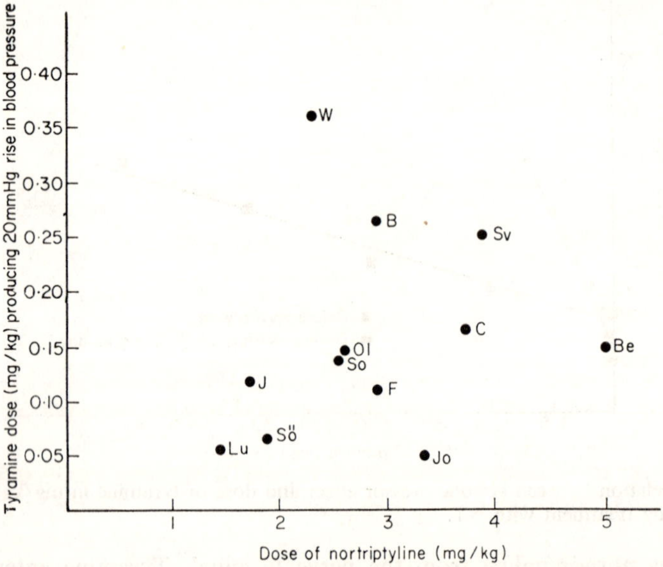


FIG. 4. Relationship between dose of NT (mg/kg) and the increase in dose of tyramine (mg/kg) producing a 20 mm Hg rise in systolic blood pressure. No correlation (= 0·18; $0{\cdot}6 > P > 0{\cdot}5$). (From Freyschuss *et al.*, 1970.) Reproduced by permission of *Pharmacologia Clinica.*

of NT in 40 inpatients with depressive disorders. Plasma levels were determined during 4 weeks of treatment with NT 50 mg t.i.d. and the patients were rated for subjective side-effects, the raters being unaware of the plasma levels of the drug. An attempt was made to separate the symptoms of depression and the placebo effects from the pharmacological side-effects in each patient by subtracting the side-effect scores recorded during a preceding placebo period from those obtained during the treatment with NT. These estimates, called corrected side-effects scores, diminished during the 4 weeks of treatment and were absent in most patients during the last week.

A regression analysis of the corrected scores of side-effect on plasma level of NT showed a positive, significant correlation during the first 3 weeks of treatment. (Table 1). During the last week most of the recorded side-effects had vanished. Table 1 also shows that no correlation was found between corrected scores of side-effects and the administered dose of NT.

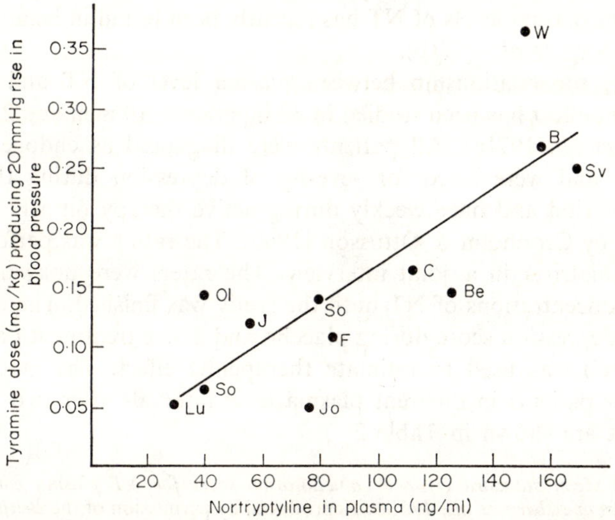


FIG. 5. Correlation between plasma level of NT and blockade of tyramine pressor effects ($y = 0{\cdot}016X + 0{\cdot}0084$; $r = 0{\cdot}81$; $P < 0{\cdot}005$). The data are the same as in Figure 4. (From Freyschuss *et al.*, 1970.) Reproduced by permission of *Pharmacologia Clinica*.

TABLE 1. *A. Regression of corrected side-effect scores* (*y*) *on plasma level of nortriptyline* (*x*)

| | *n* | *b* | *r* | *t* | level of significance |
|---|---|---|---|---|---|
| Week no. 1 | 35 | 0·04 | 0·50 | 3·3558 | p < 0·005 |
| Week no. 2 | 39 | 0·03 | 0·46 | 3·1407 | p < 0·005 |
| Week no. 3 | 36 | 0·03 | 0·42 | 2·7339 | p < 0·01 |
| Week no. 4 | 26 | 0·01 | 0·12 | 0·5899 | N.S. |

*B. Regression of corrected side-effect scores* (*y*) *on dosage of nortriptyline in mg/k body weight* (*x*)

| | *n* | *b* | *r* | *t* | level of significance |
|---|---|---|---|---|---|
| Week no. 1 | 38 | 0·99 | 0·14 | 0·8576 | N.S. |
| Week no. 2 | 39 | 0·89 | 0·12 | 0·7507 | N.S. |
| Week no. 3 | 36 | −0·05 | −0·01 | −0·0349 | N.S. |
| Week no. 4 | 28 | 1·40 | −0·18 | −0·9158 | N.S. |

*n* = number of patients (i.e. pairs of observations)
*b* = regression coefficient
*r* = correlation coefficient
N.S. = not significant
(From Åsberg *et al.*, 1970.) Reproduced by permission of the *British Medical Journal*.

There are obviously several difficulties involved in the registration of subjective side-effects. However, two observations will be emphasized: firstly, the corrected scores of side-effects did not correlate with the severity of endogenous depression in contrast to the uncorrected scores of side-effects (*loc. cit.*); and secondly, a correlation between subjective side-effects and plasma levels of NT has recently been found in healthy volunteers (Åsberg *et al.*, 1971b).

Finally, the relationship between plasma level of NT and its anti-depressant effect has been studied in 32 inpatients, 10 men and 22 women (Åsberg *et al.*, 1971a). All patients were diagnosed as endogenous depressions and were rated for severity of depression during the initial placebo period and once weekly during active therapy on a rating scale designed by Cronholm & Ottosson (1960). The rating was performed by two psychiatrists in a joint interview. The raters were unaware of the plasma concentrations of NT until the study was finished. The difference between depression score during placebo and active treatment ('amelioration score') was used to estimate therapeutic effect. The amelioration scores for patients in different plasma level intervals after two weeks of treatment are shown in Table 2.

TABLE 2. *Mean standard error or amelioration score for NT plasma concentration intervals (from Åsberg et al., 1971a)*. Reproduced by permission of the *British Medical Journal*

| NT plasma concentration interval, mμg/ml | Number of patients | Amelioration score | |
|---|---|---|---|
| | | Mean | Standard error |
| < 49 | 5 | 0·4 | 1·2 |
| 50–79 | 10 | 6·2 | 0·8 |
| 80–109 | 4 | 6·1 | 1·4 |
| 110–139 | 5 | 5·0 | 2·0 |
| ⩾ 140 | 5 | 1·2 | 1·9 |

For the three plasma level classes 'low' (< 49 mμg/ml), 'intermediate' (50–139 mμg/ml), and 'high' (> 140 mμg/ml), there is a significant difference in therapeutic effect between the groups ($\chi^2 = 10{\cdot}89$, $df = 2$, $p < 0{\cdot}01$). The anti-depressant effect is poor at a low plasma level, then increases to a plateau and finally decreases at very high plasma concentrations.

A curved relationship between plasma level of NT and therapeutic effect, with less response to both extremely low and extremely high plasma levels of the drug, could be explained on the basis of the monoamine hypothesis of depressive disorders. It is known from animal studies that these drugs have a dual action (see Sjöqvist *et al.* (1971)). It appears that the potentiation of peripheral adrenergic effects by a variety of tricyclic antidepressants, including NT and desmethylimipramine, disappear or are reversed at higher dosages. This is probably due to a blockade of the adrenergic receptor, similar to that seen with phenothiazine compounds.

Probably this latter action will tend to antagonize the primary effect on the monoamine neurons. Since very high plasma levels give rise to more side-effects and the therapeutic effect diminishes, the conventional strategy of raising the dosage when the patient does not respond to the drug may often prove unsuccessful in the case of NT.

Pharmacokinetic studies in our laboratory indicate that it will be possible to predict the steady-state plasma level of NT in any given subject from

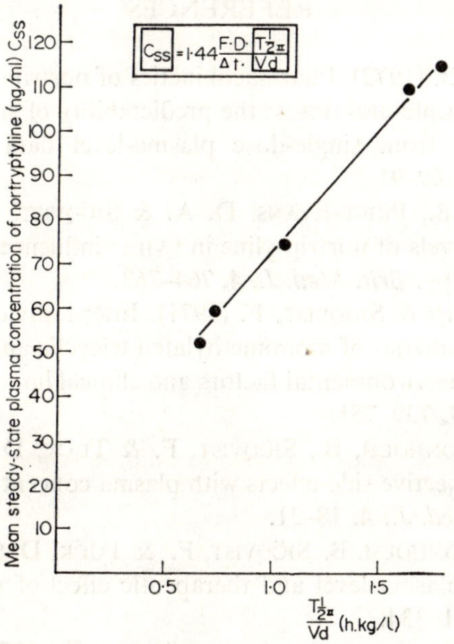


FIG. 6. Correlation between the found NT steady-state plasma concentration ($y$-axis) in 5 healthy humans treated with NT for 14 days and the reciprocal plasma clearance ($t\frac{1}{2}_{II}/V_d$) calculated in the same individuals after a single oral dose of NT. (From Alexanderson & Sjöqvist, 1971.) Reproduced by permission of the *Annals of the New York Academy of Sciences.*

single oral dose plasma level data (Alexanderson *et al.*, 1972). The five subjects represented in Figure 6 were given a single oral dose (1 mg/kg) and later a multiple dose regimen of NT (0·4 mg/kg) for two weeks. From the single-dose plasma-level data the plasma half-lives were determined from the terminal, apparent monoexponential part of the curves as well as the apparent volume of distribution, assuming complete availability of the given dose. The ratio of the plasma half-life to the volume term (equal to the inverse ratio of the plasma clearance of the drug) was plotted against the observed mean steady-state plasma level for each individual. There was a high correlation between the single-dose plasma clearances and the steady-state plasma levels which now has been confirmed in a number of patients. This predictability of the steady-state level of

NT from single-dose studies may be advantageous as most of the depressed patients undergo treatment with NT for several weeks or even months.

This study was supported by the Swedish Medical Research Council (B72–14X–1021–07A, B72–14P–3589–01 and B72–14P–3647–01), by the National Institutes of Health, Bethesda, Maryland ,USA (GM 13978), and by funds from the Karolinska Institute.

## REFERENCES

ALEXANDERSON, B. (1972). Pharmacokinetics of nortriptyline in man after single and multiple oral doses: the predictability of steady-state plasma concentrations from single-dose plasma-level data. *Europ. J. Clin. Pharmacol.*, **4**, 89–91.

ALEXANDERSON, B., PRICE-EVANS, D. A. & SJÖQVIST, F. (1969). Steady-state plasma levels of nortriptyline in twins: influence of genetic factors and drug therapy. *Brit. Med. J.*, **4**, 764–768.

ALEXANDERSON, B. & SJÖQVIST, F. (1971). Inter-individual differences in the pharmacokinetics of monomethylated tricyclic antidepressants: role of genetic and environmental factors and clinical importance. *Ann. N.Y. Acad. Sci.*, **179**, 739–751.

ÅSBERG, M., CRONHOLM, B., SJÖQVIST, F. & TUCK, D. (1970). The correlation of subjective side-effects with plasma concentrations of nortriptyline. *Brit. Med. J.*, **4**, 18–21.

ÅSBERG, M., CRONHOLM, B. SJÖQVIST, F. & TUCK, D. (1971a). Relationship between plasma level and therapeutic effect of nortriptyline. *Brit. Med. J.*, **3**, 331–334.

ÅSBERG, M., PRICE-EVANS, D. A. & SJÖQVIST, F. (1971b). Genetic control of nortriptyline kinetics in man—a study of the relatives of propositi with high plasma concentrations. *J. Med. Gen.*, **8**, 129–135.

BORGÅ, O., HAMBERGER, B., MALMFORS, T. & SJÖQVIST, F. (1970). The role of plasma protein binding in the inhibitory effect of nortriptyline on the neuronal uptake of norepinephrine. *Clin. Pharmacol. Ther.*, **11**, 581–588.

CRONHOLM, B. & OTTOSON, J. O. (1960). Experimental studies of the therapeutic action of electro-convulsive therapy in endogenous depression. *Acta Psychiat. Scandinav.*, **35**, (Suppl 145), 69.

FREYSCHUSS, U., SJÖQVIST, F. & TUCK, D. (1970). Tyramine pressor effects in man before and during treatment with nortriptyline or ECT: correlation between pharmacokinetics and effect of nortriptyline. *Pharmacologia Clinica*, **2**, 72–78.

HAMMER, W. & SJOQVIST, F. (1967). Plasma levels of monomethylated tricyclic antidepressants during treatment with imipramine-like compounds. *Life Sci.*, **6**, 1895–1903.

SJÖQVIST, F., ALEXANDERSON, B., ÅSBERG, M., BERTILSSON, L., BORGÅ, O., HAMBERGER, B. & TUCK, D. (1971). Pharmacokinetics and biological effects of nortriptyline in man. *Acta Pharmacol. Toxicol.*, **29,** (Suppl. 3), 255–280.

SJÖQVIST, F., HAMMER, W., IDESTRÖM, C-M., LIND, M., TUCK, D. & ÅSBERG, M. (1968). Plasma level of monomethylated tricyclic antidepressants and side-effects in man. *Excerpta Medica Internat. Congr. Ser.*, **145,** 246–257.

# SIXTEEN

# Action and Metabolism of Chlorpromazine

STEPHEN H. CURRY

*Department of Pharmacology and Therapeutics,*
*The London Hospital Medical College,*
*Turner Street,*
*London E1*

## Introduction

Chlorpromazine has fascinated a remarkably large number of workers in the 20 years since its introduction into medicine. The statistics alone make interesting reading. For example, 100 million people have been treated with the drug, over 10,000 investigations have been published, and several hundred of these have been concerned with chlorpromazine metabolism (Usdin, 1971). In spite of this, fundamental questions concerning relationships between the action and metabolism of chlorpromazine remain unanswered.

## Analytical Techniques

Recent developments in analytical methods for biological fluids have made possible: (1) the identification by mass fragmentography of chlorpromazine metabolites occurring in low concentrations in blood and urine (Hammer & Holmstedt, 1968); (2) the quantitative assay of chlorpromazine and its five primary demethylated and sulphoxidized metabolites in blood and urine by gas chromatography (Curry, 1968) and by radioderivative formation (Efron, Gaudette & Harris, 1968; Efron, Harris, Manian & Gaudette, 1971); and (3) the quantitative assay of 11 demethylated and hydroxylated metabolites by dansylation and fluorometry (Kaul, Conway & Clark, 1970). Additionally, methods involving microcoulometric detectors (Johnson, Rodriquez & Burchfield, 1965) and fluorescence coupling with fluorescein isothiocyanate (Usdin, 1971) have been investigated. These various techniques have now largely superseded the semiquantitative and non-specific thin-layer chromatographic and spectrophotometric techniques of earlier investigators. Gas chromatography with an electron capture detector seems to be the method of choice at present.

The greatest single advance which has followed the application of these techniques has been an increased understanding of the factors affecting concentrations of chlorpromazine and its metabolites in plasma. It is now possible to discuss concentrations of individual compounds, whereas interpretation of many earlier investigations has been complicated by the failure of authors to identify the compounds measured in their work. Non-specific assays have been described as measuring 'chlorpromazine', in spite of the fact that no unchanged drug was present in the extracts, and the term 'bound drug' has been wrongly used to designate conjugated materials. In this paper, the word 'chlorpromazine' applies only to unmetabolized drug, and all references to binding are concerned solely with chemical association with macro molecules, for example plasma proteins.

## Chlorpromazine Metabolism

Chlorpromazine undergoes extensive metabolism (Emmerson & Miya, 1963; Williams & Parke, 1964; Usdin, 1971). The initial reactions are sulphoxidation (to chlorpromazine sulphoxide), demethylation (to demonomethylchlorpromazine), hydroxylation and glucuronidation (to 7-hydroxychlorpromazine and its glucuronide) and amine oxidation (to chlorpromazine N-oxide). These metabolic pathways are shown in Figure 1. The reactions occur in combination, and hydroxylation can occur at several positions in the phenothiazine ring. In addition, it has been suggested that ring fission, deaminative oxidation and sulphone formation may occur. It has been estimated that more than 150 metabolites may occur as the result of combined reactions. Over 50 different compounds have been detected to date.

Non-specific colourimetric assays, designed mainly to detect the phenothiazine nucleus, have been used to detect about 40–50% of an administered dose in human urine. Only about 5% of the dose can be detected by these methods in faeces. The fate of the remainder of the dose is unknown. The majority of the phenothiazine material in urine and faeces consists of glucuronide conjugates, with a negligible amount of unmetabolized chlorpromazine.

Chlorpromazine metabolites vary considerably in polarity. The parent drug is the least polar material. In Figure 1, each metabolic pathway leads to more polar materials, and there is a general trend of increasing polarity reading from top to bottom of the figure. Thus chlorpromazine metabolism leads to compounds with a wide range of polarities, ranging from the extremely lipid-soluble unmetabolized drug to the highly water-soluble glucuronides. The more lipid soluble materials in each group pass the blood-brain barrier; the glucuronides apparently do not.

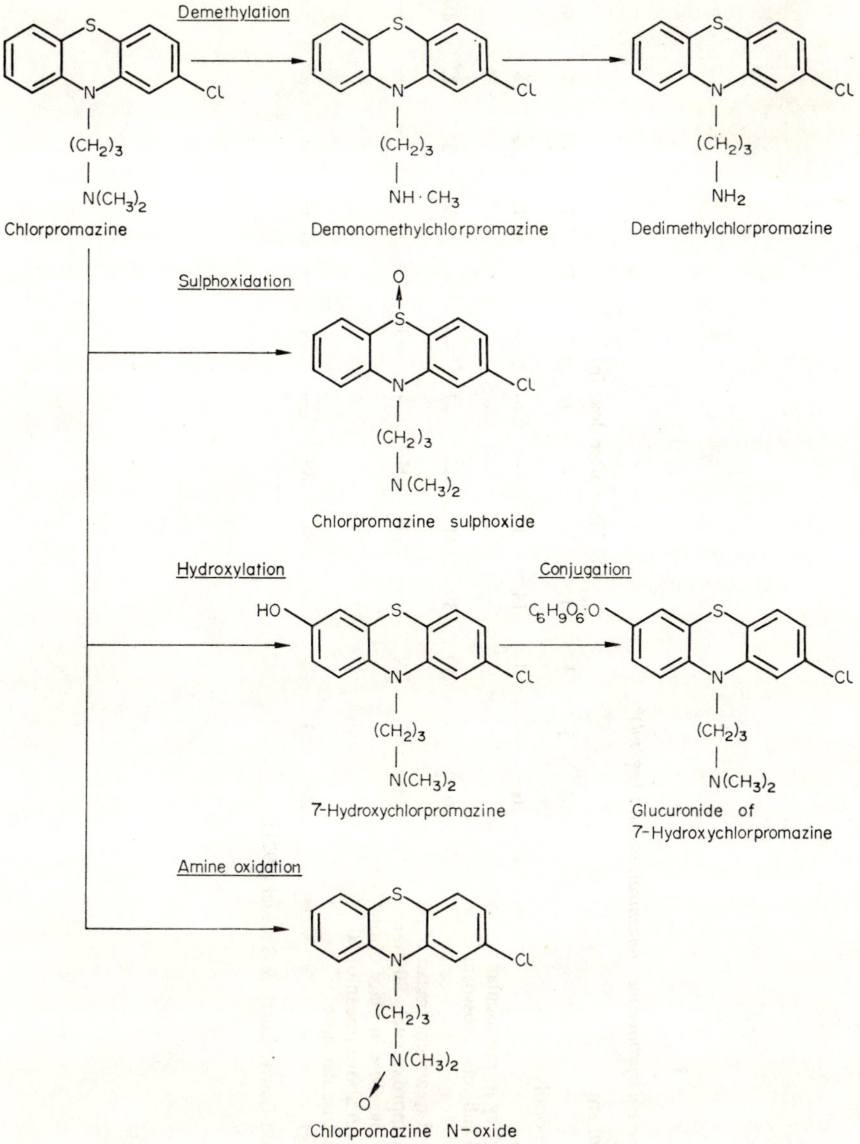


FIG. 1. Metabolic routes of chlorpromazine.

## Concentrations in Plasma

Apart from minimal reference to chlorpromazine sulphoxide, demonomethylchlorpromazine and dedimethylchlorpromazine, plasma studies have so far been solely concerned with the unmetabolized drug.

TABLE 1. *Representative chlorpromazine concentration data (ng/ml)**

| Type of study | Time after dose (h) | | | | | | | | | | | | |
|---|---|---|---|---|---|---|---|---|---|---|---|---|---|
| | 0 | $\frac{1}{4}$ | $\frac{1}{2}$ | 1 | 2 | 4 | 6 | 7 | 8 | 12 | 24 | 32 | 48 |
| (a) Single dose (100 mg) orally (mean of 5 subjects) | 0 | — | 4 | 14 | 11 | — | — | — | 4 | 13 | — | 8 | — |
| (b) Single dose (100 mg) by intramuscular injection (mean of 5 subjects; crossover with (a) above) | 0 | — | 50 | 39 | 41 | — | 47 | — | — | 36 | 35 | 22 | 10 |
| (c) During long-term oral treatment (mean of 80 subjects; mean dose approximately 80 mg) | 28 | 62 | — | — | 93 | 94 | — | 83 | — | — | — | — | — |
| (d) After one intramuscular dose in place of one routine oral dose in (c) above (mean of 80 subjects; mean intramuscular dose approximately 55 mg) | 29 | 84 | — | — | 96 | 89 | — | 94 | — | — | — | — | — |

* From Curry (1971), and Lewis, Curry & Samuel (1971).

Early studies of chlorpromazine in plasma showed that single oral doses (25–100 mg) lead to very low concentrations. Equivalent intramuscular doses lead to much higher concentrations. A similar pattern is seen during long-term treatment, but the oral doses used and the concentrations achieved are higher. During long-term oral treatment the concentration is low before each dose. There is approximately a three-fold increase to a peak concentration about 2 h after the dose and the concentration then declines rapidly, reaching the predosage level at about 12 h. Representative concentration data of these types are listed in Table 1.

TABLE 2. *Concentrations of chlorpromazine (ng/ml) in one patient treated for six weeks with* 100 *mg three times a day. The first dose was by intramuscular injection and the others were oral (syrup preparation). Samples were collected after the first dose of the sampling days.*

| | Time after dose (h) | | | |
|---|---|---|---|---|
| Day | 0 | 2 | 4 | 6 |
| 1 | 30* | 61 | 48 | 24 |
| 4 | 79 | 118 | 91 | 119 |
| 8 | 82 | 193 | 176 | 89 |
| 15 | 30 | 96 | 67 | 65 |
| 22 | 17 | 37 | 15 | 16 |
| 29 | 21 | 22 | 14 | 25 |
| 36 | 6 | 34 | 13 | 6 |

* Immediately following administration of the dose; data from Curry, Lader, Mould & Sakalis (1972).

During the first six weeks of treatment, if the oral dose is kept constant at, for example, 100 mg three times a day, and plasma samples from representative days are assayed, a pattern of the type shown in Table 2 is observed. After an initial rise in the first 8–15 days, concentrations drop markedly. It is presumed that enzyme induction plays a part in this phenomenon. This pattern has been observed in more than a dozen subjects, and no exceptions have been observed.

## Concentrations and Effects

The relationship between chlorpromazine concentration and effect has been studied in three separate investigations. In the first investigation, 10 drug-free patients requiring phenothiazine treatment received oral chlorpromazine 100 mg 8-hourly in solution. No other drug was given except nitrazepam at night if needed. The patients were first evaluated on a day before treatment, at 10 a.m. Testing was then carried out on the 4th, 8th, 15th, 22nd, 29th and 36th or 43rd days of treatment, and consisted of: (a) blood samples for chlorpromazine analysis at 0, 2, 4 and 6 h after the dose; (b) blood pressure and pulse rate (sitting and standing), pupil size, sweat gland activity and electroencephalogram (EEG) at these times;

(c) salivary secretion, EEG auditory evoked response, simple auditory reaction time and handwriting tests at the two-hour point only (10 a.m.); and (d) clinical ratings between the 2nd and 4th hours.

The drug concentration pattern was as discussed in the earlier section. The changes were paralleled by some of the peripheral measures, including pupil size, pulse rate (in part), blood pressure (in part), sweat gland activity, salivary secretion and EEG 4·0–7·5 Hz percentage. Clinical improvement over the first fortnight showed a tenuous relationship with drug concentration, but there was no correlation during the later phases of the study. This is illustrated by the fact that improvement continued during the six-week period, during a phase of falling drug concentration (Sakalis, Lader, Curry & Mould, 1972).

In the second study, 29 chronically hospitalized psychiatric patients considered suitable for treatment with phenothiazines were given a course of oral chlorpromazine lasting at least one month. In a chosen dosage period, blood samples were collected for chlorpromazine assay at 0, 2, 4 and 7 h after the dose. One week later, one of the oral doses was replaced by an intramuscular dose, and another set of four blood samples was collected. A number of psychomotor tests were applied at the time of the peak drug concentration after oral and intramuscular doses. Although the drug concentrations were significantly higher following the intramuscular doses, and significant differences were observed in performances in the reaction time, porteus maze and pursuit rotor tests, no relationship between the psychomotor tests and the concentrations was observed.

The third study was an investigation into the potential clinical significance of the divergence of drug concentration data following injected and oral doses in long-term psychiatric in-patients. Studies in animals and man have shown that the relatively low concentrations seen in certain patients during long-term oral treatment probably result from decomposition of chlorpromazine in the intestinal wall before absorption. The products resulting appear to be freely absorbed (Curry, D'Mello & Mould, 1971; Hollister & Curry, 1971). One way of testing the clinical significance of this would have been to compare oral and intramuscular chlorpromazine as treatments, but for practical reasons it seemed more appropriate to compare oral doses, and a single intramuscular dose, of chlorpromazine, with intramuscular injections of the long-acting analogue, fluphenazine decanoate. The single injection of chlorpromazine facilitated evaluation of individual capacities for absorption of orally administered chlorpromazine. The fluphenazine injections facilitated evaluation of long-term treatment with intramuscular phenothiazines. The comparison thus concerned absorption of, and response to, the standard oral phenothiazine (chlorpromazine) and the response to the standard long-acting intramuscular phenothiazine (fluphenazine decanoate).

In the study, 39 chronically hospitalized patients considered suitable for treatment with phenothiazines were given an initial course of oral chlorpromazine and no other drugs lasting at least one month. All had a history of poor response to orally administered drugs. As in the previous study, in a chosen dosage period, blood samples were collected at 0, 2, 4 and 7 h after the dose. Oral chlorpromazine was then continued, and one week later one of the oral doses was replaced by an intramuscular dose, and another set of blood samples was collected. Before disclosure of the analytical results, the patients were treated for two months with fluphenazine decanoate and rated for change in condition using the seven-point improvement scale of the United States National Institute of Mental Health Collaborative Research Group (1964). The patients who had the deficiencies in chlorpromazine absorption were the ones who showed the improvement when treated with the intramuscular drug. There thus appeared to be a group of schizophrenic patients, with a phenothiazine-sensitive disease, who failed to effectively absorb chlorpromazine, because of a remarkable capacity to metabolize the drug in the intestinal wall, and these patients apparently benefited from fluphenazine decanoate.

## General Considerations

The various studies relating concentration and effect are listed in Table 3. It appears that, in general, peripheral effects of chlorpromazine relate to the concentration of the unmetabolized drug. Thus effects of this

TABLE 3. *Pharmacological measurements which have shown good correlations with concentrations of chlorpromazine in plasma*

Pupil size
Pulse rate (standing)
Blood pressure (sitting diastolic)
Sweat gland activity
Salivary secretion
EEG 4·0–7·5 Hz percentage
(Curry, Lader, Mould & Sakalis, 1972)

Outcome of treatment with an intramuscular phenothiazine (fluphenazine decanoate)
(Lewis, Curry & Samuel, 1971; Curry & Adamson, 1972).

*Pharmacological measurements which have failed to show good correlations with concentrations of chlorpromazine in plasma*

Psychomotor tests:
- Reaction time
- Porteus maze
- Pursuit rotor

(Ratner & Curry, 1971).

Clinical rating:
(Curry, Lader, Mould & Sakalis, 1971).

type are probably mediated by chlorpromazine, as opposed to metabolites. Additionally, it is known that early somnolence, to which tolerance develops rapidly, is also mediated by the unmetabolized drug (Curry, 1971).

In contrast, in long-term psychiatric patients, changes in psychomotor test scores and in clinical rating did not relate directly to changes in chlorpromazine concentration, and this *may* indicate that these effects are mediated through metabolites of the drug. In support of this is the long-established idea that schizophrenic relapse occurs when chlorpromazine metabolites cease to be detectable in urine. The outcome of future studies of the relationship between metabolite concentrations in plasma and schizophrenic relapse will be awaited with great interest.

The observation that those patients who achieved very low plasma concentrations of chlorpromazine after oral dosing responded well to intra-muscular fluphenazine decanoate suggests that the decomposition of chlorpromazine in the gut leads to inactive metabolites. This decomposition apparently prevents the drug reaching the general circulation, and by inference the central nervous system, in its active form. The lack of direct correlation between improvement and plasma levels of chlorpromazine suggests that the active form is a metabolite of chlorpromazine formed in the liver.

A word of caution however. At this stage, it would be unwise to reach, from these plasma studies, the *definitive* conclusion that the antipsychotic effect of chlorpromazine is mediated through a metabolite of the drug. Of particular interest in this context is the fact that the majority of the body content of chlorpromazine-derived material appears to be eliminated within 48 h of withdrawal of drug treatment, although relapse may take many months. This conclusion, which conflicts with the popular idea that these materials persist in the body for long periods, is derived from the knowledge that drug concentrations in plasma decline rapidly during this period, and that the rate of metabolite excretion also falls off quickly. It is probable that the turnover of the majority of the chlorpromazine and chlorpromazine metabolites in the body is much more rapid than is commonly supposed, as tissue concentrations, including concentrations in brain in the rat and dog, are proportional to plasma concentrations (Curry, Derr & Maling, 1970). However, *low* concentrations of chlorpromazine and its metabolites *do* persist for long periods. This probably indicates retention of a small proportion of the administered material for a long period. It is therefore important to note that a number of important phenomena, apart from action through metabolites, can cause drug effects to fail to relate directly to the plasma concentration of the unmetabolized drug. These phenomena include influences from pre-equilibrium distribution situations, non-reversible binding at receptors, active transport of drug molecules to or at receptors, tolerance, and effects on complex physiological systems in which the measurable parameter represents the balance of a number of processes, affected differently by any one drug type (Curry, 1971).

## REFERENCES

CURRY, S. H. (1968) Determination of nanogram quantities of chlorpromazine and some of its metabolites in plasma using gas-liquid chromatography with an electron capture detector. *Anal. Chem.*, **40,** 1251–1255.

CURRY, S. H. (1970). Drug distribution and effect. *J. Roy. Coll. Phycns. Lond.*, **4,** 315–334.

CURRY, S. H. (1971). Chlorpromazine concentrations in plasma, excretion in urine and duration of effect. *Proc. Roy. Soc. Med.* **64,** 285–289.

CURRY, S. H. & ADAMSON, L. (1972). Double blind trial of fluphenazine decanoate. *Lancet*, **2,** 543–544.

CURRY, S. H., DERR, J. E. & MALING, H. M. (1970). The physiological disposition of chlorpromazine in the rat and dog. *Proc. Soc. Exp. Biol. and Med.*, **134,** 314–318.

CURRY, S. H., D'MELLO, A. & MOULD, G. P. (1971). Destruction of chlorpromazine during absorption in the rat *in vivo* and *in vitro*. *Brit. J. Pharmacol.*, **42,** 403–411.

CURRY, S. H., LADER, M. H., MOULD, G. P. & SAKALIS, G. (1972). Clinical pharmacology of chlorpromazine. *Brit. J. Pharmacol.* (in press).

EFRON, D. H., GAUDETTE, L. E. & HARRIS, S. R. (1968). A new method for measuring minute amounts of chlorpromazine and some of its metabolites in plasma. *Agressologie*, **9,** 103–107.

EFRON, D. H., HARRIS, S. R., MANIAN, A. A. & GAUDETTE, L. E. (1971). Radioassay of chlorpromazine and its metabolites in plasma. *Psychopharmacologia*, **19,** 207–211.

EMMERSON, J. L. & MIYA, T. S. (1963) Metabolism of phenothiazine drugs. *J. Pharm. Sci.*, **52,** 411–419.

HAMMER, C. G. & HOLMSTEDT, B. (1968). The identification of chlorpromazine metabolites in human blood by gas liquid chromatography. *Experientia*, **24,** 98–102.

HOLLISTER, L. E. & CURRY, S. H. (1971). Urinary excretion of chlorpromazine metabolites following single doses and in steady-state conditions. *Res. Comm. in Chem. Path. and Pharmacol.*, **2,** 330–338.

JOHNSON, D. E., RODRIGUEZ, C. F. & BURCHFIELD, H. P. (1965). Determination by microcoulometric gas chromatography of chlorpromazine metabolites in human urine. *Biochem. Pharmacol.*, **14,** 1453–1455.

KAUL, P. N., CONWAY, M. W. & CLARK, M. L. (1970). Sensitive quantitative determination of chlorpromazine metabolism. *Nature*, **226,** 372.

KAUL, P. N., CONWAY, M. W., CLARK, M. L. & HUFFINE, J. (1970). Chlorpromazine metabolism. 1: quantitative fluorometric method for 11 chlorpromazine metabolites. *J. Pharm. Sci.*, **59,** 1745–1749.

LEWIS, D. M., CURRY, S. H. & SAMUEL, G. (1971). Long-acting phenothiazines in schizophrenia. *Brit. Med. J.*, **1,** 671–672.

RATNER, L. & CURRY, S. H. (1971). Unpublished data.

SAKALIS, G., LADER, M. H., CURRY, S. H. & MOULD, G. P. (1972). Plasma levels and physiological effects of chlorpromazine in patients. *Clin. Pharmacol. Ther.*, **13,** 931–946.

UNITED STATES NATIONAL INSTITUTE OF MENTAL HEALTH COLLABORATIVE RESEARCH GROUP (1966). *Arch. Gen. Psych.*, **10,** 246.

USDIN, E. (1971). The assay of chlorpromazine and metabolites in blood, urine and other tissues. *Critical Reviews in Clinical Laboratory Sciences*, **2,** 347–391.

WILLIAMS, R. T. & PARKE, D. V. (1964). The metabolic fate of drugs. *Ann. Rev. Pharmacol.*, **4,** 85–114.

SEVENTEEN

# The Significance of Measuring Blood Levels of Benzodiazepines

S. GARATTINI, F. MARCUCCI,
P. L. MORSELLI AND E. MUSSINI

*Istituto di Ricerche Farmacologiche 'Mario Negri'*
*Via Eritrea, 62–20157 Milano, Italy*

## Introduction

Diazepam belongs to the chemical class of benzodiazepines, a group of very powerful anticonvulsant, muscle relaxant and tranquillizing agents (Zbinden & Randall, 1967). After parenteral administration, diazepam leaves the blood stream slowly and accumulates in tissues, particularly the brain (Marcucci, Fanelli, Mussini & Garattini, 1970a; Marcucci, Guaitani, Fanelli, Mussini & Garattini, 1971b) and fat (Van der Kleijn, 1969; Marcucci, Fanelli, Frova & Morselli, 1968b). Diazepam, as such, is not appreciably excreted in urine (Ruelius, Lee & Alburn, 1965) or in bile (Bertagni, Marcucci, Mussini & Garattini, 1972).

A number of studies indicated that diazepam undergoes three major metabolic processes: $N_1$-demethylation, $C_3$-hydroxylation (Schwartz, Koechlin, Postma, Palmer & Krol, 1965; Schwartz, Bommer & Vane, 1967; Kvetina, Marcucci & Fanelli, 1968) and *p*-hydroxylation of the 5-phenyl ring (Schwartz *et al.*, 1967) (see Figure 1 for chemical structures). N-demethyldiazepam and N-methyloxazepam, two of the known metabolites of diazepam, can be respectively $C_3$-hydroxylated and $N_1$-demethylated to form a common metabolite, oxazepam (Marcucci, Mussini, Fanelli & Garattini, 1970b; Mussini, Marcucci, Fanelli & Garattini, 1971). The hydroxylated metabolites, particularly N-methyloxazepam and oxazepam, can be conjugated with glucuronic acid. The glucuronides are excreted in urine (Schwartz *et al.*, 1967; Kvetina *et al.*, 1968) or in bile (Bertagni *et al.*, 1972).

The glucuronides excreted in bile are reabsorbed from the intestine, probably following hydrolysis by the gut flora, thus establishing an enterohepatic circulation which may be responsible for sustained blood levels (Marcucci *et al.*, 1970b; Marcucci *et al.*, 1971b; Mussini, Marcucci, Fanelli & Garattini, 1972). Enterohepatic circulation of oxazepam has

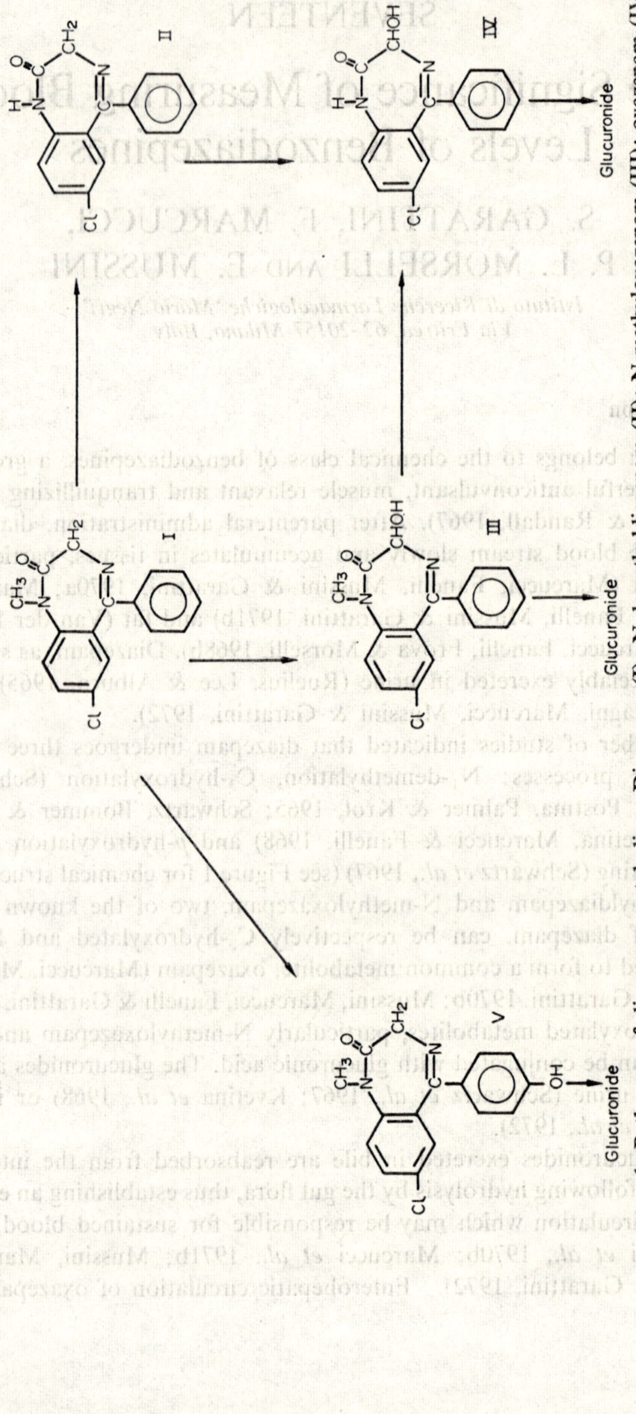


FIG. 1. Pathways of diazepam metabolism. Diazepam (I); N-demethyldiazepam (II); N-methyloxazepam (III); oxazepam (IV) and 50 H-diazepam (V).

been found in various animal species including man (unpublished results). These studies were made possible by the development of gas chromatographic methods (Garattini, Marcucci & Mussini, 1969; Marcucci, Fanelli & Mussini, 1968a), combined when necessary with mass spectrometry (Forgione, Martelli, Marcucci, Fanelli, Mussini & Jommi, 1971), for the detection in plasma and tissues of low levels of benzodiazepines with high sensitivity and specificity. It was important to measure the metabolites of diazepam since N-demethyldiazepam, N-methyloxazepam and oxazepam have pharmacological activities comparable to the parent compound (Marcucci, Mussini, Guaitani, Fanelli & Garattini, 1971c). Findings from this laboratory, which concern the importance of animal species and age in determining diazepam metabolism, were previously summarized (Garattini, Marcucci & Mussini, 1972).

### Blood Levels of Diazepam in Man

As shown in Figure 2, diazepam given orally in a single dose (capsules) to human subjects is rapidly absorbed from the intestine but leaves the blood stream slowly.

It is also evident that peak levels are achieved more rapidly in children than in adults, while the rate of disappearance is slower in elderly subjects. Figure 3 shows the plasma levels obtained after intra-muscular administration of diazepam to premature and infants and older children who received the drug for therapeutic reasons. It is clear that plasma levels of

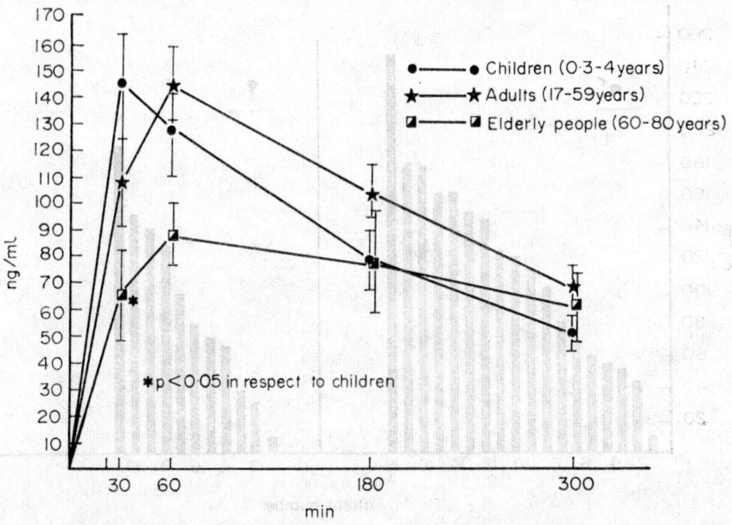


FIG. 2. Diazepam blood levels in children, adults and elderly people after a single oral dose (0·25 mg/kg).

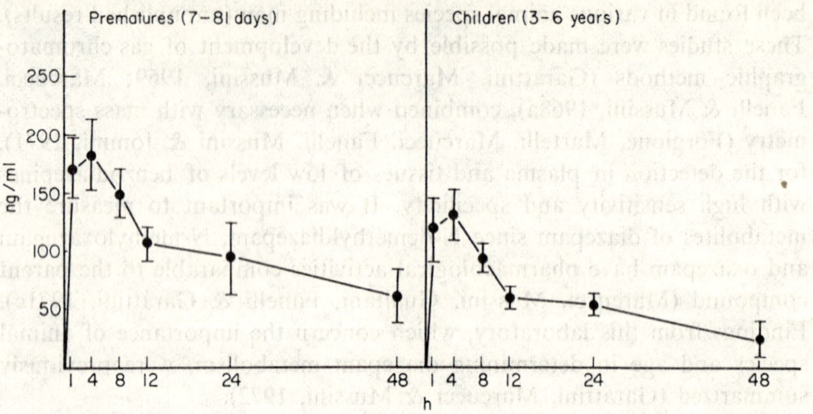


FIG. 3. Diazepam plasma levels in premature infants and children after an i.m. administration of 0·30 mg/kg.

diazepam are higher in premature subjects than children. Further studies have shown that the recovery of diazepam metabolites in urine is lower in premature newborn infants than in children (Morselli, Principi, Tognoni, Reali, Belvedere & Sereni, 1973b). Other studies have shown that the liver metabolism of diazepam is slower in newborn than in adult rats (Garattini *et al.*, 1972) and this may be the explanation of our results in humans. There is a great individual variability in blood levels after the oral administration of diazepam to adult humans (Figure 4). This is not entirely due to

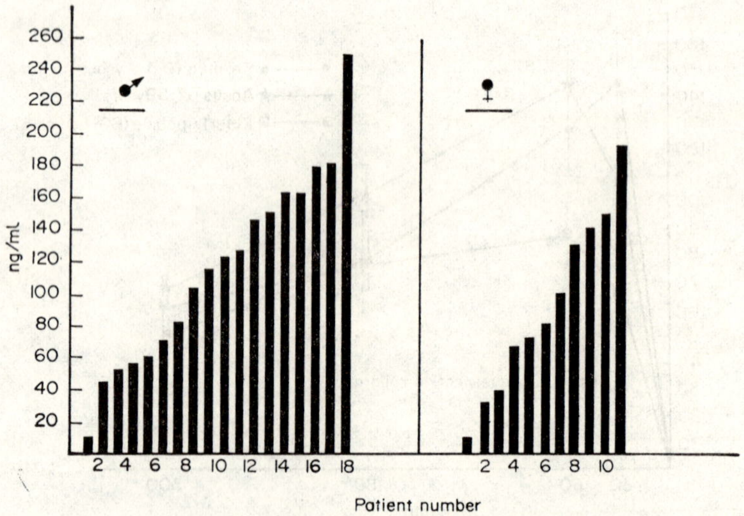


FIG. 4. Individual variability of diazepam blood levels 180 min after an oral administration of 15 mg.

TABLE 1. *Blood half-lives of diazepam after an intravenous injection of* 0·2 *mg/kg*

| Subject | Age (years) | Sex | B.W. (kg) | Apparent First $T\frac{1}{2}$ (min) |
|---|---|---|---|---|
| B. A. | 26 | ♀ | 87 | 38 |
| G. P. | 23 | ♀ | 65 | 92 |
| L. F | 33 | ♀ | 57 | 45 |
| T. L. | 52 | ♀ | 60 | 50 |
| B. C. | 48 | ♀ | 65 | 62 |

a variability in rate of absorption, because after an intravenous administration of diazepam the $T\frac{1}{2}$ of diazepam in blood may range from 38 to 92 min (Table 1).

These blood levels are useful in adults but not in children, because they correlate with the presence of drowsiness (Table 2). If diazepam is given

TABLE 2. *Relationship between diazepam blood levels and drowsiness*

| Blood Levels (ng/ml) | Adults | | | Children | | |
|---|---|---|---|---|---|---|
| | No. of subjects | No. of subjects with drowsiness | | No. of subjects | No. of subjects with drowsiness | |
| < 100 | 11 | 2 | 18% | 3 | 1 | 33% |
| 100–180 | 15 | 5 | 33% | 8 | 4 | 50% |
| > 180 | 16 | 14 | 87% | 4 | 0 | 0% |

$\chi^2 < 180/ > 180 = p < 0{\cdot}001$.

for several days (5 mg × 3 daily), a metabolite, which has been identified as N-demethyldiazepam (De Silva, Koechlin & Bader, 1966), accumulates in blood. This metabolite exceeds the level of the parent compound in all cases studied after 48 days of treatment (Table 3).

TABLE 3. *Diazepam blood levels after chronic administration* (3 × 5 *mg day for* 48 *days*)

| Subject | Age (years) | Sex | B.W. (kg) | Blood Levels (ng/ml) DZ* | DM† | DZ/DM |
|---|---|---|---|---|---|---|
| M. F. | 36 | ♀ | 60 | 104 | 120 | 0·86 |
| S. G. | 48 | ♀ | 69 | 106 | 144 | 0·73 |
| B. I. | 37 | ♀ | 78 | 123 | 184 | 0·66 |
| C. L. | 47 | ♀ | 45 | 152 | 243 | 0·62 |
| G. R. | 64 | ♀ | 46 | 180 | 247 | 0·72 |
| P. D. | 37 | ♀ | 46 | 194 | 226 | 0·85 |
| V. R. | 61 | ♀ | 73 | 231 | 281 | 0·82 |
| B. E. | 20 | ♀ | 45 | 243 | 314 | 0·77 |
| | | | | 166·2 | 219·8 | 0·75 |
| | | | S.E. | ±19·1 | ±23·5 | ±0·03 |

Samples were taken at 8 a.m., 12 h after the last dose.
* DZ = Diazepam.
† DM = N-demethylated metabolite.

**Blood Levels of N-demethyldiazepam in Man**

Since N-demethyldiazepam accumulates in blood following dosing with diazepam it was of interest to investigate the absorption of this metabolite and its persistence in blood. This compound was given orally to humans in a single capsular dose of 20 mg. Table 4 shows that, although there is a

TABLE 4. *N-demethyldiazepam (DZ) blood levels (μg/ml) after a single oral administration of DZ (20 mg)*

| Case | Time after Administration (h) | | | | | |
|---|---|---|---|---|---|---|
| | 0 | 1 | 2 | 4 | 8 | 24 | 48 |
| A | 0 | 0·54 | 0·56 | 0·74 | 0·48 | 0·47 | 0·40 |
| B | 0 | 0·0 | 0·23 | 0·25 | 0·21 | 0·18 | 0·05 |
| C | 0 | 0·16 | 0·18 | n.c.* | 0·18 | 0·06 | 0·02 |
| D | 0 | 0·52 | 0·62 | n.c. | 0·85 | 0·42 | n.c. |
| E | 0 | 0·25 | 0·28 | n.c. | 0·27 | 0·16 | n.c. |
| Mean | 0 | 0·294 ±0·104 | 0·374 ±0·090 | n.c. | 0·398 ±0·125 | 0·258 ±0·079 | n.c. |

* n.c. = blood sampling not carried out.

great variability in blood levels, N-demethyldiazepam persists longer than diazepam. This explains why N-demethyldiazepam accumulates when diazepam or N-demethyldiazepam are given chronically (Table 3 and Table 5). This finding is important because N-demethyldiazepam shows

TABLE 5. *Plasma levels of N-demethyldiazepam in humans after repeated administration* (2 × 10 *mg/day*)

| Case | Days of treatment | | |
|---|---|---|---|
| | 4 | 4 | 7 |
| 1 | 380 | 700 | 460 |
| 2 | 540 | 450 | 450 |
| 3 | 280 | 280 | 320 |
| 4 | 89 | 159 | 267 |
| 5 | 182 | 315 | 430 |
| 6 | 94 | 61 | 162 |
| $\chi$ | 260 | 327 | 348 |
| S.E. | ±72 | ±92 | ±47 |

pharmacological activities (for instance anticonvulsant effect: Marcucci *et al.*, 1971c) similar to diazepam, although it may be an antagonist of the muscle relaxing effect of diazepam (Barnett & Fiore, 1971).

Other metabolites of diazepam, such as N-methyloxazepam and oxazepam, could not be detected in blood ( < 50 ng/ml) after diazepam administration. This may be due to the rapid formation and removal of the glucuronides of both N-methyloxazepam (Morselli *et al.*, 1973b) and oxazepam (Schwartz *et al.*, 1965) that were found in human urine.

**Is there a Relationship between Blood and Brain Levels?**

To answer this question we must refer to experimental work carried out on animals. In mice, rats and guinea pigs it was found that diazepam accumulated very rapidly in brain, so that even one minute after intravenous administration the levels always exceeded those in blood (Marcucci *et al.*, 1970a; Marcucci *et al.*, 1971b). Also the concentration of metabolites in rats (Marcucci *et al.*, 1970a) and in guinea pigs (Marcucci *et al.*, 1971b) was always higher in brain than in blood. Therefore, depending on the time of the determinations, diazepam or its metabolites could be found in brain but not in blood. As shown in Table 6, the ratio between brain and blood is not constant and it tends to change with time of determination. When the dose of diazepam is relatively low (1 mg/kg), it is possible to detect oxazepam in the brain of cats, but not in their plasma (Morselli, Cassano, Placidi, Muscettola & Rizzo, 1973a).

Studies were performed to determine whether doses of benzodiazepines, exerting well-defined pharmacological effects, as for example the $ED_{50}$ against metrazol (1,5-pentamethylentetrazole) convulsions, induce always the same brain levels and whether in these conditions there is a constant ratio between brain and blood levels. Oxazepam was chosen from this investigation in order to avoid the presence of other active metabolites. Table 7 shows that the brain levels of oxazepam present after the administration of an $ED_{50}$ against metrazol are different according to the animal species. Rats, for instance, require about six times the brain oxazepam levels in respect to mice to produce the same degree of protection. However, the ratios between brain and blood levels are quite similar in both animal species and are independent from the time at which the $ED_{50}$ was determined. It should be noted also that previous studies indicated metrazol levels in brain as being similar in rats and mice (Marcucci, Airoldi, Mussini & Garattini, 1971a) and that benzodiazepines at anticonvulsant doses do not influence the brain metrazol concentrations (unpublished results).

In guinea pigs the situation is different because the brain concentration of oxazepam is higher at the $ED_{50}$ determined at shorter, rather than longer times. This may indicate that oxazepam is stored in the brain of guinea pigs also in sites which are not important for the anticonvulsant activity and that from these sites oxazepam disappears faster than from the sites associated with its anticonvulsant effect.

In any case, it is remarkable that the ratio between brain and blood remains constant despite the differences observed in the brain concentrations in relation to time.

TABLE 6. *Brain levels of several benzodiazepines after their administration* (5 *mg/kg i.v.*) *to mice, rats and guinea pigs, and ratio between brain and blood drug levels*

| Drug | Time after Adminis-tration | Benzodiazepine levels in brain ($\mu$g/g ± S.E.) | | | Drug level ratio: brain/blood | | |
|---|---|---|---|---|---|---|---|
| | | Mouse | Rat | Guinea pig | Mouse | Rat | Guinea pig |
| Diazepam | 1 min | 7·04 ±0·37 | 4·28 ±0·14 | | 5·17 | 1·83 | |
| | 5 min | 3·06 ±0·12 | 3·64 ±0·15 | 6·28 ±0·30 | 3·40 | 2·75 | 9·81 |
| | 30 min | 0·74 ±0·09 | 1·01 ±0·02 | 1·13 ±0·06 | 7·40 | 3·60 | 4·03 |
| | 1 h | 0·13 ±0·007 | 0·42 ±0·02 | 0·45 ±0·02 | 2·60 | 4·66 | 2·81 |
| | 3 h | <0·01 | 0·23 ±0·01 | 0·13 ±0·02 | — | 5·75 | 3·25 |
| | 5 h | <0·01 | 0·08 ±0·01 | 0·08 ±0·008 | — | >8 | 4·00 |
| | 10 h | <0·01 | <0·01 | 0·01 ±0·002 | — | — | — |
| | 20 h | <0·01 | — | 0·01 ±0·002 | — | — | — |
| N-de-methyl-diazepam | 1 min | 8·16 ±0·21 | 7·82 ±0·37 | | 2·05 | 1·52 | |
| | 5 min | 6·52 ±0·12 | 6·35 ±0·09 | 5·23 ±0·13 | 3·70 | 1·93 | 4·39 |
| | 30 min | 5·55 +0·05 | 3·01 ±0·07 | 5·12 ±0·04 | 4·24 | 1·90 | 5·33 |
| | 1 h | 4·52 ±0·18 | 0·59 ±0·07 | 2·20 ±0·11 | 9·61 | 6·02 | 2·34 |
| | 3 h | 0·62 ±0·01 | 0·02 ±0·001 | 1·06 ±0·05 | 5·16 | 3·00 | 5·88 |
| | 5 h | <0·01 | 0·01 ±0·0005 | 0·76 ±0·06 | — | 3·00 | 5·42 |
| | 10 h | <0·01 | <0·01 | 0·50 ±0·05 | — | — | 5·00 |
| | 20 h | — | — | 0·06 ±0·001 | — | — | 2·35 |
| N-methyl-oxazepam | 1 min | 6·98 ±0·54 | 9·40 ±0·26 | | 1·97 | 1·64 | |
| | 5 min | 5·25 ±0·63 | 8·04 ±0·34 | 6·06 ±0·20 | 3·77 | 4·62 | 6·37 |
| | 30 min | 2·63 ±0·20 | 1·20 ±0·19 | 5·97 ±0·21 | 3·13 | 0·93 | 8·65 |
| | 1 h | 0·44 +0·01 | 0·52 ±0·02 | 3·96 ±0·16 | 2·93 | 2·16 | 6·18 |
| | 3 h | 0·21 ±0·02 | <0·03 | 0·78 ±0·03 | >2·33 | — | 9·75 |
| | 5 h | <0·03 | — | 0·07 ±0·007 | — | — | >3·5 |
| | 10 h | <0·03 | — | 0·05 ±0·004 | — | — | >2·5 |
| | 20 h | — | — | 0·039 ±0·003 | — | — | >1·9 |

| Drug | Time after Adminis-tration | Benzodiazepine levels in brain (μg/g ± S.E.) Mouse | Rat | Guinea pig | Drug level ratio: brain/blood Mouse | Rat | Guinea pig |
|---|---|---|---|---|---|---|---|
| Oxazepam | 1 min | 3·59 ±0·05 | 3·06 ±0·05 | | 1·13 | 1·87 | |
| | 5 min | 14·30 ±0·17 | 4·50 ±0·03 | 3·47 ±0·47 | 6·87 | 3·00 | 1·91 |
| | 30 min | 6·84 ±0·12 | 2·90 ±0·02 | 3·21 ±0·08 | 4·52 | 5·27 | 2·11 |
| | 1 h | 5·21 ±0·03 | 1·43 ±0·05 | 2·84 ±0·08 | 4·73 | 6·21 | 3·73 |
| | 3 h | 3·12 ±0·01 | 0·20 ±0·0005 | 1·37 ±0·04 | 4·39 | 3·33 | 6·52 |
| | 5 h | 2·78 ±0·02 | <0·03 | 0·80 ±0·06 | 5·91 | — | 8·88 |
| | 10 h | 2·25 ±0·02 | | 0·48 ±0·08 | 11·25 | — | 6·80 |
| | 20 h | 0·11 ±0·01 | — | 0·15 ±0·07 | >5·5 | — | 3·00 |

TABLE 7. *Brain levels of oxazepam after administration of an $ED_{50}$ against metrazol in different animal species*

| Species | Time (min)* | $ED_{50}$ mg/kg i.v. antimetrazol | Brain ng/g ± S.E. (A) | Plasma ng/g ± S.E. (B) | Brain/Plasma ratio (A/B) |
|---|---|---|---|---|---|
| Rat | 5 | 0·470 | 624 ± 18 | 289 ± 15 | 2·1 |
| | 30 | 0·833 | 618 ± 12 | 362 ± 16 | 1·7 |
| | 180 | 10·000 | — | — | — |
| Mouse | 5 | 0·342 | 96 ± 2 | — | — |
| | 30 | 0·380 | 113 ± 13 | 79 ± 10 | 1·4 |
| | 720 | 4·850 | 117 ± 12 | 76 ± 12 | 1·5 |
| Guinea pig | 5 | 0·645 | 275 ± 7 | 226 ± 12 | 1·2 |
| | 30 | 0·520 | 242 ± 13 | 175 ± 14 | 1·3 |
| | 180 | 0·818 | 118 ± 12 | 74 ± 14 | 1·5 |
| | 720 | 4·400 | 91 ± 4 | 64 ± 4 | 1·5 |

* Minutes between drug and metrazol administration (120 mg/kg i.p.).

## Is there any Relation between Blood Levels and Levels in Different Parts of the Brain?

The answer to this question is negative because diazepam is unevenly distributed in brain. The determination of diazepam levels in various parts of the rat brain at one minute after intravenous administration indicates that the olfactory bulbs contain about 50% of the concentration of diazepam present in the hemispheres (unpublished results). These studies were extended to cats, thus permitting a better analysis of the various parts of the brain (Morselli *et al.*, 1973a).

The results in Table 8 confirm that diazepam accumulates quite differ-

TABLE 8. *Diazepam concentrations in different areas of the brain* 1 *min after i.v. administration of* $C^{14}$ *diazepam* (1 *mg/kg*). *From* The Benzodiazepines, *ed. S. Garattini, E. Mussini and L. O. Randall* (*Raven Press* © 1973)

| Brain area | Diazepam μg/g ± S.E. |
|---|---|
| Frontal grey matter | 2·68 ± 0·33 |
| Occipital grey matter | 2·60 ± 0·69 |
| Temporal grey matter | 2·51 ± 0·25 |
| Parietal grey matter | 2·50 ± 0·47 |
| Olfactory bulb | 2·46 ± 0·37 |
| Cerebellar grey matter | 2·41 ± 0·17 |
| Thalamus | 2·95 ± 0·38 |
| Hyppocampus | 1·88 ± 0·21 |
| Hypothalamus | 2·08 ± 0·24 |
| Mesencephalon | 2·65 ± 0·19 |
| Pons | 2·24 ± 0·17 |
| Bulb | 2·13 ± 0·21 |
| Hypophysis | 2·90 ± 0·26 |
| Frontal white matter | 1·04 ± 0·14 |
| Temporal white matter | 1·48 ± 0·44 |
| Occipital white matter | 1·07 ± 0·09 |
| Cerebellar white matter | 1·62 ± 0·24 |

ently in various areas of the brain. The early uptake of diazepam, as well as the rate of removal, seems to correlate directly with the regional blood flow in the brain (Figure 5). There is also a redistribution of diazepam

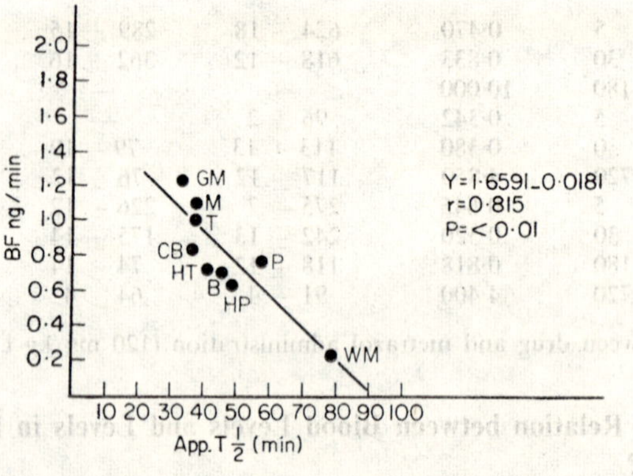


FIG. 5. Relationship between diazepam apparent half-life (T½ min) and blood flow in the various areas of cat brain. (GM = cortical grey matter, M = mesencephalon, T = thalamus, P = pons, CB = cerebellum, HT = hypothalamus, B = bulb, HP = hyppocampus, WM = subcortical white matter.) After Morselli *et al.* (1973a).

within the brain between the white and grey matters, which is in agreement with autoradiographic studies performed by Cassano, Ghiozzi & Ghetti (1969) with other benzodiazepines. The data in Table 9 show that the ratio between the concentration of diazepam or N-demethyldiazepam in the white or grey matter and the plasma changes with time.

TABLE 9. *Ratio between diazepam (DZ) and N- demethyldiazepam (DDZ) levels in white or grey matter and plasma of cats given $C^{14}$ diazepam (1 mg/kg i.v.)*

| Time | Grey Cortex DZ | Grey Cortex DDZ | White matter DZ | White matter DDZ |
|---|---|---|---|---|
| 1 min | 6·3 | — | 2·0 | — |
| 15 min | 13·0 | 5·8 | 15·0 | 1·7 |
| 30 min | 6·7 | 7·3 | 10·0 | 7·3 |
| 1 h | 4·6 | 9·2 | 9·9 | 11·0 |
| 4 h | 5·0 | 7·2 | 8·0 | 10·5 |

## Are Different Pharmacological Effects Achieved at the Same Blood or Brain Level?

Since benzodiazepines exert different pharmacological effects, it is important to ascertain whether these effects are associated with different brain or blood levels. Diazepam was given by intravenous injection to mice to determine blood and brain levels of diazepam and its metabolites. In other groups of mice, under the same experimental conditions, the presence and the duration of the following effects were recorded: (a) antimetrazol activity, (b) muscle relaxation (rotarod test), and (c) antiaggressive activity (measured according to Valzelli, 1973). The results of

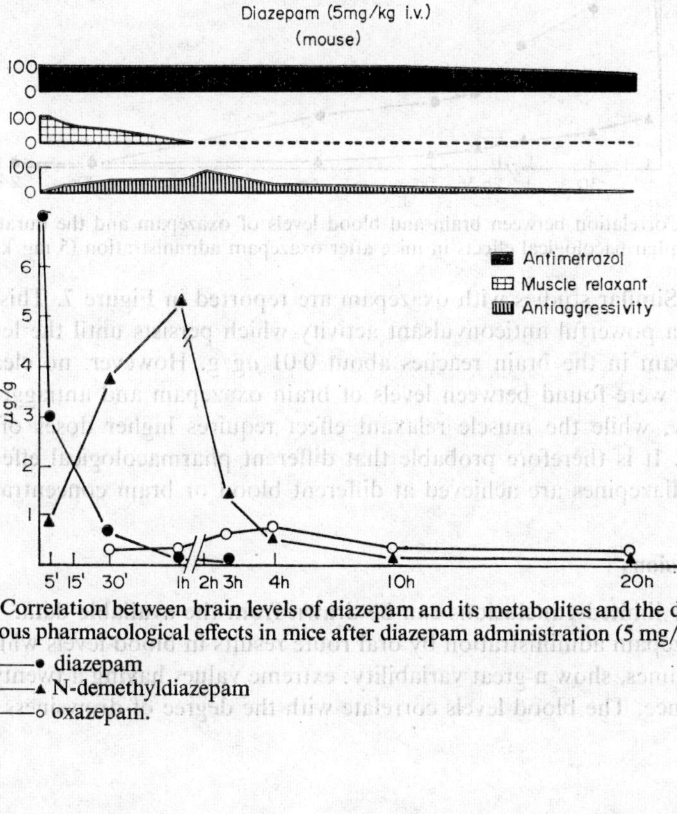


FIG. 6. Correlation between brain levels of diazepam and its metabolites and the duration of various pharmacological effects in mice after diazepam administration (5 mg/kg i.v.).
•——• diazepam
▲——▲ N-demethyldiazepam
○——○ oxazepam.

this investigation are reported in Fig. 6. It is evident that the various pharmacological effects terminate at different times. The duration of the anticonvulsant activity is not related to the brain level of diazepam, or to the level of a single metabolite, but rather to the sum of diazepam plus N-demethyldiazepam and oxazepam.

The muscle relaxant effect is short and seems to be best related to the brain or blood level of diazepam, while the anti-aggressive activity apparently parallels the accumulation and removal of N-demethyldiazepam in the

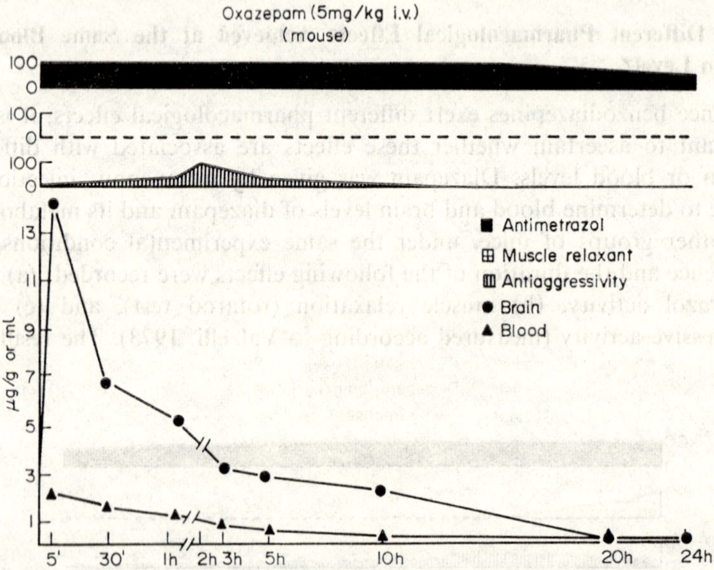


FIG. 7. Correlation between brain and blood levels of oxazepam and the duration of various pharmacological effects in mice after oxazepam administration (5 mg/kg i.v.).

brain. Similar studies with oxazepam are reported in Figure 7. This drug exerts a powerful anticonvulsant activity which persists until the level of oxazepam in the brain reaches about 0·01 μg/g. However, no clear relations were found between levels of brain oxazepam and antiaggressive activity, while the muscle relaxant effect requires higher doses of oxazepam. It is therefore probable that different pharmacological effects of benzodiazepines are achieved at different blood or brain concentrations.

## Conclusions

Only limited conclusions can be drawn from the available data.

Diazepam administration by oral route results in blood levels which, at given times, show a great variability: extreme values having a twenty-fold difference. The blood levels correlate with the degree of drowsiness when the drug is taken for the first time in a single dose. During chronic administration a metabolite of diazepam, N-demethyldiazepam, accumulates in the blood of patients. This is an important finding since N-demethyldiazepam possesses much of the pharmacological activity of diazepam.

For several reasons it is not possible to correlate blood levels of diazepam with therapeutic effect: 1. several metabolites of diazepam show powerful pharmacological effects; 2. the relationship between brain and blood levels is not always constant, and in any case the distribution of benzodiazepines in different parts of the brain is uneven; 3. different pharmacological effects of benzodiazepines require different blood or brain levels.

Further studies are needed to determine whether blood levels can be meaningfully related to therapeutic responses. However, the determination of blood benzodiazepines in man may be justified by the necessity (a) to obtain information about the bioavailability of benzodiazepines in different pharmaceutical preparations; (b) to investigate the accumulation of metabolites; and (c) to study how other drugs may influence the absorption, distribution and metabolism of various benzodiazepines.

The experimental work presented in this paper has been supported by the National Institutes of Health, Bethesda, Maryland, USA (Contract No. PH/NIH/43-67-83 and Grant No. 1 POI GMI 8376-01 PTR).

## REFERENCES

BARNETT, A. & FIORE, J. W. (1971). Acute tolerance to diazepam in cats and its possible relationship to diazepam metabolism. *Eur. J. Pharmac.*, **13**, 239–243.

BERTAGNI, P., MARCUCCI, F., MUSSINI, E. & GARATTINI, S. (1972). Biliary excretion of conjugated hydroxyl benzodiazepines after administration of several benzodiazepines to rats, guinea pigs and mice. *J. Pharm. Sci.*, **61**, 965–966.

CASSANO, G. B., GLIOZZI, E. & GHETTI, B. (1969). The relationship between dynamic features of the brain distribution of $C^{14}$-chlordiazepoxide and motor behaviour changes in mice. In: *The Present Status of Psychotropic Drugs. Pharmacological and Clinical Aspects*, ed. by Cerletti A. & Bové, F. J., pp. 342–346. Amsterdam: Excerpta Medica Foundation.

DE SILVA, J. A. F., KOECHLIN, B. A. & BADER, G. (1966). Blood level distribution patterns of diazepam and its major metabolite in man. *J. Pharm. Sci.*, **55**, 692–702.

FORGIONE, A., MARTELLI, P., MARCUCCI, F., FANELLI, R., MUSSINI, E. & JOMMI, G. C. (1971). Gas liquid chromatography and mass spectrometry of several benzodiazepines. *J. Chromat.*, **59**, 163–168.

GARATTINI, S., MARCUCCI, F. & MUSSINI, E. (1969). Gas-chromatographic analysis of benzodiazepines. In: *Gas Chromatography in Biology and Medicine*, ed. by Porter, R., pp. 161–172. London: Churchill.

GARATTINI, S., MARCUCCI, F. & MUSSINI, E. (1972). Benzodiazepine metabolism *in vitro*. *Drug Metabolism Reviews* (in press).

KLEIJN, E. VAN DER (1969). Kinetics of distribution and metabolism of diazepam and chlordiazepoxide in mice. *Archs. int. Pharmacodyn. Thér.*, **178,** 193–215.

KVETINA, J., MARCUCCI, F. & FANELLI, R. (1968). Metabolism of diazepam in isolated perfused liver of rat and mouse. *J. Pharm. Pharmac.*, **20,** 807–808.

MARCUCCI, F., AIROLDI, L., MUSSINI, E. & GARATTINI, S. (1971a). Brain levels of metrazol determined with a new gas chromatographic procedure. *Eur. J. Pharmac.*, **16,** 219–221.

MARCUCCI, F., FANELLI, R., FROVA, M. & MORSELLI, P. L. (1968b). Levels of diazepam in adipose tissue of rats, mice and man. *Eur. J. Pharmac.*, **4,** 464–466.

MARCUCCI, F., FANELLI, R. & MUSSINI, E. (1968a). A method for gas-chromatographic determination of benzodiazepines. *J. Chromat.*, **37,** 318–320.

MARCUCCI, F., FANELLI, R., MUSSINI, E. & GARATTINI, S. (1970a). Further studies on species difference in diazepam metabolites. *Eur. J. Pharmac.*, **9,** 253–256.

MARCUCCI, F., GUAITINI, A., FANELLI, R., MUSSINI, E. & GARATTINI, S. (1971b). Metabolism and anticonvulsant activity of diazepam in guinea pigs. *Biochem. Pharmac.*, **20,** 1711–1713.

MARCUCCI, F., MUSSINI, E., FANELLI, R. & GARATTINI, S. (1970b). Species differences in diazepam metabolism. I. Metabolism of diazepam metabolites. *Biochem. Pharmac.*, **19,** 1847–1851.

MARCUCCI, F., MUSSINI, E., GUAITINI, A., FANELLI, R. & GARATTINI, S. (1971c). Anticonvulsant activity and brain levels of diazepam and its metabolites in mice. *Eur. J. Pharmac.*, **16,** 311–314.

MORSELLI, P. L., CASSANO, G. B., PLACIDI, G. F., MUSCETTOLA, G. B. & RIZZO, M. (1973a). Kinetics of the distribution of $C^{14}$-diazepam and its metabolites in various areas of cat brain. In: *The Benzodiazepines*, ed. by Garattini, S., Mussini, E. & Randall, L. O., pp. 129–143. New York: Raven Press.

MORSELLI, P. L., PRINCIPI, N., TOGNONI, G., REALI, E., BELVEDERE, G. & SERENI, F. (1973b). Diazepam disposition in premature and full term infants and children. *J. Perinat. Med.* (in press).

MUSSINI, E., MARCUCCI, F., FANELLI, R. & GARATTINI, S. (1971). Metabolism of diazepam and its metabolites by guinea pig liver microsomes. *Biochem. Pharmac.*, **20,** 2529–2531.

MUSSINI, E., MARCUCCI, F., FANELLI, R. & GARATTINI, S. (1972). Metabolism of diazepam metabolites in guinea pigs. *Chem. Biol. Interactions*, **5**, 73–76.

RUELIUS, H. W., LEE, J. M. & ALBURN, H. E. (1965). Metabolism of diazepam in dogs: transformation to oxazepam. *Archs. Biochem. Biophys.*, **111**, 376–380.

SCHWARTZ, M. A., BOMMER, P. & VANE, F. M. (1967). Diazepam metabolites in the rat: characterization by high-resolution mass spectrometry and nuclear magnetic resonance. *Archs. Biochem. Biophys.*, **121**, 508–516.

SCHWARTZ, M. A., KOECHLIN, B. A., POSTMA, E., PALMER, S. & KROL, G. (1965). Metabolism of diazepam in rat, dog and man. *J. Pharmac. exp. Ther.*, **149**, 423–435.

VALZELLI, L. (1973). Activity of benzodiazepines on aggressive behaviour in rats and mice. In: *The Benzodiazepines*, ed. by Garattini, S., Mussini, E. & Randall, L. O., pp. 405–417. New York: Raven Press.

ZBINDEN, G. & RANDALL, L. O. (1967). Pharmacology of benzodiazepines: laboratory and clinical correlations. In: *Advances in Pharmacology*, vol. 5, ed. by Garattini, S. & Shore, P. A., pp. 213–291. New York: Academic Press.

EIGHTEEN

# Effects of Phenytoin in Patients with Epilepsy in Relation to its Concentration in Plasma

LARS LUND

*Departments of Neurology, Karolinska Hospital,*
*and Clinical Pharmacology, Huddinge Hospital,*
*S-104 01 Stockholm 60, Sweden*

## Introduction

Phenytoin has been used in the treatment of epilepsy since 1938, when it was introduced by Merritt & Putnam (1938a, b). It has become the most widely used antiepileptic drug and is effective in the prevention of generalized or partial epileptic seizures.

No method for the measurement of phenytoin was available before 1956. In that year two spectrophotometric methods were published (Plaa & Hine, 1956, Dill, Kazenko, Wolf & Glazko, 1956) which were sufficiently specific to allow studies of the pharmacokinetics of phenytoin. Buchthal, Svensmark & Schiller (1960) were the first to correlate clinical and electro-encephalographic data to the concentration of phenytoin in plasma. In a group of 12 in-patients they showed that clinical improvement did not occur until the plasma concentration was above 10 $\mu$g/ml. These patients were observed over two months.

In another group consisting of 51 out-patients a decrease in seizure frequency to about 50% or less was not seen until the plasma concentration was 10 $\mu$g/ml or more. By contrast, Triedman, Fishman & Yahr (1960) found no differences in plasma concentration between two groups of patients with good and poor seizure control respectively. However, they neither defined these groups clinically nor reported the length of the observation period.

In both these studies simplified modifications of Dill's method were used. which may give misleading values when drugs other than phenytoin or phenobarbitone are given (*cf.* Buchthal *et al.*, 1960). A further simplification of Dill's method (Svensmark & Kristensen, 1963) has also been shown to be non-specific (Kristensen, Mølholm Hansen, Hansen & Lund, 1967).

Buchthal *et al.* (1960) reported pronounced side-effects in 50% of the patients with plasma concentrations of phenytoin above 30 μg/ml. Kutt, Winters, Kokenge, & McDowell (1964) stated that nystagmus appeared at 20, ataxia at 30 and mental symptoms at 40 μg/ml. Lascelles, Kocen & Reynolds (1970), however, did not find such a clear relationship between plasma concentrations and side-effects of phenytoin, especially not in cases with insidiously developing symptoms.

Lund, Jørgensen & Kühl (1964) compared the plasma concentration of phenytoin in ambulatory patients. In one group of patients the plasma concentration was determined in connection with check-ups in the out-patient clinic 2, 6 and 12 weeks after discharge from the hospital, while the other group consisted of patients who had their first check-up after 12 weeks. In the first group 17 of 22 patients had plasma levels above 10 μg/ml at 12 weeks compared to only 10 of 29 in the other group. Gibberd, Dunne, Handley & Hazleman (1970) found a mean plasma concentration in 15 out-patients of $15{\cdot}7 \pm 12{\cdot}9$ μg/ml compared with $28{\cdot}0 \pm 8{\cdot}1$ in 14 in-patients with comparable doses. Kutt, Haynes & McDowell (1966) showed that 12 of 16 patients with poor seizure control in spite of high doses of phenytoin increased their plasma concentrations when the drug intake was supervised.

The studies reviewed above suggest that it might be useful to measure the plasma concentration of phenytoin. However, it was felt that further studies were necessary to answer the following problems. (1) How often is unreliable drug intake the reason for low plasma concentrations? (2) At which plasma levels is the drug most effective in preventing seizures without giving disturbing side-effects? (3) Are there any differences in this regard between patients treated only with phenytoin and those treated with additional antiepileptic drugs?

This study was undertaken partly to elucidate these questions and partly to get patient material suitable for longitudinal monitoring of phenytoin plasma levels.

## Patients

A total of 294 ambulatory patients treated for generalized epileptic seizures (excluding *petit mal*) or various forms of partial epilepsy, or combinations thereof, were studied. They had been treated with phenytoin for at least 6 months. The same pharmaceutical formulation (Difhydan®, Leo), containing the acid of phenytoin, was used in all cases.

No other selection was made at this stage, which means that the aetiology of the epilepsy and the frequency of seizures vary considerably. 148 patients were treated only with phenytoin. This group was analysed separately. The remaining patients had additional treatment with other antiepileptic drugs, usually phenobarbitone, primidon or carbamazepine.

## Methods

Blood was drawn in heparinized tubes during a routine visit to the out-patient clinic. The blood was centrifuged within an hour and 5 ml of plasma was kept frozen until analysis. The patients had not been informed about the investigation in advance and as a rule they had therefore already taken their morning dose of phenytoin (and any other antiepileptic drug prescribed) when the blood was drawn. The total number of seizures and side-effects during the last two months were recorded. A neurological examination was performed by the author in each case, with special reference to the occurrence of nystagmus, ataxia and somnolence, i.e. the most common signs of dose-dependent side-effects of phenytoin.

In a group of patients with at least one seizure during the last two months and with a concentration of phenytoin in plasma below 10 $\mu$g/ml, the reliability of the drug intake was checked during a stay in the ward for at least seven days with unchanged oral dose of phenytoin in the same pharmaceutical formulation. All other medication was kept unchanged. Phenytoin was given at the same time and with the same intervals as before hospitalization. The patients were closely supervised and observed to swallow their medicine. Plasma samples were taken each morning before the first daily dose of phenytoin was given. If the plasma level was at least 25% higher on the seventh than on the first day, unreliable drug intake was considered as a main reason for the low concentration in plasma.

Phenytoin in plasma was determined using the spectrophotometric method described by Dill *et al.* (1956). The selectivity of this method has been investigated (Borgå, Lund & Sjöqvist, 1969). The results with this method when used in patients under strict clinical control agree well with those obtained with a recently developed gas chromatographic procedure (Sjöqvist & Bertilsson, this symposium pp. 25–40; and Berlin, Agurell, Borgå, Lund & Sjöqvist, 1972).

## Results

The relation between the concentration of phenytoin in plasma and the prescribed daily dose in the whole patient material is shown in Figure 1. In Table 1 the material has been divided according to the number of seizures during the last two months. Eighteen patients (6%) in the whole material were unable to give an accurate account of their seizure frequency. The mean prescribed dose and the mean plasma concentration of this group did not differ significantly from the whole material.

Of the remaining 276 patients 167 (60·5%) reported absence of seizures during the last two months, while the rest had had one seizure or more. There was no difference in the mean prescribed dose between these groups. By contrast, the mean concentration of phenytoin in plasma was significantly lower ($p < 0.01$) in the seizure group as a whole than in the seizure-free group.

Table 2 shows in a similar way the patients treated only with phenytoin.

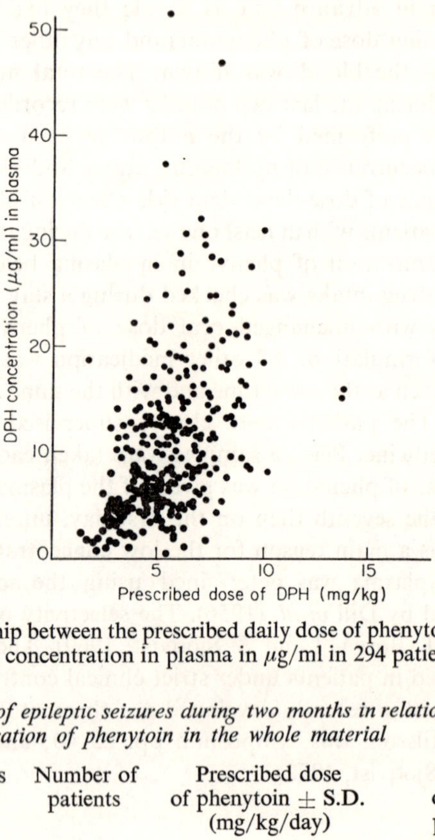


FIG. 1. The relationship between the prescribed daily dose of phenytoin (DPH) in mg/kg body-weight and the concentration in plasma in μg/ml in 294 patients with epilepsy.

TABLE 1. *Number of epileptic seizures during two months in relation to prescribed dose and plasma concentration of phenytoin in the whole material*

| Number of seizures during the last two months | Number of patients | Prescribed dose of phenytoin ± S.D. (mg/kg/day) | Concentration of phenytoin in plasma ± S.D. (μg/ml) |
|---|---|---|---|
| 0 | 167 | 5·5 ± 1·9 | 12·6 ± 8·8 |
| 1 | 48 | 5·8 ± 1·5 | 8·0 ± 4·1 |
| 2 | 18 | 5·2 ± 1·6 | 7·3 ± 4·0 |
| 3–5 | 17 | 5·7 ± 1·2 | 11·2 ± 6·0 |
| >5 | 26 | 5·8 ± 1·5 | 8·9 ± 4·6 |
| unknown | 18 | 5·6 ± 2·4 | 12·0 ± 6·1 |
| whole seizure group | 109 | 5·7 ± 1·5 | 8·6 ± 4·6 |
| total material | 294 | 5·6 ± 1·8 | 11·1 ± 7·6 |

Also in this material the mean plasma concentration of phenytoin was significantly lower ($p < 0{\cdot}001$) in the seizure-group as a whole than in the group without seizures. In Table 3 patients with unknown seizure-frequency have been excluded and the remainder (276 patients) has been divided into three groups according to the plasma concentration. Only 36·6% fell in the range between 10·0 and 19·9 μg/ml, while 51·8% had lower and 11·6% higher plasma concentrations.

The corresponding percentages for the group treated only with phenytoin was 22·3, 64·2 and 13·5 respectively (Table 4). In the whole material

TABLE 2. *Number of epileptic seizures during two months in relation to prescribed dose and plasma concentration of phenytoin in the group treated only with phenytoin*

| Number of seizures during the last two months | Number of patients | Prescribed dose of phenytoin ± S.D. (mg/kg/day) | Concentration of phenytoin in plasma ± S.D. (μg/ml) |
|---|---|---|---|
| 0 | 84 | 5·0 ± 1·7 | 13·4 ± 11·2 |
| 1 | 19 | 5·7 ± 1·6 | 8·8 ± 3·9 |
| 2 | 23 | 4·8 ± 1·7 | 7·3 ± 3·7 |
| 3–5 | 11 | 4·4 ± 1·2 | 4·5 ± 2·9 |
| >5 | 11 | 6·4 ± 1·6 | 6·2 ± 5·6 |
| whole seizure group | 64 | 5·1 ± 1·7 | 7·1 ± 4·2 |
| total material | 148 | 5·3 ± 1·7 | 10·6 ± 9·4 |

TABLE 3. *Number of patients without seizures in various plasma concentration intervals for the whole material*

| Concentration of phenytoin in plasma (μg/ml) | 0–9·9 | 10·0–19·9 | above 20·0 |
|---|---|---|---|
| Number of patients | 143 | 101 | 32 |
| % of total material | 51·8 | 36·6 | 11·6 |
| Number of patients without seizures during the last two months | 69 | 67 | 31 |
| % seizure-free in each group | 48·3 | 66·3 | 96·9 |

TABLE 4. *Number of patients without seizures in various plasma concentration intervals. Patients treated only with phenytoin.*

| Concentration of phenytoin in plasma (μg/ml) | 0–9·9 | 10·0–19·9 | above 20·0 |
|---|---|---|---|
| Number of patients | 95 | 33 | 20 |
| % of total material | 64·2 | 22·3 | 13·5 |
| Number of patients without seizures during the last two months | 41 | 24 | 19 |
| % seizure-free in each group | 43·2 | 72·5 | 95·0 |

the seizure-free fraction of each group was 48·3%, 67·3% and 96·9% respectively compared to 43·2%, 72·5% and 95·0% in the group treated only with phenytoin.

The reliability of drug intake was investigated in the patients who had had at least one epileptic seizure during the two-month's period and plasma levels between 0 and 9·9 μg/ml. This group consisted of 74 patients, corresponding to 67·9% of all patients with seizures. Ten patients did not participate in the study. In one case the medication had to be stopped due

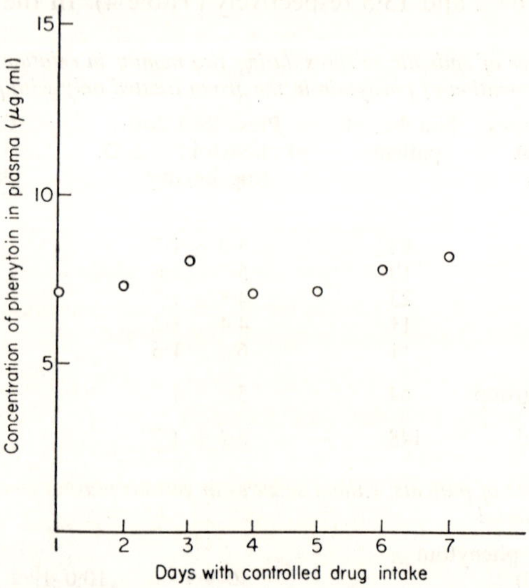


FIG. 2. Effect of controlled drug intake on the plasma concentraton of phenytoin in a patient with epilepsy. Example of reliable drug intake.

to a rash presumably caused by phenytoin, the other nine refused to cooperate. There was evidence of alcohol abuse in all these cases, either admitted by the patient or shown in the records.

In 48 (75·0%) of the participating 64 patients the plasma concentration did not change or increased with less than 25% of the initial value during seven days of supervised drug intake. In the remaining 16 (25·0%) the

TABLE 5. *Effect of controlled intake of phenytoin on the plasma concentration*

| | Number of patients | % |
|---|---|---|
| Less than 25% increase in the concentration of phenytoin in plasma ('reliable drug intake') | 48 | 75·0 |
| More than 25% increase in the concentration of phenytoin in plasma ('unreliable drug intake') | 16 | 25·0 |

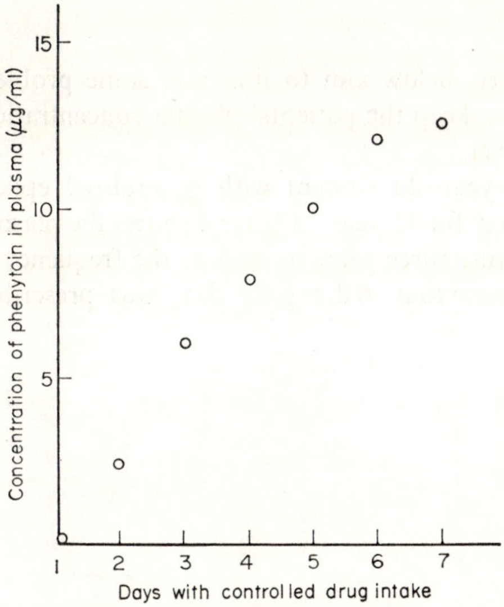


FIG. 3. Effect of controlled drug intake on the plasma concentration of phenytoin in a patient with epilepsy. Example of unreliable drug intake.

plasma concentration rose to a value which was at least 25% higher than that recorded on the first day (see Table 5).

Only five of these patients had admitted irregular drug intake before the investigation. The rest did so after having been confronted with their own plasma concentration values. Examples of 'reliable' and 'unreliable' drug intake are given in Figures 2–3.

## Side-effects

Table 6 summarizes data from those six patients (2·0%) who showed side-effects, i.e. nystagmus, ataxia or somnolence. The prescribed daily

TABLE 6. *Prescribed dose of phenytoin, plasma concentration and clinical data from six patients with side-effects*

| Patient | Prescribed dose of phenytoin (mg/kg/day) | Concentration of phenytoin in plasma (µg/ml) | Nystagmus | Ataxia | Somnolence |
|---|---|---|---|---|---|
| A. J. | 5·2 | 27·5 | + | − | − |
| J. H. | 6·8 | 31·8 | + | − | + |
| H. N. | 4·5 | 32·0 | + | + | + |
| A. G. | 10·0 | 33·0 | − | + | − |
| E. G. | 7·4 | 38·5 | + | + | + |
| H. E. | 5·8 | 52·8 | + | + | + |

dose varied from 4·5 to 10·0 mg/kg and the plasma concentrations from 27·5 to 52·8 µg/ml. Plasma levels above 20 µg/ml were found in 35 of the 294 patients (11·9%).

## Case Reports

The case reports below aim to illustrate some problems encountered in our attempts to keep the patients' plasma concentrations of phenytoin at an effective level.

*Case 1.* A 44-year-old woman with generalized epileptic seizures of unknown aetiology for 15 years. Figure 4 shows the plasma concentration of phenytoin during three years as well as the frequency of seizures. The same dose of phenytoin, 6·8 mg/kg/day, was prescribed during these

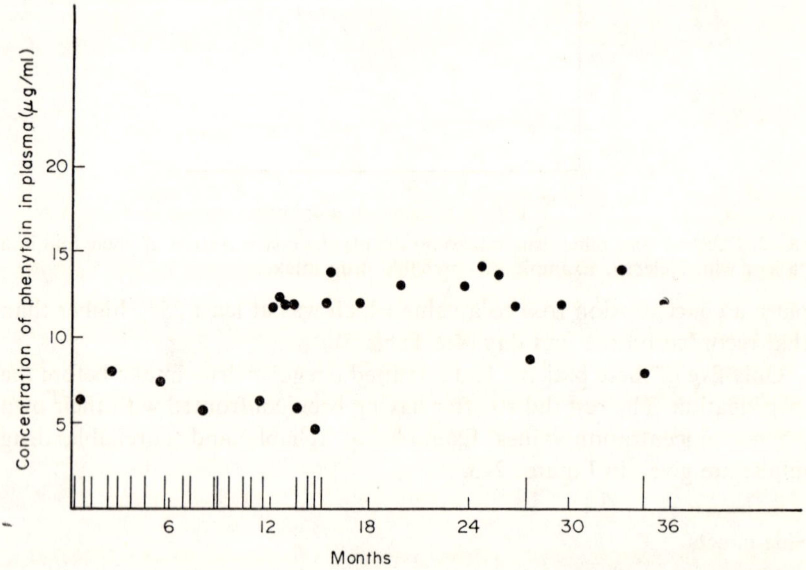


FIG. 4. Case 1. The plasma concentration of phenytoin and the seizure frequency in a patient with epilepsy treated with 6·8 mg phenytoin/kg body weight. Each bar represents one generalized seizure.

years, but no particular attention was paid to the low plasma concentrations during the first year. A lot of other antiepileptic drugs were tried with unsatisfactory results. After a stay in the hospital (month 12 in Figure 4.), during which unreliable drug intake was found, the plasma concentration has remained between 12 and 15 μg/ml and the number of seizures has diminished markedly. There have been two seizures during the last two years. On both occasions the plasma concentration had dropped due to irregular drug intake.

*Case 2.* A 33-year-old man with generalized and psychomotor seizures for six years of unknown aetiology. The result of ambulatory treatment with phenytoin and carbamazepine was disappointing. Figure 5 shows the plasma concentrations of phenytoin during a six-weeks' stay in the hospital.

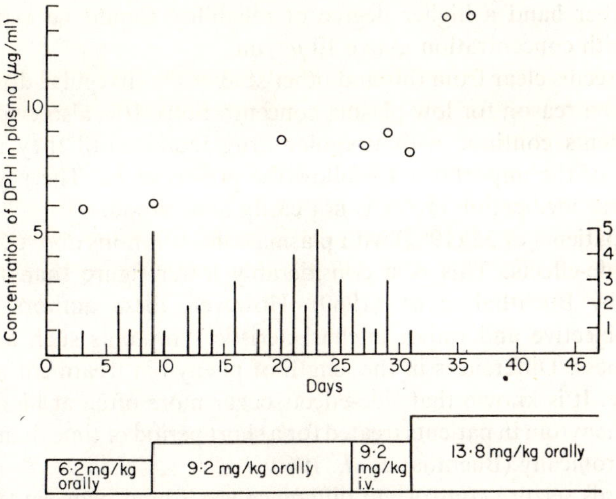


FIG. 5. Case 2. The plasma concentration of phenytoin and the seizure frequency in a patient with generalized and psychomotor seizures in the relation one to two.

The dose of carbamazepine, 1·2 g/day, was not changed. In this case there was no change in seizure-frequency until the plasma concentration of phenytoin was about 15 µg/ml. The seizure control after discharge from hospital has been very good as regards the generalized seizures (three seizures during ten months) and satisfactory as regards the psychomotor seizures (one to two seizures each week.)

## Discussion

The wide scatter of phenytoin plasma levels found in our ambulatory patient material agrees well with the findings of other authors (Stensrud & Palmer, 1964; Haerer & Grace, 1969; Gibberd *et al.*, 1970; Lascelles *et al.*, 1970). Buchthal *et al.* (1960) found that 47% of a group consisting of 51 out-patients had levels below 10 µg/ml. The corresponding figure in our material is 52%. Only 37% have values between 10 and 19·9 µg/ml. This figure compares well with that of Lascelles *et al.* who found that 45% of their patients fell within this range.

One reason for the great interindividual variations in plasma concentrations of phenytoin seems to be unreliable drug intake, which in this study occurred in 25% of patients with plasma concentrations below 10 µg/ml and with poor seizure control. This figure is considerably lower than that reported by Kutt *et al.* (1966), probably due to different selection principles. The frequency of irregular drug intake in the whole material is difficult to estimate. Presumably at least the same frequency should be found in the group with concentrations lower than 10 µg/ml but without seizures.

On the other hand a higher degree of reliability should be expected in patients with concentration above 10 μg/ml.

Thus it seems clear from this and other studies that irregular drug intake is a common reason for low plasma concentrations. It is also evident that many patients continue with irregular drug intake until they are fully convinced of the importance to follow the prescriptions. The psychology behind these medication errors is not easily understood.

Only 6 patients of 32 (19%) with plasma concentrations above 20 μg/ml showed side-effects. This is a considerably lower figure than the 50% reported by Buchthal *et al.* (1960). However, these authors also recorded subjective and rather uncharacteristic symptoms such as fatigue and giddiness. Differences in the length of phenytoin treatment may also play a role. It is known that side-effects occur more often at high plasma levels of phenytoin in patients treated for a short period of time than in those treated chronically (Buchthal *et al.*, 1960).

As regards seizure control, no difference was found between the entire material and those treated only with phenytoin. Of the latter, however, only 22·3% had plasma concentrations between 10 and 19·9 μg/ml compared with 36·6% in the whole material. This difference is difficult to explain.

No statistically significant difference in plasma concentration was found between the group without seizures and that with one seizure or more. However, there is a clear tendency towards lower plasma levels in the seizure groups especially in patients treated only with phenytoin. The percentage of seizure-free patients is much higher in the groups with plasma concentration above 10 μg/ml than in those with concentrations below this level (Tables 3 and 4).

In this non-selected material, where many patients had a mild epilepsy with only one or two generalized seizures every year, the length of the observation period is too short. Some patients may therefore have been wrongly classified as seizure-free. However, a longer retrospect observation period than two months might have increased the risk for invalid reports on the seizure frequency.

It is also obvious that the plasma concentrations determined at the end of the observation period are not necessarily the same as those occurring at the time of the seizure. To avoid such disadvantages of a retrospective study, a longitudinal investigation has been started where the plasma concentration of phenytoin is determined monthly or bimonthly and the seizure frequency is recorded at the same time. Our experience so far (*cf.* case 1) suggests that this is the most accurate way to assess the therapeutic range of phenytoin plasma concentrations. Already it is possible to state that the monitoring of phenytoin plasma concentrations in patients with epilepsy is an invaluable complement to clinical examination.

**Summary**

The plasma concentration of phenytoin was determined according to Dill's method in 294 ambulatory patients with various forms of epilepsy except *petit mal.* Other antiepileptic drugs (phenobarbitone, primidone, carbamazepine) were often given at the same time, but 148 cases were treated only with phenytoin.

The number of seizures during the last two months were noted as well as symptoms and signs of side-effects of phenytoin. Eighteen patients (6%) could not give an accurate account of the number of seizures. Among the remaining patients 109 (40%) had had seizures. The plasma concentration was lower in this group than in the group without seizures ($8{\cdot}6 \pm 4{\cdot}6$ $\mu$g/ml versus $12{\cdot}6 \pm 8{\cdot}8$ $\mu$g/ml). The prescribed dose of phenytoin did not differ significantly between the two groups.

In the group treated only with phenytoin essentially the same results were found.

The explanations of the low plasma concentrations of phenytoin in patients with poor seizure control include irregular drug intake, which was shown to occur in 25% of 64 patients with plasma concentrations below 10 $\mu$g/ml.

Thirty-five patients (12%) had plasma concentrations above 20 $\mu$g/ml. Six of them showed side-effects of phenytoin at plasma concentrations from 27·5 to 52·8 $\mu$g/ml.

**Acknowledgements**

This study was supported by the Swedish Medical Research Council (B73–14X–3902–01), Föreningen Margarethahemnet and Karolinska Institutet.

## REFERENCES

BERLIN, A., AGURELL, S., BORGÅ, O., LUND, L. & SJÖQVIST, F. (1972). Micromethod for the determination of diphenylhydantoin in plasma and cerebrospinal fluid—a comparison between a gas chromatographic and a spectrophotometric method. *Scand. J. Lab. Clin. Invest.*, **29,** 281–287.

BORGÅ, O., LUND, L. & SJÖQVIST, F. (1969). Bestämning av difenylhydantoin (DFH) i plasma hos patienter med epilepsi. *Läkartidningen*, **66,** 89–98.

BUCHTHAL, F., SVENSMARK, O. & SCHILLER, P. J. (1960). Clinical and electroencephalographic correlations with serum levels of diphenylhydantoin. *Arch. Neurol.*, **2,** 624–630.

DILL, W. A., KAZENKO, A., WOLF, L. M. & GLAZKO, A. J. (1956). Studies on 5, 5-diphenylhydantoin (Dilantin) in animals and man. *J. Pharmacol. Exp. Ther.*, **118,** 270–279.

GIBBERD, F. B., DUNNE, J. F., HANDLEY, A. J. & HAZLEMAN, B. L. (1970). Supervision of epileptic patients taking phenytoin. *Brit. Med. J.*, **1,** 147–149.

HAERER, A. F. & GRACE, J. B. (1969). Studies of anticonvulsant levels in epileptics. *Acta Neurol. Scand.*, **45,** 18–31.

KRISTENSEN, M., MØLHOLM HANSEN, J., HANSEN, O. E. & LUND, V. (1967). Sources of error in the determination of phenytoin (Dilantin) by Svensmark & Kristensen's method. *Acta Neurol. Scand.*, **43,** 447–450.

KUTT, H., HAYNES, J. & MCDOWELL, F. (1966). Some causes of ineffectiveness of diphenylhydantoin. *Arch. Neurol.*, **14,** 489–492.

KUTT, H., WINTERS, W., KOKENGE, R. & MCDOWELL, F. (1964). Diphenylhydantoin metabolism, blood levels and toxicity. *Arch. Neurol,* **11,** 642–648.

LASCELLES, P. T., KOCEN, R. S. & REYNOLDS, E. H. (1970). The distribution of plasma phenytoin levels in epileptic patients. *J. Neurol. Neurosurg. Psychiat.*, **33,** 501–505.

LUND, M., JÖRGENSEN, R. S. & KÜHL, V. (1964). Serum diphenylhydantoin (phenytoin) in ambulant patients with epilepsy. *Epilepsia.*, **5,** 51–58.

MERRITT, H. & PUTNAM, T. J. (1938a). A new series of anticonvulsant drugs tested by experiments on animals. *Arch. Neurol. Psychiat.*, **39,** 1003–1015.

MERRITT, H. & PUTNAM, T. J. (1938b). Sodium diphenyl hydantoinate in the treatment of convulsive disorders. *J.A.M.A.*, **111,** 1068.

PLAA, G. L. & HINE, C. H. (1956). A method for the simultaneous determinations of phenobarbital and diphenylhydantoin in blood. *J. Lab. Clin. Med.*, **47,** 649–657.

STENSRUD, P. A. & PALMER, H. (1964). Serum phenytoin determinations in epileptics. *Epilepsia,* **5,** 364–370.

SVENSMARK, O. & KRISTENSEN, P. (1963). Determination of diphenylhydantoin and phenobarbital in small amounts of serum. *J. Lab. Clin. Med.*, **61,** 501–507.

TRIEDMAN, H. M., FISHMAN, R. A. & YAHR, M. D. (1960). Determination of plasma and cerebrospinal fluid levels of Dilantin in the human. *Trans. Amer. Soc. Neurol.*, **85,** 166–170.

# Discussion: Therapeutic Use of Drugs Acting on the Central Nervous System

PROFESSOR PRICE EVANS Dr. Alexanderson has shown that you can predict steady-state plasma levels from a single dose of nortriptyline. I would like to know if any similar manœuvre can be done with diphenylhydantoin?

DR. LUND Not as yet, but we hope that we can do the same thing as Dr. Alexanderson has done, namely to give the patient a single, oral dose, or, perhaps, a parenteral dose, and then calculate the dose which you must give in order to achieve the correct steady-state level.

**Session 5**

Chairman: Professor C. T. Dollery

When Ought We to Measure Plasma Concentrations in Clinical Practice?

General Discussion

# General discussion: When Ought We to Measure Plasma Concentrations in Clinical Practice?

PROFESSOR DOLLERY I propose to put some of the questions that are in all our minds to the panel to try and get an answer to them.

I suppose that the extreme pharmacckinetic view would be that if there was a close relationship between plasma concentration and drug effect that we could, by measuring plasma concentration after a known dose, simply send a report back giving the plasma concentration and predicting what dose would be necessary to achieve an optimal therapeutic effect. Do the members of the panel consider that there are any drugs where one can do better by measuring the plasma concentration and controlling the therapy in that way, than by the usual clinical methods. Would you like to begin, Professor Sjöqvist?

PROFESSOR SJÖQVIST Yes, indeed, I think that there are a few drugs where the present state of knowledge is such that we know that we can improve drug therapy considerably by measuring the drug plasma concentration under control conditions. I take it for granted that we are measuring the drug specifically, and that no nonsense is going on in the laboratory! I would like to quote an early paper by Dr. Bruck and co-workers (*Lancet*, Jan. 30th, 1954, p. 225) who showed that phenylbutazone may be one of these drugs. They gave evidence that the effective therapeutic plasma concentration is in the range of 50 to 100 $\mu$g/ml and we are therefore monitoring phenylbutazone in our hospital. I am also convinced about the importance of monitoring digoxin. I have also been convinced by the data of Dr. Lund for diphenylhydantoin, and I can tell you that the Swedish Medical Board is also convinced, especially when the drug is used in the treatment of retarded children. There are two very interesting cases where such children have been hospitalized for long periods of time, and where diphenylhydantoin intoxication has been missed. We know that diphenylhydantoin in a high concentration in the brain inhibits the intellectual ability, and this is specially alarming in retarded children.

I also feel convinced that procaine amide should be monitored if it is going to be used in the future at all. I am also convinced by the work of Dr. Schou on lithium especially as far as its toxicity is concerned. I think that as regards the data of therapeutic effect in relation to plasma concentration we need more information. Thus, you have about six drugs for which plasma concentrations may be important.

PROFESSOR DOLLERY There is something like a six-fold variation in the plasma concentrations producing a given effect for a number of drugs discussed today. If there is such a large range of concentration that will give the desired therapeutic effect, I, personally, am a little sceptical whether measuring plasma concentrations routinely is really going to be of very much value for such drugs. Dr. Levy, where do you stand on this, which drugs should we routinely monitor?

PROFESSOR LEVY As an academician and not a clinician, I would like to evade this question. I would rather address myself to the question posed in the programme: when ought we to measure plasma concentrations in clinical practice? The answer to this is so simple, that it is extremely difficult namely whenever it helps in the management of the patient.

I can tell you how we are about to try to answer this question. We have seven affiliated hospitals in the university, where we have university medical personnel involved in the management of the patients. The first decision that we made was to stay away from them and to go into an eighth hospital, which is more representative of the common or garden variety of hospital. We have arranged to obtain laboratory facilities there, and to start to collect blood samples from patients receiving certain types of drugs, which we select. We do not make this information available to the clinicians. We are undertaking what might be called a 'dry run'. In other words, we are collecting these data and we are noting down what we would recommend at a certain time, based on the history of the patient, his medication history, concomitant therapy, the symptomatology and any other relevant factors. We make a notation of what we would recommend in terms of dosage adjustment, and then we look at two things: whether in due time the clinician does make such an adjustment; whether there is a lag time, and, if so, how long was that lag time, and how much trouble did it get the patient into; or, whether he does not make the adjustment at all, and whether this has made any difference to the patient. This requires, incidentally, yet another clinical monitor, who is going to keep a watch on the patient and evaluate the patient but in a passive capacity, without getting involved in the actual patient management. That, I think, will give us the answer. We do not know whether we can earn our keep in clinical pharmacokinetics, only time will tell. I suspect that with a number of drugs, it will be worth while; with a number of other drugs, the background noise will be so great that our contribution will not be significant and not worth the investment.

PROFESSOR DOLLERY What drugs are you measuring in this study?

PROFESSOR LEVY A very important consideration in the choice of drugs to be studied is the availability of specific analytical methods. Thus, we are looking at the cardiac glycosides; at phenylbutazone, even salicylate for that matter, because we feel that physicians tend to be overly conservative in dosages of anti-inflammatory agents. We are not looking at anticoagulants, because I think that the pharmacological effect is easily measured.

PROFESSOR DOLLERY You bring out the important point, that it is easier to measure a plasma concentration than it is to quantitate the effect. It is no coincidence that clinical pharmacology grew up largely in cardiovascular disease and it is precisely in these areas that it is relatively easy to measure drug effects. One of the things that we need is very much better methods of measuring the therapeutic and pharmacological action of many sorts of drugs in man. One point in Dr. Lund's paper interested me, namely how a longitudinal study in the individual patient may be helpful in the control of therapy. Such a concept could be helpful in the control of therapy, even with a drug where there are quite wide interindividual differences in the concentration causing the desired pharmacological effect. In an individual, once you have determined the concentration that gave the right sort of effect, it is probable that the concentration–effect relation will be constant.

PROFESSOR LEVY I am glad that you make this point. We are now starting to determine the plasma concentration of diphenylhydantoin in patients to establish the plateau concentration at which they are apparently well controlled. This value becomes part of a record which one day could be useful as, for example, when there might be need for concomitant administration of drugs which are enzyme inducers.

PROFESSOR DOLLERY This information could also be of value in explaining why a patient who was well controlled, suddenly does not respond. The first doubt that comes to mind is that the patient has not taken the drug and patients are not always truthful about this. To know that the plasma concentration is low, and therefore that it is most likely that the drug has not been taken, would be of value, Otherwise one might increase the dose and perhaps give the patient a bawling out into the bargain. He then takes the increased dose and may get a toxic effect.

DR. BRAITHWAITE (LONDON) Professor Sjöqvist made the point that in the bear-garden of normal medical practice the correlation of the pharmacological effects of an anti-depressant drug, with its steady state plasma concentration in the depressed patient may be difficult to elucidate. The results of a pilot study in which 50 depressed patients had been taking nortriptyline for an average of three weeks seem to substantiate Professor Sjöqvist's views. For this study psychiatrists were asked simply to make a decision as to whether their patients were making satisfactory progress or not. A blood sample was taken at that point, and the plasma nortriptyline level was estimated using a new specific gas chromatographic procedure. Low and high plasma levels were equally often associated with a satisfactory and an unsatisfactory response. No doubt, there are very many variables involved, but, clearly, there are several limitations to the general application of plasma nortriptyline levels to general clinical practice in the treatment of depression.

PROFESSOR LEVY I think that there is an important point to be made here and that is that one has to distinguish between obtaining a plasma concentration response relationship in one individual, or in a group of individuals as opposed to a whole collection of people pulled from all over, with different baseline conditions and different pathologies. Let us not mix up those two.

PROFESSOR PRICE EVANS I would like to add another answer to the question of when to estimate plasma levels. That is, when suitable methods are available. Our list is quite short—some half-dozen drugs—and I think that this is due to the great scarcity of good analytical methods. Somebody mentioned diuretics. I do not think that there is a suitable, relatively simple method for measuring diuretic levels, is there? It is no good having methods that require a mass spectrometer! This is just not on for ordinary hospital practice. One wants simple methods, and perhaps some new techniques like radio-immune assay may provide simple, economical measurements.

Another factor which may limit the usefulness of plasma measurement, is the nature of the disease. In the very fast-moving, dangerous situations for the patient, you really have to know quickly and fairly accurately what is happening.

PROFESSOR DOLLERY On that note, we will draw this discussion to a close. The measurement of plasma concentrations can certainly be helpful in understanding why some patients have toxic responses to drugs and others do not respond to them. But if there are any indications for routine measurement of drug concentrations in plasma they are as yet very few. However, this may not apply in the future as we know more about the relationship between concentrations and drug effect.

It remains for me to thank the speakers, many of whom came long distances across the oceans to speak at this first symposium organized by the Clinical Pharmacology Section of the British Pharmacological Society. We have had a very good day, and we are very grateful to them.

# Index of Authors

Entries in bold type refer to papers, other entries to contributions to discussions.

# Index of Subjects